GERIATRIC
SLEEP
MEDICINE

SLEEP DISORDERS

Advisory Board

GERIATRIC SLEEP MEDICINE

Edited by
Alon Y. Avidan
University of California
Los Angeles, California, USA

Cathy A. Alessi
Veterans Administration Greater Los Angeles
University of California
Los Angeles, California, USA

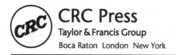

CRC Press
Taylor & Francis Group
Boca Raton London New York

CRC Press is an imprint of the
Taylor & Francis Group, an **informa** business

CRC Press
Taylor & Francis Group
6000 Broken Sound Parkway NW, Suite 300
Boca Raton, FL 33487-2742

First issued in paperback 2019

ISBN-13: 978-1-4200-5868-0 (hbk)
ISBN-13: 978-0-367-38678-8 (pbk)

This book contains information obtained from authentic and highly regarded sources. While all reasonable efforts have been made to publish reliable data and in formation, neither the author[s] nor the publisher can accept any legal responsibility or liability for any errors or omissions that may be made. The publishers wish to make clear that any views or opinions expressed in this book by individual editors, authors or contributors are personal to them and do not necessarily reflect the views/opinions of the publishers. The information or guidance contained in this book is intended for use by medical, scientific or healthcare professionals and is provided strictly as a supplement to the medical or other professional's own judgement, their knowledge of the patient's medical history, relevant manufacturer's instructions and the appropriate best practice guidelines. Because of the rapid advances in medical science, any information or advice on dosages, procedures or diagnoses should be independently verified. The reader is strongly urged to consult the relevant national drug formulary and the drug companies' and device or material manufacturers' printed instructions, and their websites, before administering or utilizing any of the drugs, devices or materials mentioned in this book. This book does not indicate whether a particular treatment is appropriate or suitable for a particular individual. Ultimately it is the sole responsibility of the medical professional to make his or her own professional judgements, so as to advise and treat patients appropriately. The authors and publishers have also attempted to trace the copyright holders of all material reproduced in this publication and apologize to copyright holders if permission to publish in this form has not been obtained. If any copyright material has not been acknowledged please write and let us know so we may rectify in any future reprint.

Library of Congress Cataloging-in-Publication Data

Geriatric sleep medicine / edited by Alon Y. Avidan, Cathy A. Alessi.
   p. ; cm. – (Sleep disorders ; 6)
Includes bibliographical references and index.
ISBN-13: 978-1-4200-5868-0 (hardcover : alk. paper)
ISBN-10: 1-4200-5868-1 (hardcover : alk. paper)
   1. Sleep disorders–Age factors.   2. Older people–Diseases.   I. Avidan, Alon Y.
II. Alessi, Cathy.   III. Series: Sleep disorders (New York, N.Y.); 6.
   [DNLM: 1. Sleep Disorders.   2. Aged.   WM 188 G369 2008]

RC547.G47 2008
618.97'68498 – dc22   2008025107

Visit the Informa Web site at
www.informa.com

and the Informa Healthcare Web site at
www.informahealthcare.com

Foreword

Approximately 37 million Americans are 65 years of age or older, representing 12.5% of the national population. The next 20 plus years will see a remarkable shift in the older adult population (Fig. 1). By 2030, 20% of the U.S. population, one in five persons, will be aged 65 or older, a near doubling of the present ratio of one in nine persons. This radical population shift in the proportion of older adults will have a massive negative impact on our already strained health-care systems.

Of the many major physiological changes that accompany the aging process, one change that is typically problematic for many is an often profound disruption of an older adult's daily sleep–wake cycle. Epidemiological studies have consistently shown that the prevalence of significant sleep complaints grows steadily with advancing age. Some 57% of adults over the age of 60 complain of significant sleep disruption, 45% have periodic limb movements during sleep (PLMS), 29% have insomnia, 24% have obstructive sleep apnea (OSA), 19% complain of early morning awakening, and 12% have restless legs syndrome (RLS). Only a minority of patients described no sleep complaints in survey of over 9000 participants aged 65 years and older in the National Institute on Aging's multicentered study entitled "Established Populations for Epidemiologic Studies of the Elderly" (EPESE). The majority of patients described difficulties initiating sleep, nocturnal awakenings, insomnia, daytime napping, troubles falling asleep, waking up too early in the morning, and waking up too early without feeling rested (Fig. 2) (Foley DJ, Monjan AA, et al. Sleep complaints among elderly persons: An epidemiologic study of three communities. Sleep 1995; 18(6):425–432.). While sleep disturbances can have profound implications for an individual's health, the nature of these disruptions is complex.

The most striking change in sleep in older adults is the repeated and frequent interruption of sleep by long periods of wakefulness, possibly the result of an age-dependent intrinsic change in sleep homeostatic processes. This age-dependent increase of nighttime wakefulness, as well as other well-characterized sleep–wake changes, is mirrored by increases in daytime fatigue, excessive daytime sleepiness and increased likelihood of napping, or falling asleep during the day. Aging is also associated with a tendency to both fall asleep and awaken earlier and to be less tolerant of phase shifts in time of the sleep–wake schedule such as those produced by jet lag and shift work. These changes suggest an age-dependent breakdown of the normal adult circadian sleep–wake cycle.

However, when age-related comorbidities, such as the medical and psychiatric illnesses, that typically accompany the aging process are controlled for and "optimal" aging examined, then the bulk of age-dependent sleep changes occurs in early and middle adulthood (years 19–60), such that after age 60, assuming one is in good health, further age-dependent sleep changes are, at most, modest. Conversely,

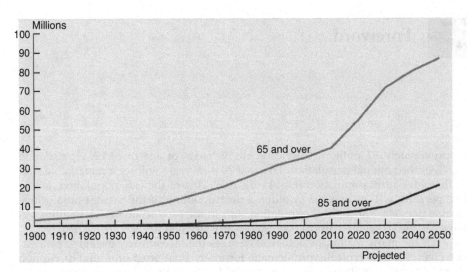

FIGURE 1 Projected population increased in millions between the time interval 2010 and 2050 for patients over 65 years of age and for patients over 85 years of age. *Source:* U.S. Department of Decennial Census and Projections. *Note:* Reference population: these data refer to the resident population.

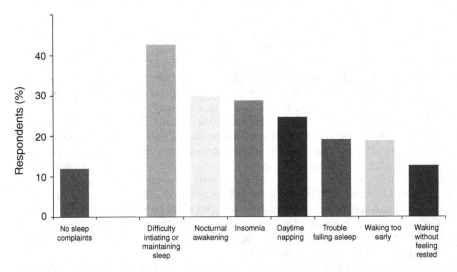

FIGURE 2 Frequency of sleep disorders in older adults. *Source:* From Foley DJ, Monjan AA, et al. Sleep complaints among elderly persons: An epidemiologic study of three communities. Sleep 1995; 18(6):425–432.

if comorbidities are present, it is clear that normal age-dependent sleep disruption may be exacerbated, often extremely.

In addition to the impact of age-dependent sleep changes and age-associated comorbidities, the sleep of older adults can be further adversely impacted by primary sleep disorders, such as insomnia, OSA and RLS, and other factors such as prescription medications, over-the-counter medications, social drug use, and psychosocial and environmental factors including poor sleep hygiene. Indeed, the sleep of a given older adult can be adversely impacted by any and, more often than not, several of these factors. These disturbances in sleep and increases in daytime sleepiness can have significant impact, not only on quality of life, but are also being implicated in increased morbidity and mortality in older adults.

It is in this context that Avidan and Alessi's *Geriatric Sleep Medicine* is a welcome, indeed necessary, resource supporting the worthy effort to improve the health and well-being of the nation's burgeoning older population. This excellent and comprehensive guide to the effective practice of sleep medicine in older adults appears at a very exciting time for sleep research and sleep medicine, especially in the area of geriatrics. In 2006, the Institute of Medicine (IOM) of the National Academy of Sciences released its report, "Sleep Disorders and Sleep Deprivation: An Unmet Public Health Problem," which recognized that sleep disorders and sleep deprivation are significant public health problems that have a wide range of deleterious health and safety consequences. The IOM report called for increased awareness among healthcare professionals about the physiology of healthy sleep and sleep disorders across the life span and the development and implementation of programs to promote the early diagnosis and treatment of sleep disorders.

The last ten years have been marked by significant and rapid advances in our ability to diagnose and treat, both behaviorally and pharmacologically, sleep disorders generally and in older adults in particular. *Geriatric Sleep Medicine* admirably summarizes this new knowledge and puts it readily in the hands of geriatric healthcare providers.

Geriatric Sleep Medicine is organized into four logical sections. The first describes sleep and sleep disturbances in the context of both aging and disease. These chapters provide the foundation for an appreciation of how sleep changes with aging and how it is impacted by the large number of comorbid illnesses, medical, psychiatric, and neurological, that occur with increasing prevalence in older adult populations. The second section focuses on insomnia and provides descriptions of its epidemiology and treatment, both pharmacological and behavioral. The third section addresses the other sleep disorders common in older adults and their treatments. These include both obstructive and central sleep apnea, circadian rhythm disorders, and motor disorders, such as restless legs syndrome. Finally, section four focuses on issues of sleep quality and disturbance in special older populations; addressing sleep in peri- and postmenopausal women, napping, and sleep in nursing home and end-of-life populations. Each chapter of *Geriatric Sleep Medicine* is authored by recognized experts in the topic being covered. These authors, typically both researchers and practitioners, carefully evaluate the relevant literature, which more often than not involves their own work, and provide state-of-the-art guidance in the diagnosis and management of the many disturbances of sleep–wake experienced by older adults.

Geriatric Sleep Medicine is a comprehensive, authoritative, and extremely valuable guide in treating sleep disorders in older adults. It will prove an invaluable resource not only for practitioners of sleep medicine but also for all health-care practitioners who regularly work with older adults.

Michael V. Vitiello, PhD
Professor of Psychiatry and Behavioral Sciences, Medicine,
and Biobehavioral Nursing
University of Washington, Seattle WA
Editor-in-Chief (for the Americas) *Sleep Medicine Reviews*

The frequencies of five common sleep complaints—trouble falling asleep, waking up, awaking too early, needing to nap, and not feeling rested—were assessed in over 9000 participants aged 65 years and older in the National Institute on Aging's multicentered study entitled "Established Populations for Epidemiologic Studies of the Elderly" (EPESE). Less than 20% of the participants in each community rarely or never had any complaints, whereas over half reported at least one of these complaints as occurring most of the time. Between 23% and 34% had symptoms of insomnia, and between 7% and 15% rarely or never felt rested after waking up in the morning. In multivariate analyses, sleep complaints were associated with an increasing number of respiratory symptoms, physical disabilities, nonprescription medications, depressive symptoms, and poorer self-perceived health. Sleep disturbances, particularly among older persons, oftentimes may be secondary to coexisting diseases. Determining the prevalence of specific sleep disorders, independent of health status, will require the development of more sophisticated and objective measures of sleep disturbances.

Preface

The management of sleep complaints among older adults is both rewarding and challenging. Given the high prevalence of sleep disorders in this population and the ever expanding knowledge about the impact of sleep disturbances on quality of life, life expectancy, mental health, and cardiovascular and neurologic morbidity, healthcare providers are increasingly asked to address sleep problems in older people. Unfortunately, sleep disorders in older people may go unrecognized and/or untreated, contributing to refractory neurological, psychiatric, and medical conditions. For example, obstructive sleep apnea can contribute to considerable cardiovascular disease and may be viewed as a reversible cause of dementia in elderly patients. Despite that, little time is spent in medical and postgraduate education describing the key elements of the evaluation of the sleepy patient. With these issues in mind, we now present one of the first textbooks in sleep disorders focusing on the geriatric patient. The purpose of this educational tool is to review common sleep problems in this group and provide the reader with an updated, easily read, and practical approach to their evaluation, diagnosis, and management in a busy clinical practice. We also hope that researchers with a focus in geriatric sleep research will find this book resourceful.

We have compiled outstanding and distinguished authorities in sleep medicine for this text, representing key leaders in the field of geriatric sleep medicine. Many of them have co-authored their work with more junior faculty and trainees in the field, which offers a unique outlook on these important topics. In addition, our author list represents wide geographic distribution. While many of our authors are geriatricians and internists, we also were fortunate to include psychiatrists, neurologists, psychologists, clinical researchers, nurses, and pulmonologists. In fact, we hope our author list parallels the diversity of sleep medicine as a field that is probably the most interdisciplinary "subspecialty" in existence.

Chapters in this text are organized to cover the range of topics of greatest importance providers involved in the recognition and management of sleep problems in the older adult. First, a forward by Dr. Vitiello summarizes important aspects of sleep in aging, and sets the stage for the remaining chapters of the textbook. Then, there are several chapters addressing key concepts in the understanding of sleep in aging and disease. This includes a chapter by Drs. Wright and Frey that summarizes important issues in sleep physiology in the geriatric patient. Next, Dr. Barczi provides a comprehensive summary of sleep problems associated with medical illness and comorbidities in the older adult. Drs. Pigeon and Perlis then provide a careful review of sleep and psychiatric illness, followed by a review of sleep in neurological and neurodegenerative disorders by Dr. Avidan.

The next several chapters focus on the important topic of insomnia in aging. First, Drs. Choi and Irwin provide a comprehensive review of key aspects of insomnia in aging, followed by a careful review of pharmacological treatment of insomnia in the older adult by Drs. Lee-Chiong and Harrington. This is followed by a careful review of behavioral treatment of insomnia by Drs. Morin and Belanger.

The textbook then addresses several additional important sleep disorders in the older adult, including a review of sleep-related breathing disorders in aging by Dr. Gooneratne and a comprehensive review of central sleep apnea by Drs. Chowdhuri and Badr. This is followed by a comprehensive review of circadian rhythm disorders in aging by Drs. Naylor and Zee, and a careful discussion of periodic limb movement disorder and restless legs syndrome by Dr. Bliwise.

Finally, the textbook addresses several special topics of sleep in aging. First, Drs. Martin and Alessi review sleep in nursing home residents. Then, Drs. Misra and Malow provide a careful summary of sleep in the older woman. The next chapter, by Drs. Stone and Ancoli-Israel, reviews the literature on napping in older adults. Finally, Drs. Nazir and Richards review sleep in late-stage dementia and end of life.

We would like to conclude by providing our sincerest thanks to the authors for their dedication and outstanding contributions to this textbook. We have had the pleasure of working with many of them as colleagues and good friends for many years in this ever evolving and exciting field, and we sincerely appreciate their contributions to this textbook. Finally, we would like to thank Ms. Dana Bigelow, Development Editor, U.S. Books Informa Healthcare for her direction and guidance as this project evolved from an idea into an indispensible educational product.

Alon Y. Avidan, MD, MPH
Cathy A. Alessi, MD

Contents

Contributors

Cathy A. Alessi   Veterans Administration Greater Los Angeles Healthcare System, Geriatric Research, Education and Clinical Center and David Geffen School of Medicine at UCLA, Department of Medicine, University of California, Los Angeles, California, U.S.A.

Sonia Ancoli-Israel   Department of Psychiatry, University of California, San Diego, California, U.S.A.

Alon Y. Avidan   Department of Neurology, David Geffen School of Medicine at UCLA, University of California, Los Angeles, California, U.S.A.

M. Safwan Badr   John D. Dingell Veterans Affairs Medical Center and Wayne State University, Detroit, Michigan, U.S.A.

Steven R. Barczi   Department of Medicine, Section of Geriatrics, University of Wisconsin School of Medicine and Public Health, and The Madison V.A. Geriatric Research, Education and Clinical Center, William S. Middleton Veterans Administration Hospital, Madison, Wisconsin, U.S.A.

Lynda Bélanger   École de Psychologie, Université Laval Québec, Québec, Canada

Donald L. Bliwise   Program in Sleep, Aging and Chronobiology, Department of Neurology, Emory University Medical School, Atlanta, Georgia, U.S.A.

Octavio Choi   UCLA Semel Institute of Neuroscience, Los Angeles, California, U.S.A.

Susmita Chowdhuri   John D. Dingell Veterans Affairs Medical Center and Wayne State University, Detroit, Michigan, U.S.A.

Danielle J. Frey   Sleep and Chronobiology Laboratory, Department of Integrative Physiology, Center for Neuroscience, University of Colorado at Boulder, Boulder, Colorado, U.S.A.

Nalaka S. Gooneratne   Division of Geriatric Medicine and the Center for Sleep and Respiratory Neurobiology, University of Pennsylvania School of Medicine, Philadelphia, Pennsylvania, U.S.A.

John Harrington   National Jewish Medical and Research Center, Denver, Colorado, U.S.A.

Michael R. Irwin   UCLA Semel Institute of Neuroscience, Los Angeles, California, U.S.A.

Teofilo Lee-Chiong   National Jewish Medical and Research Center, Denver, Colorado, U.S.A.

Beth Malow   Department of Neurology, Vanderbilt University Medical Center, and Vanderbilt Sleep Disorders Center, Vanderbilt University Medical Center, Nashville, Tennessee, U.S.A.

Jennifer L. Martin   Veterans Administration Greater Los Angeles Healthcare System, Geriatric Research, Education and Clinical Center and David Geffen School of Medicine at UCLA, Department of Medicine, University of California, Los Angeles, California, U.S.A.

Sumi Misra   Division of General Internal Medicine, Vanderbilt University Medical Center, and Geriatric Primary Care Clinic, Tennessee Valley Health Care System, Veterans Affairs Hospital, Nashville, Tennessee, U.S.A.

Charles M. Morin   École de Psychologie, Université Laval Québec, Québec, Canada

Erik Naylor   Department of Neurology, Northwestern University Medical School, Chicago, Illinois, U.S.A.

Shoab A. Nazir   Division of Pulmonary, Critical Care and Sleep Medicine, University of Arkansas for Medical Sciences, and Central Arkansas Veterans Health Care System, Little Rock, Arkansas, U.S.A.

Michael L. Perlis   Sleep and Neurophysiology Research Laboratory, Department of Psychiatry, University of Rochester School of Medicine and Dentistry, Rochester, New York, U.S.A.

Wilfred R. Pigeon   Sleep and Neurophysiology Research Laboratory, Department of Psychiatry, University of Rochester School of Medicine and Dentistry, Rochester, New York, U.S.A.

Kathy C. Richards   Polisher Research Institute, Madlyn and Leonard Abramson Center for Jewish Life, and School of Nursing, University of Pennsylvania, Philadelphia, Pennsylvania, U.S.A.

Katie L. Stone   Research Institute, California Pacific Medical Center, San Francisco, California, U.S.A.

Kenneth P. Wright Jr.   Sleep and Chronobiology Laboratory, Department of Integrative Physiology, Center for Neuroscience, University of Colorado at Boulder, Boulder, Colorado, U.S.A.

Phyllis C. Zee   Department of Neurology, Northwestern University Medical School, Chicago, Illinois, U.S.A.

1

Age Related Changes in Sleep and Circadian Physiology: From Brain Mechanisms to Sleep Behavior

Kenneth P. Wright Jr. and Danielle J. Frey

Sleep and Chronobiology Laboratory, Department of Integrative Physiology, Center for Neuroscience, University of Colorado at Boulder, Boulder, Colorado, U.S.A.

INTRODUCTION

Sleep and circadian physiology change in healthy older adults independent of medical conditions or medications (1–3). In general, deep nonrapid eye movement (NREM) sleep is reduced, there are more awakenings from sleep, and the time spent awake in bed trying to sleep is increased. Such sleep disruptions are exacerbated by age-related diseases such as cardiovascular disease (4), cancer (5,6), nocturia (7), pain (4,8), diabetes (8,9), and depression (10,11). It is estimated that 40% to 70% of older adults experience chronic sleep problems, and that about 50% of the cases are untreated by primary care physicians (12). Sleep problems are even more common in geriatric patients with dementia (13,14). Aging with and without associated medical problems is also associated with changes in the physiology of the internal circadian timekeeping system that regulates near-24-hour rhythms in human physiology and behavior; and age-related changes in circadian physiology are thought to contribute to sleep problems (14–17). This chapter will first review sleep–wakefulness and circadian neurophysiology. Knowledge of the brain regions involved in promoting sleep and wakefulness states can provide perspective on how medications commonly used in the geriatric patient can affect daytime and nighttime function. This discussion will be followed by a review of how sleep and circadian brain regulatory systems change with aging. Knowledge of age-related changes in sleep and circadian systems may promote a better understanding of potential mechanisms underlying sleep problems in the geriatric patient and may help to inform the development of pharmacological and nonpharmacological treatment strategies.

NEUROPHYSIOLOGY OF SLEEP–WAKEFULNESS AND CIRCADIAN SYSTEMS

Sleep and wakefulness states are actively promoted by the brain. Ascending brain arousal systems serve to promote wakefulness and inhibition of these systems promotes sleep. Central nervous system control of transitions between sleep and wakefulness states can be modeled as a "flip-flop" switch (18). In the "flip-flop switch" model, sleep and wakefulness-generating neural networks are mutually inhibitory, such that when sleep networks are active, they inhibit wakefulness networks, and when wakefulness networks are active, they inhibit sleep networks (18,19). The sleep switch is modulated by the internal circadian timekeeping system and by orexin cells in the hypothalamus, both of which are thought to be important for stabilizing the switch to promote consolidated sleep and wakefulness.

Wakefulness Mechanisms

Wakefulness-generating systems include neurons in the brainstem and forebrain, which stimulate cortical activation. The brain stem reticular formation (20) contains neurons that through ascending projections via the thalamus, hypothalamus, and basal forebrain inhibit sleep-generating neurons and activate cortical neurons. In addition, descending projections from the reticular formation to the spinal cord are important for maintaining postural control and muscle tone. Several neurotransmitters are involved in wakefulness-generating neural networks, including glutamate, acetylcholine, norepinephrine, dopamine, histamine, orexin, and serotonin. Noradrenergic (norepinephrine) neurons, localized primarily in the locus coeruleus, project to the forebrain and cerebral cortex and are involved in attention and maintaining and enhancing cortical activation. Activities of locus coeruleus neurons are higher during wakefulness than during sleep (21,22). Dopaminergic neurons, located primarily in the substantia nigra and ventral tegmental areas, project to the striatum and frontal cortex, which when activated are important for behavioral arousal and movement. Although dopamine neurons are reported to show similar firing rates across sleep–wakefulness states (23), inputs to dopamine neurons from other arousal systems may influence sleep and wakefulness (24). Cholinergic cells, located in the brain stem, excite thalamocortical cells, which results in arousal and information transfer to the cerebral cortex. Cholinergic cells, located in neurons in the basal forebrain, promote behavioral and cortical arousal (21,25–28). Histamine neurons are localized in the tuberomammillary nucleus of the caudal hypothalamus and provide excitatory input to the cerebral cortex; antihistamines that cross the blood brain barrier produce drowsiness (29,30). Glutamate and aspartate are excitatory amino acids localized within many neurons projecting to the cerebral cortex, the forebrain, and brainstem. Glutamate and aspartate are released in the largest amounts during wakefulness and their antagonists produce sleep (31,32). Orexin/hypocretin cells are localized in the lateral hypothalamus and project to widespread areas of the brain stem, thalamus, hypothalamus, and cerebral cortex (33–35) and are reported to have a role in brain arousal (36).

Sleep Mechanisms

Sleep physiology can be divided into NREM and REM sleep stages, and sleep-generating networks vary between these stages.

NREM Sleep

During the transition from wakefulness to NREM sleep in healthy adult humans, the electroencephalographic (EEG) pattern changes from a fast, low-amplitude desynchronized waveform to a slower, high-amplitude synchronized wave (37–40). NREM sleep is divided into stages 1 and 2 and stages 3 and 4. Stage 1 is a transitional stage typically observed at sleep onset. Stage 2 sleep consists of a dominant theta pattern with the presence of sleep spindles and K-complexes. Stage 2 sleep is distributed equally across the night. Deep NREM stage 3/4 sleep (referred to as slow-wave sleep [SWS]) is defined by a slow, high-amplitude, synchronized EEG waveform, which is often quantified by the amount of delta (0.5–2.5 Hz) or slow-wave activity (SWA) (41,42). Slow wave sleep occurs mostly during the first half of the night.

The transition from wakefulness to NREM sleep is associated with the inhibition of the reticular activating system and thalmocortical disassociation mediated through the inhibitory neurotransmitter gamma-aminobutyric acid (GABA) (21). Locus coeruleus neurons decrease their discharge frequency during the transition from wakefulness to sleep (22). The diminished release of acetylcholine and norepinephrine activity affects the activities of thalamocortical and cortical cells, most notably to reduce responsiveness to afferent signals. GABAergic neurons are responsible for the production of sleep spindles, which are inhibitory oscillations between the thalamus and cortex (43,44). Sleep-active neurons in the ventrolateral preoptic nucleus (VLPO) of the hypothalamus (45) via GABAergic projections inhibit excitatory histaminergic cells of the hypothalamus (46) and also inhibit excitatory noradrenergic and serotoninergic cells of the brain stem (47,48). Lesion of the VLPO is reported to decrease the total sleep time (49). NREM sleep is primarily an aminergic state, which involves activation neurons located in the VLPO, basal forebrain, nucleus of the solitary tract, and raphe nuclei that project to and inhibit wakefulness-generating areas and areas of the cortex (50). While the exact neurobiological mechanisms underlying sleep homeostasis are poorly understood, the neuromodulator adenosine has been reported to build up with time awake in brain regions associated with sleep–wakefulness regulation and to dissipate with sleep (26,51–54). Adenosine is a byproduct of cellular metabolism (i.e., a breakdown of ATP). Adenosine is reported to inhibit wakefulness-promoting neurons in the basal forebrain (28,51,55) and to activate sleep-promoting neurons in the hypothalamus (26,56–58). Cerebral adenosine receptors are also reported to be upregulated following sleep deprivation in humans (59). Endogenous immune factors such as prostaglandin D2 (PGD2), interleukin-1 (IL-1), and muramyl peptides also are reported to promote sleep (56,60,61).

REM Sleep

REM sleep is defined by a low-amplitude fast theta desynchronized EEG waveform with characteristic saw tooth waves and inhibition of skeletal muscle activity, referred to as muscle atonia. Rapid eye movements and other phasic activity may or may not be present during REM sleep. In healthy adult humans, NREM and REM sleep alternate throughout the night approximately every 80 to 120 minutes. The duration of REM episodes increases across the night.

REM sleep is primarily a cholinergic (acetylcholine) state during which neurons in the reticular formation are active, primarily those located in the pontine tegmentum (62,25), leading to cortical activation. Firing rates and synaptic excitability of cholinergic neurons are higher during wakefulness and REM sleep compared with NREM sleep (63,64). GABAergic REM-on neurons are located in the sublaterodorsal nucleus and the periventricular grey matter, and GABAergic REM-off neurons are located in the ventrolateral part of the periaqueductal grey matter and the lateral pontine tegmentum (65). REM-on neurons are reported to inhibit REM-off neurons (65,66) and thus promote REM sleep. Reciprocal inhibitory interactions between REM-on and REM-off neurons are thought to be involved in REM sleep regulation. In addition, monoamine neurons are relatively quiescent during REM sleep (22,23), and stimulation of serotoninergic, noradrenergic, or histaminergic cells will inhibit REM sleep (67–70). Loss of orexin/hypocretin neurons is reported to result in abnormal regulation of REM sleep (71,72). These cells may influence REM sleep via activation of the locus coeruleus (36). Related, orexin/hypocretin cells/levels are diminished in patients with narcolepsy, a sleep disorder of REM sleep regulation (73). Release from inhibitory actions of GABAergic neurons in the pons may also be involved in the generation of REM sleep (64,74).

REM state-specific activation of brain stem cholinergic neuronal cells groups and reductions in brain stem serotonergic and noradrenergic activity are reported to contribute to muscle atonia during REM sleep (75,76). Glutamatergic cells within the sublaterodorsal tegmental nucleus of the brain stem are reported to project to spinal cord interneurons (65), and to actively inhibit alpha motor neuron action potentials though release of glycine and GABA (65,76,77). In addition, an increase in small-amplitude spontaneous as well as sensory-stimulated inhibitory postsynaptic potentials (IPSPs) in the motorneurons occurs during REM sleep. Inhibitory drives generally predominate during REM sleep. However, phasic muscle twitches occur during REM sleep because of temporary dominance of excitatory over inhibitory drives.

Circadian Mechanisms

A master clock, located in the mammalian suprachiasmatic nucleus (SCN) of the hypothalamus (78–80), regulates near-24-hour rhythms in physiology and behavior. Lesion of the SCN leads to the disruption of a number of circadian rhythms, including rhythms of sleep and wakefulness, hormone secretion, and activity (81–84). Afferent projections to the SCN are predominantly from specialized retinal ganglion cells via the monosynaptic retinohypothalamic tract (RHT) and a multisynaptic pathway involving the geniculohypothalamic tract (GHT) (85–87). These retinal and SCN structures have been described in humans (88–90) and represent the primary input pathway for photic environmental time cues. Efferent projections from the human SCN project to nearby structures such as the paraventricular nucleus and the dorsomedial nucleus in the hypothalamus, and to the SCN itself (91,92). Afferent and efferent connections between the SCN and brain areas involved in the regulation of sleep and wakefulness have been described (47,93–97).

Circadian physiology in humans is commonly assessed by measuring various circadian rhythms that are considered to be outputs of the SCN, including core body temperature, melatonin, and cortisol. Assessment of the period (duration), amplitude, phase (timing), and phase relationships (timing of one circadian rhythm relative to another) of such rhythms provides information about the function of the circadian system. The period and phase measures reflect stability and precision of the circadian system (98,99), while the amplitude reflects the strength of the circadian system or resistance to change (99–101).

Circadian period in humans is reported to be near, but on an average, longer than 24 hours (98). The range of circadian periods in sighted humans is reported to be from ~23.5 hours to 24.5 hours, with a mode of ~24.2 (98,102–104). Circadian period is genetically determined and is reported to influence such factors as morning-eveningness behavioral preferences (105) and habitual circadian time of sleep (106).

Circadian phase of the melatonin, body temperature, and cortisol rhythms are used to describe internal biological time. Low melatonin and high body temperature levels represent the biological day, and high melatonin and low body temperature levels represent the biological night. During the biological day, the clock system promotes wakefulness and its associated functions (e.g., activity, energy intake), and during the biological night, the clock system promotes sleep and its associated functions (e.g., rest, energy conservation). When the circadian timekeeping system is properly entrained to the 24-hour day, melatonin levels rise on an average ~2 hours before habitual bedtime, body temperature levels are near their circadian minimum ~2.5 hours before habitual wake time, and cortisol levels peak near habitual wake time.

The primary environmental time cue that entrains the circadian system to the 24-hour day is exposure to light (99,104). In humans, light exposure across the day influences the phase of the circadian clock. In general, light exposure in the morning shifts the clock earlier (eastward), whereas light exposure in the evening shifts the clock later (westward) (99,104). In humans, light exposure is integrated across the day to influence circadian phase (99,104,107).

AGE-RELATED CHANGES IN SLEEP TIMING AND QUALITY

Sleep Characteristics That Change with Age and Possible Neurophysiological Mechanisms

Age-associated changes in sleep EEG include reductions in SWS and total sleep time and increases in WASO (wake after sleep onset) and the number and duration of arousals (Fig. 1) (17,108–110,110–122). Even exceptionally healthy older adults are reported to show reduced SWS and sleep efficiency and increased arousals and WASO compared with younger adults (1–3,3,16,123).

In studies using computer quantification of SWA, older males are reported to show larger reductions in SWA across all ages, whereas females are reported to show relatively stable levels of SWA until the time of menopause, at which time, an age related decline is reported (121). However, the SWA of males is reported to be significantly lower than that of females throughout the lifespan (109,121). The percentage of SWS in a sleep episode has been reported to be less in older adults versus young adults (3). For example, a ~50% reduction in SWS has been reported in older adults compared with young controls (124). In addition, sleep efficiencies have been reported to be lower in older adults versus young adults (3). Furthermore, the percentage stage 2 is reported to be increased in older adults (17). The frequency and duration of nocturnal awakenings is also increased in older adults (17,109,110,115,116,118). REM sleep changes with age are less consistent. Changes in REM density and REM onset latency have been reported (110,118,122,125–128), but others report that REM sleep structure remains stable with aging (2,114,120).

The reduction of SWS in older adults is thought to reflect changes in sleep homeostasis, such that older adults have an overall lower homeostatic drive for sleep (41,129). Dijk et al. (3) reported a significant interaction between SWS and age across the sleep episode, such that older adults had less SWS during the first third of the sleep episode, but a similar amount of SWS as compared with young adults by the last two-thirds of the sleep episode. The first third of a sleep episode corresponds to the time when the homeostatic drive for sleep is strongest, and suggests that since the older adults had a lower amount of SWS during this time, they have a lower sleep homeostatic drive. Older adults continue to respond to sleep deprivation with an increased amount of SWS during recovery sleep (1,130), suggesting that the sleep homeostatic process remains functional. However, while older adults showed

(A)

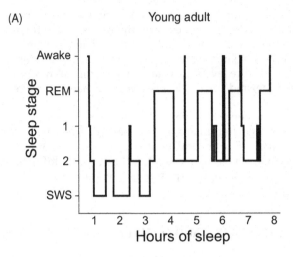

(B)

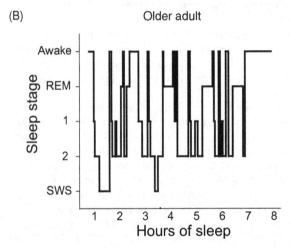

FIGURE 1 Hypnograms of sleep architecture in young (a) and older adults (b). Stages 1, 2, and SWS represent NREM sleep. Horizontal lines represent time spent in the sleep stage on the y-axis. The normal sleep episode begins with progression through the NREM stages followed by a brief REM episode. This cycle through NREM and REM typically takes ~90 minutes. As the sleep episode advances, REM comprises longer amounts of the 90-minute cycle, and SWS disappears. The pattern of sleep across the night has been reported to be maintained in older adults, including ~90 minute cycles through the sleep stages with SWS predominating in the first half of the night, and REM sleep predominating in the second half of the night. However, as can be seen, older adults have a greater number of awakenings, of longer duration, compared with young adults. Older adults often sleep less than young adults.

the same percentage of SWS increase during recovery sleep as young adults, the SWS increase was not large enough to restore SWS levels to that seen in young adults during a normal night of sleep (1,130). In addition, Drapeau and Carrier (131) reported no age difference in the rise in theta activity across wakefulness, another

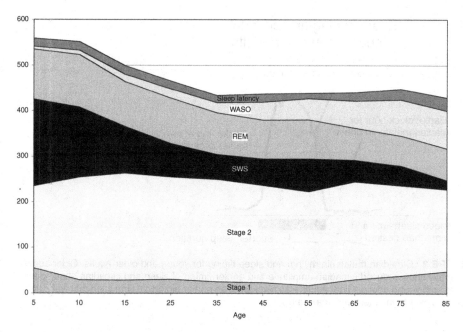

FIGURE 2 Age-related changes in sleep architecture. The most dramatic changes include a reduction in slow-wave sleep (delta sleep) and REM sleep and an increase in stage 1 and stage 2 sleep. Sleep efficiency and sleep continuity also decrease. *Source*: From Ref. 176.

EEG marker reported to reflect homeostatic sleep drive, but that the older adults had less of a rebound of SWA. The authors suggested that these results indicate that sleep need (waking theta rise) does not decline with age, but that sleep ability (SWA rebound) does show age-related decrements.

Mechanistically, changes in sleep homeostasis in older adults may be related in part to changes in adenosine physiology. Older animals are reported to show higher basal forebrain adenosine levels than younger rats (132), higher adenosine metabolic enzymes (133), fewer adenosine receptor numbers (134), and larger increases in adenosine levels during sleep loss, yet a reduced responsiveness to adenosine administered to the basal forebrain region (132). Taken together, these changes suggest that aging may be associated with the development of adenosine resistance, perhaps similar to the insulin and leptin resistance that occurs with diabetes and obesity in aging. Specifically, normal amounts of adenosine in the basal forebrain appear to be insufficient to produce a young sleep phenotype in older animals. When cells are exposed to higher adenosine levels associated with older age, the cells may downregulate their adenosine receptor numbers and the receptors that remain may be desensitized to adenosine (132). In fact, age-related decreases in adenosine receptor binding have been reported to occur in older humans (135). Age-related changes in sleep architecture are summarized in Figure 2.

Circadian Characteristics that Change with Age
Age-related changes in the circadian system have been reported to include an advance in circadian timing and a reduction in circadian amplitude (Fig. 3). These

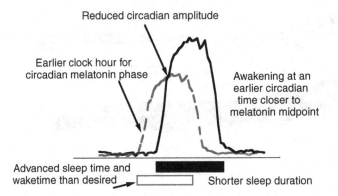

FIGURE 3 Circadian melatonin rhythm and sleep timing for young and older adults. Older adults generally show reduced circadian amplitude and earlier timing of sleep and circadian phase compared with young adults. Older adults also awaken at an earlier biological time such that wake time occurs closer to the melatonin maximum.

changes may be related to changes in the master circadian clock in the SCN and/or to changes in input and output pathways of the SCN.

One of the most commonly reported age-related changes in sleep is that older individuals often wake up at an earlier environmental time than desired (1,4,15,16,100,108,109,116,136–141). The early morning awakening that older adults experience may be in part explained by the advance in circadian phase. Phase advances of core body temperature, cortisol, and melatonin rhythms in older relative to young adults have been reported (15,100,136,138,142,143). In addition, Duffy et al. (142) reported that there are changes in the phase relationships between circadian rhythms in older adults versus young adults. Older adults not only awaken at an earlier clock hour but they also awaken at an earlier biological time. Specifically, older adults are reported to awaken closer to their body temperature minimum than do young adults (142). Such a change in the phase relationship between the time of awakening and internal biological time would be hypothesized to promote a phase advance of the circadian clock. Specifically, when older adults awaken early in the morning and are exposed to light, their circadian phase will be advanced and thus continue to promote early awakening (99,104). It should also be noted that many of the age-related changes in circadian timing reported above can be observed in middle-aged adults (144,145).

Older adults are reported to show a reduced amplitude in several circadian rhythms, including cognitive performance, melatonin, cortisol, core body temperature, and sleep spindles (15,100,110,142,143,146–150). However, healthy older adults do not always show a significant reduction in circadian amplitude compared with young adults (139). The general finding of reduced circadian amplitude with age could reflect decreased clock amplitude, clock output, and/or reduced downstream activity. Lower circadian amplitudes in output rhythms are most often (100,147,151), but not always (152), reported to be related to poor sleep quality. Indeed, age-related changes in circadian temperature amplitude may have implications for age-related sleep disruption (12). Age-related reductions in circadian amplitude have been reported in the electrical rhythm of SCN slices (153), individual SCN neurons (154), and in the circadian rhythms of spontaneous action potentials in culture (155).

Light exposure is the strongest input into the circadian system (99), and age-related circadian changes in the sensitivity to light exposure have been hypothesized to contribute to the earlier wake times seen in older adults. Although, older adults are reported to show a similar responsiveness to the phase delaying effects of bright light exposure as young adults (156–158), Duffy et al. (157) reported that older adults were less sensitive to low-to-moderate levels of light of ~50–1000 lux, as compared with findings previously reported in young adults (159). It is unknown how much age-related changes in the human visual system, such as changes in ocular lens transmittance (160,161), contribute to the reported reduced sensitivity to light with older age. Evidence from studies of nonhumans support that older animals show a decreased sensitivity to phase-resetting agents such as light exposure (162) and exogenous melatonin (163). Furthermore, older animals are reported to show lower light exposure-induced immediate early gene expression in the SCN (164). Light exposure is reported to induce smaller induction clock gene Per1 expression, thought to be involved in phase shifting, in the SCN of older versus younger hamsters (165). Resetting of clock gene expression in the SCN versus peripheral tissues is reported to be faster in some peripheral tissues and slower in others when comparing older versus young rats (166).

It has also been hypothesized that a shortening of the period of the circadian clock may contribute to earlier sleep and wake times. Expression of a circadian clock gene in SCN culture is reported to show a shorter circadian period in SCN from older versus younger rats (167). Studies assessing the circadian period of older human adults have been conflicting. Shorter (128,168) or no change (98) in period in older versus younger adults has been reported. Methodological differences may explain the conflicting reports as the masking effects were not controlled in the earlier studies (128,168). Czeisler et al. (98) reported an average circadian period of 24:10 and 24:11 for core body temperature and melatonin, respectively, in young adults, and 24:10 and 24:13 for core body temperature and melatonin, respectively, in older adults using a forced desynchrony protocol. These data suggest that the circadian period in humans remains relatively stable with age; and therefore, changes in circadian period likely have a small influence on the earlier morning awakening of older adults. However, the available studies assessing age changes in circadian period are cross-sectional. Therefore, there have been no prospective studies to assess changes in circadian period across the lifespan.

Age-Related Sleep Disruption and Changes in the Interaction Between Sleep Homeostasis and the Circadian Clock

The brain arousal systems discussed earlier are under homeostatic (18,47,55,169) and circadian control (94,97). In general, sleep homeostasis builds up with increased duration of wakefulness. When daily sleep need is not met, homeostatic sleep drive is increased resulting in impaired alertness and performance. The internal circadian clock influences the likelihood of falling asleep (170) and the timing of REM sleep. When sleep occurs at night, the circadian drive for wakefulness progressively increases across the biological day and peaks near habitual bedtime, whereas the

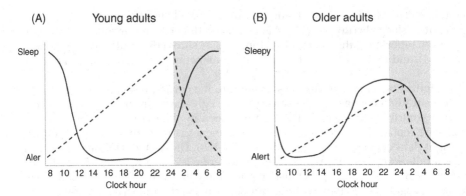

FIGURE 4 Two-process model of sleep and alertness regulation. Dashed lines represent the sleep homeostatic process and solid lines represent the circadian process. Dark gray shadings represent a sleep episode. During the day, as the homeostatic drive for sleep increases with time awake, the circadian signal promoting wakefulness increases to counteract the homeostatic drive for sleep so as to maintain a relatively high level of wakefulness across the day. During the night, as the homeostatic drive for sleep is dissipated, the circadian signal promoting sleep increases to maintain sleep. Older adults (B, *right*) generally show reduced circadian amplitude and earlier timing of sleep and circadian phase compared with young adults (A, *left*). Older adults also appear to show a reduced sensitivity or responsiveness to the buildup of homeostatic sleep drive during wakefulness. Clock hour is in military time.

circadian drive for wakefulness decreases during the biological night reaching a minimum near habitual wake time (137,171,172). The circadian and sleep homeostatic processes interact in an opponent process manner to promote consolidated wakefulness during the biological day and consolidated sleep during the biological night (137,173). The circadian drive for sleep is strongest just after the circadian temperature minimum. Subsequently, the circadian drive for wakefulness increases across the day until it peaks approximately just before habitual bedtime (Fig. 4). The circadian drive for REM sleep is highest in the early morning hours. Sleep homeostasis and circadian phase interact to regulate the sleep timing and structure (136,137,174,175). Sleep initiation and sleep maintenance are dependent on an appropriate phase relationship between the circadian timing system and the sleep–wake schedule. Sleep efficiency in young adults can be maintained at high levels for 8 hours only when sleep is initiated ~4 to 6 hours before the endogenous circadian minimum of core body temperature (136,174), whereas sleep efficiency in older adults can be maintained at high levels for less time (3).

CONCLUSIONS

The primary sleep and wakefulness centers are located in the brain stem and midbrain. Active inhibition of wakefulness centers promotes sleep, whereas active inhibition of sleep centers promotes wakefulness. Modification in function of these brain regions has impact on the quality of sleep and wakefulness. Research has shown that sleep and circadian physiology are altered with age. Sleep is lighter and more fragmented with older age, as evidenced by less SWS, increased number and duration of EEG arousals, and more stage 2 sleep. Total sleep time is reduced, yet it is unclear if this reduction in sleep time represents a reduction in sleep need or sleep ability. Adenosine levels increase with age, suggesting that increased sleep drive yet aging also appears to be associated with adenosine resistance which might reflect reduced sleep ability. Age-related sleep disturbance appears to occur regardless of comorbid health problems. Changes in circadian physiology with age include earlier sleep and wake times than desirable, earlier clock hour of internal circadian time, a change in the phase relationship between sleep and internal circadian time, a reduction in circadian amplitude, and a reduction in sensitivity to low to moderate light levels. Changes in the electrophysiology of the SCN and/or SCN degeneration may be responsible for age-related changes in circadian physiology. Given the complexity of sleep–wakefulness and circadian systems, and possible targets for treatments of age-related sleep and wakefulness disruption, additional research is needed to identify other age-related changes in these fundamental regulatory systems.

REFERENCES

1. Dijk DJ, Duffy JF, Czeisler CA. Contribution of circadian physiology and sleep homeostasis to age-related changes in human sleep. Chronobiol Int 2000; 17(3):285–311.
2. Dijk DJ, Duffy JF, Czeisler CA. Age-related increase in awakenings, impaired consolidation of nonrem sleep at all circadian phases. Sleep 2001; 5:565–582.
3. Dijk DJ, Duffy JF, Riel E, et al. Ageing and the circadian and homeostatic regulation of human sleep during forced desynchrony of rest, melatonin and temperature rhythms. J Physiol 1999; 516(Pt 2):611–627.
4. Prinz PN. Sleep and sleep disorders in older adults. J Clin Neurophysiol 1995; 12(2):139–146.
5. Anderson KO, Getto CJ, Mendoza TR, et al. Fatigue and sleep disturbance in patients with cancer, patients with clinical depression, and community-dwelling adults. J Pain Symptom Manage 2003; 25(4):307–318.
6. Asplund R. Sleep disorders in the elderly. Drugs Aging 1999; 14(2):91–103.
7. Asplund R. Nocturia in relation to sleep, health, and medical treatment in the elderly. BJU Int 2005; 96:15–21.
8. Foley D, Ancoli-Israel S, Britz P, et al. Sleep disturbances and chronic disease in older adults, results of the 2003 National Sleep Foundation Sleep in America Survey. J Psychosom Res 2004; 56(5):497–502.
9. Asplund R. Daytime sleepiness and napping amongst the elderly in relation to somatic health and medical treatment. J Intern Med 1996; 239(3):261–267.
10. Ancoli-Israel S. Insomnia in the elderly, a review for the primary care practitioner. Sleep 2000; 23(suppl 1):S23–S30.
11. Vitiello MV. Sleep disorders and aging, understanding the causes. J Gerontol A Biol Sci Med Sci 1997; 52(4):M189–M191.
12. Van Someren EJW. More than a marker, interaction between the circadian regulation of temperature and sleep, age-related changes, and treatment possibilities. Chronobiol Int 2000; 17(3):313–354.
13. Bliwise DL. Sleep in normal aging and dementia. Sleep 1993; 16(1):40–81.
14. Van Someren EJ. Circadian rhythms and sleep in human aging. Chronobiol Int 2000; 17(3):233–243.
15. Czeisler CA, Dumont M, Duffy JF, et al. Association of sleep–wake habits in older people with changes in output of circadian pacemaker. Lancet 1992; 340(8825):933–936.
16. Duffy JF, Czeisler CA. Age-related change in the relationship between circadian period, circadian phase, and diurnal preference in humans. Neurosci Lett 2002; 318(3):117–120.

17. Carrier J, Monk TH, Reynolds CF, et al. Are age differences in sleep due to phase differences in the output of the circadian timing system? Chronobiol Int 1999; 16(1):79–91.
18. Saper CB, Chou TC, Scammell TE. The sleep switch, hypothalamic control of sleep and wakefulness. Trends Neurosci 2001; 24(12):726–731.
19. Mcginty D, Szymusiak R. Sleep-promoting mechanisms in mammals. In: Kryger MH, Roth T, Dement WC, eds. Principles and Practice of Sleep Medicine, 4th edn. Philadelphia: Elsevier Saunders, 2005:169–184.
20. Moruzzi G, Magoun HW. Brain stem reticular formation and activation of the EEG. Electroenceph Clin Neurophysiol 1949; 1:455–473.
21. Steriade M. Basic mechanisms of sleep generation. Neurology 1992; 42(7 suppl 6):9–17.
22. Aston-Jones G, Bloom FE. Activity of norepinephrine-containing locus coeruleus neurons in behaving rats anticipates fluctuations in the sleep–waking cycle. J Neurosci 1981; 1(8):876–886.
23. Shouse MN, Staba RJ, Saquib SF, et al. Monoamines and sleep, microdialysis findings in pons and amygdala. Brain Res 2000; 860(1–2):181–189.
24. Monti JM, Monti D. The involvement of dopamine in the modulation of sleep and waking. Sleep Med Rev 2007; 11(2):113–133.
25. Rye DB. State of the art review, contributions of the pedunculopontine region to normal and altered REM sleep. Sleep 1997; 20(9):757–788.
26. Strecker RE, Morairty S, Thakkar MM, et al. Adenosinergic modulation of basal forebrain and preoptic/anterior hypothalamic neuronal activity in the control of behavioral state. Behav Brain Res 2000; 115(2):183–204.
27. Panksepp J. The neurochemistry of behavior. Annu Rev Psychol 1986; 37:77–107.
28. Alam MN, Szymusiak R, Gong H, et al. Adenosinergic modulation of rat basal forebrain neurons during sleep and waking, neuronal recording with microdialysis. J Physiol 1999; 521(Pt 3):679–690.
29. Nicholson AN, Stone BM. Antihistamines, impaired performance and the tendency to sleep. Eur J Clin Pharmacol 1986; 30:27–32.
30. Culebras A. The neurology of sleep. Introduction. Neurology 1992; 42(7 suppl 6):6–8.
31. Jones BE. Basic mechanisms of sleep–wake states. In: Kryger MH, Roth T, Dement WC, eds. Principles and Practice of Sleep Medicine, 3rd edn. Philadelphia: W.B. Saunders Company, 2000:134–154.
32. Nitz D, Siegel J. GABA release in the dorsal raphe nucleus, role in the control of REM sleep. Am J Physiol 1997; 273(1 Pt 2):R451–R455.
33. Date Y, Ueta Y, Yamashita H, et al. Orexins, Orexigenic Hypothalamic Peptides, Interact With Autonomic, Neuroendocrine And Neuroregulatory Systems. Proc Natl Acad Sci U S A 1999; 96(2):748–753.
34. De Lecea L, Kilduff TS, Peyron C, et al. The hypocretins, hypothalamus-specific peptides with neuroexcitatory activity. Proc Natl Acad Sci U S A 1998; 95(1):322–327.
35. Peyron C, Tighe DK, Van Den Pol AN, et al. Neurons containing hypocretin (orexin) project to multiple neuronal systems. J Neurosci 1998; 18(23):9996–10015.
36. Hagan JJ, Leslie RA, Patel S, et al. Orexin A activates locus coeruleus cell firing and increases arousal in the rat. Proc Natl Acad Sci U S A 1999; 96(19):10911–10916.
37. Davis H, Davis PA, Loomis AL, et al. Human brain potentials during the onset of sleep. J Neurophysiol 1938; 1:34–38.
38. Wright KP Jr., Badia P, Wauquier A. Topographical and temporal patterns of brain activity during the transition from wakefulness to sleep. Sleep 1995; 18(10):880–889.
39. Ogilvie RD, Wilkinson RT, Allison S. The detection of sleep onset, behavioral, physiological, and subjective convergence. Sleep 1989; 12(5):458–474.
40. Ogilvie RD, Simons I. Falling asleep and waking up, a comparison of EEG spectra. Sleep Arousal Performance 1992:73–87.
41. Achermann P, Dijk DJ, Brunner DP, et al. A model of human sleep homeostasis based on EEG slow-wave activity, quantitative comparison of data and simulations. Brain Res Bull 1993; 31(1–2):97–113.
42. Dijk DJ, Beersma DG. Effects of SWS deprivation on subsequent EEG power density and spontaneous sleep duration. Electroencephalogr Clin Neurophysiol 1989; 72(4):312–320.

43. Steriade M, Domich L, Oakson G, et al. The deafferented reticular thalamic nucleus generates spindle rhythmicity. J Neurophysiol 1987; 57(1):260–273.

44. Lancel M. Role of GABAA receptors in the regulation of sleep, initial sleep responses to peripherally administered modulators and antagonists. Sleep 1999; 22:33–42.

45. Szymusiak R, Alam N, Steininger TL, et al. Sleep–waking discharge patterns of ventrolateral preoptic/anterior hypothalamic neurons in rats. Brain Res 1998; 803:178–188.

46. Sherin JE, Elmquist JK, Torrealba F, et al. Innervation of histaminergic tuberomammillary neurons by GABAergic and galaninergic neurons in the ventrolateral preoptic nucleus of the rat. J Neurosci 1998; 18(12):4705–4721.

47. Chou TC, Bjorkum AA, Gaus SE, et al. Afferents to the ventrolateral preoptic nucleus. J Neurosci 2002; 22(3):977–990.

48. Gallopin T, Fort P, Eggermann E, et al. Identification of sleep-promoting neurons in vitro. Nature 2000; 404(6781):992–995.

49. Lu J, Greco MA, Shiromani P, et al. Effect of lesions of the ventrolateral preoptic nucleus on NREM and REM sleep. J Neurosci 2000; 20(10):3830–3842.

50. Jones BE. Basic mechanisms of sleep–wake states. In: Kryger MH, Roth T, Dement WC, eds. Principles and Practice of Sleep Medicine, 4th edn. Philadelphia: Elsevier Saunders, 2005:36–153.

51. Alanko L, Heiskanen S, Stenberg D, et al. Adenosine kinase and 5'-nucleotidase activity after prolonged wakefulness in the cortex and the basal forebrain of rat. Neurochem Int 2003; 42(6):449–454.

52. Basheer R, Rainnie DG, Porkka-Heiskanen T, et al. Adenosine, prolonged wakefulness, and A1-activated NF-kappab DNA binding in the basal forebrain of the rat. Neuroscience 2001; 104(3):731–739.

53. Porkka-Heiskanen T, Strecker RE, Mccarley RW. Brain site-specificity of extracellular adenosine concentration changes during sleep deprivation and spontaneous sleep, an in vivo microdialysis study. Neuroscience 2000; 99(3):507–517.

54. Dunwiddie TV, Masino SA. The role and regulation of adenosine in the central nervous system. Annu Rev Neurosci 2001; 24:31–55.

55. Basheer R, Strecker RE, Thakkar MM, et al. Adenosine and sleep–wake regulation. Prog Neurobiol 2004; 73(6):379–396.

56. Szymusiak R, Gvilia I, Mcginty D. Hypothalamic control of sleep. Sleep Med 2007; 8(4):291–301.

57. Scammell TE, Gerashchenko DY, Mochizuki T, et al. An adenosine A2a agonist increases sleep and induces FOS in ventrolateral preoptic neurons. Neuroscience 2001; 107(4):653–663.

58. Chamberlin NL, Arrigoni E, Chou TC, et al. Effects of adenosine on gabaergic synaptic inputs to identified ventrolateral preoptic neurons. Neuroscience 2003; 119(4):913–918.

59. Elmenhorst D, Meyer PT, Winz OH, et al. Sleep deprivation increases A1 adenosine receptor binding in the human brain, a positron emission tomography study. J Neurosci 2007; 27(9):2410–2415.

60. Krueger JM, Majde JA. Humoral links between sleep and the immune system, research issues. Ann N Y Acad Sci 2003; 992:9–20.

61. Alam MN, Mcginty D, Bashir T, et al. Interleukin-1beta modulates state-dependent discharge activity of preoptic area and basal forebrain neurons, role in sleep regulation. Eur J Neurosci 2004; 20(1):207–216.

62. Siegel JM. Brainstem mechanisms generating REM sleep. In: Kryger MH, Roth T, Dement WC, eds. Principles and Practice of Sleep Medicine, 3rd edn. Philadelphia: W.B. Saunders Company, 2000:112–133.

63. Thakkar MM, Strecker RE, Mccarley RW. Behavioral state control through differential serotonergic inhibition in the mesopontine cholinergic nuclei, a simultaneous unit recording and microdialysis study. J Neurosci 1998; 18(14):5490–5497.

64. Maloney KJ, Mainville L, Jones BE. C-Fos expression in gabaergic, serotonergic, and other neurons of the pontomedullary reticular formation and raphe after paradoxical sleep deprivation and recovery. J Neurosci 2000; 20(12):4669–4679.

65. Lu J, Sherman D, Devor M, et al. A putative flip-flop switch for control of REM sleep. Nature 2006; 441(7093),589–594.
66. Fuller PM, Saper CB, Lu J. The pontine REM switch, past and present. J Physiol 2007; 584(Pt 3):735–741.
67. Crochet S, Sakai K. Effects of microdialysis application of monoamines on the EEG and behavioural states in the cat mesopontine tegmentum. Eur J Neurosci 1999; 11(10):3738–3752.
68. Aston-Jones G, Rajkowski J, Cohen J. Role of locus coeruleus in attention and behavioral flexibility. Biol Psychiatry 1999; 46(9):1309–1320.
69. Cirelli C, Pompeiano M, Tononi G. Neuronal gene expression in the waking state, a role for the locus coeruleus. Science 1996; 274:1211–1215.
70. Benington JH, Heller HC. Restoration of brain energy metabolism as the function of sleep. Prog Neurobiol 1995; 45:347–360.
71. Lin L, Faraco J, Li R, et al. The sleep disorder canine narcolepsy is caused by a mutation in the hypocretin (orexin) receptor 2 gene. Cell 1999; 98(3):365–376.
72. Chemelli RM, Willie JT, Sinton CM, et al. Narcolepsy in orexin knockout mice, molecular genetics of sleep regulation. Cell 1999; 98(4):437–451.
73. Siegel JM. Narcolepsy, a key role in *Hypocretins* (*Orexins*). Cell 1999; 98(4):409–412.
74. Xi MC, Morales FR, Chase MH. Evidence that wakefulness and REM sleep are controlled by a gabaergic pontine mechanism. J Neurophysiol 1999; 82(4):2015–2019.
75. Fenik VB, Davies RO, Kubin L. Noradrenergic, serotonergic and gabaergic antagonists injected together into the XII nucleus abolish the REM sleep-like depression of hypoglossal motoneuronal activity. J Sleep Res 2005; 14(4):419–429.
76. Chase MH, Morales FR. Control of motoneurons during sleep. In: Kryger MH, Roth T, Dement WC, eds. Principles and Practice of Sleep Medicine. Philadelphia: Elsevier Saunders, 2005:154–168.
77. Lai YY, Kodama T, Siegel JM. Changes in monoamine release in the ventral horn and hypoglossal nucleus linked to pontine inhibition of muscle tone, an in vivo microdialysis study. J Neurosci 2001; 21(18):7384–7391.
78. Moore RY. The suprachiasmatic nucleus and the circadian timing system. In: Klein DC, Moore RY, Reppert SM, eds. Suprachiasmatic Nucleus, The Mind's Clock, 1st edn. New York, Oxford: Oxford University Press, 1991:13–15.
79. Albers HE, Lydic R, Moore-Ede MC. Role of the suprachiasmatic nuclei in the circadian timing system of the squirrel monkey. II. Light–dark cycle entrainment. Brain Res 1984; 300(2):285–293.
80. Schwartz WJ, Davidsen LC, Smith CB. In vivo metabolic activity of a putative circadian oscillator, the rat suprachiasmatic nucleus. J Comp Neurol 1980; 189:157–167.
81. Moore RY, Eichler VB. Loss of a circadian adrenal corticosterone rhythm following suprachiasmatic lesions in the rat. Brain Res 1972; 42:201–206.
82. Edgar DM, Dement WC, Fuller CA. Effect of SCN lesions on sleep in squirrel monkeys, evidence for opponent processes in sleep–wake regulation. J Neurosci 1993; 13(3):1065–1079.
83. Wurts SW, Edgar DM. Circadian and homeostatic control of rapid eye movement (REM) sleep, promotion of REM tendency by the suprachiasmatic nucleus. J Neurosci 2000; 20(11):4300–4310.
84. Ibuka N, Kawamura H. Loss of circadian rhythm in sleep–wakefulness cycle in the rat by suprachiasmatic nucleus lesions. Brain Res 1975; 96:76–81.
85. Moore RY. Organization of the mammalian circadian system. In: Waterhouse JM, ed. Circadian Clocks and Their Adjustment. Chichester (Ciba Foundation Symp 183): John Wiley and Sons, Inc., 1994:88–99.
86. Moore RY, Speh JC, Card JP. The retinohypothalamic tract originates from a distinct subset of retinal ganglion cells. J Comp Neurol 1995; 352:351–366.
87. Gooley JJ, Lu J, Chou TC, et al. Melanopsin in cells of origin of the retinohypothalamic tract. Nat Neurosci 2001; 4(12):1165.
88. Lydic R, Schoene WC, Czeisler CA, et al. Suprachiasmatic region of the human hypothalamus, homolog to the primate circadian pacemaker? Sleep 1980; 2:355–361.

89. Swaab DF, Fliers E, Partiman TS. The suprachiasmatic nucleus of the human brain in relation to sex, age and senile dementia. Brain Res 1985; 342:37–44.
90. Weaver DR, Stehle JH, Stopa EG, et al. Melatonin receptors in human hypothalamus and pituitary, implications for circadian and reproductive responses to melatonin. J Clin Endocrinol Metab 1993; 76:295–301.
91. Watts AG. The efferent projections of the suprachiasmatic nucleus, anatomical insights into the control of circadian rhythms. In: Klein DC, Moore RY, Reppert SM, eds. Suprachiasmatic Nucleus, The Mind's Clock, 1st edn. New York, Oxford: Oxford University Press, 1991:77–106.
92. Dai J, Swaab DF, Buijs RM. Distribution of vasopressin and vasoactive intestinal polypeptide (VIP) fibers in human hypothalamus with special emphasis on suprachiasmatic nucleus effect projections. J Comp Neurol 1997; 383:397–414.
93. Saper CB, Scammell TE, Lu J. Hypothalamic regulation of sleep and circadian rhythms. Nature 2005; 437(7063):1257–1263.
94. Aston-Jones G, Chen S, Zhu Y, et al. A neural circuit for circadian regulation of arousal. Nat Neurosci 2001; 4(7):732–738.
95. Aston-Jones G. Brain structures and receptors involved in alertness. Sleep Med 2005; 6(suppl 1):S3–S7.
96. Deboer T, Overeem S, Visser NA, et al. Convergence of circadian and sleep regulatory mechanisms on hypocretin-1. Neuroscience 2004; 129(3):727–732.
97. Deurveilher S, Semba K. Indirect projections from the suprachiasmatic nucleus to major arousal-promoting cell groups in rat, implications for the circadian control of behavioural state. Neuroscience 2005; 130(1):165–183.
98. Czeisler CA, Duffy JF, Shanahan TL et al. Stability, precision, and near-24-hour period of the human circadian pacemaker. Science 1999; 284(5423):2177–2181.
99. Czeisler CA, Wright KP Jr. Influence of light on circadian rhythmicity in humans. In: Turek FW, Zee PC, eds. Regulation of Sleep and Circadian Rhythms. New York: Marcel Dekker, Inc., 1999:149–180.
100. Myers BL, Badia P. Changes in circadian rhythms and sleep quality with aging, mechanisms and interventions. Neurosci Biobehav Rev 1995; 19(4):553–571.
101. Winfree AT. The Geometry of Biological Time. New York: Springer-Verlag, 1980.
102. Wright KP Jr., Hughes RJ, Kronauer RE, et al. Intrinsic near-24-hour pacemaker period determines limits of circadian entrainment to a weak synchronizer in humans. Proc Natl Acad Sci U S A 2001; 98(24):14027–14032.
103. Gronfier C, Wright KP Jr., Kronauer RE, et al. Entrainment of the human circadian pacemaker to longer-than-24-h days. Proc Natl Acad Sci U S A 2007; 104(21):9081–9086.
104. Duffy JF, Wright KP Jr. Entrainment of the human circadian system by light. J Biol Rhythms 2005; 28(4):326–338.
105. Duffy JF, Rimmer DW, Czeisler CA. Association of intrinsic circadian period with morningness–eveningness, usual wake time, and circadian phase. Behav Neuroscience 2001; 115(4):895–899.
106. Wright KP Jr., Gronfier C, Duffy JE, et al. Intrinsic period and light intensity determine the phase relationship between melatonin and sleep in humans. J Biol Rhythms 2005; 20(2):168–177.
107. Jewett ME, Rimmer DW, Duffy JF, et al. Human circadian pacemaker is sensitive to light throughout subjective day without evidence of transients. Am J Physiol 1997; 273:R1800–R1809.
108. Larsen LH, Moe KE, Vitiello MV, et al. Age trends in the sleep EEG of healthy older men and women. J Sleep Res 1995; 4(3):160–172.
109. Bliwise D. Normal aging. In: Kryger MH, Roth T, Dement WC, eds. Principles and Practice of Sleep Medicine, 3rd edn. Philadelphia: W.B. Saunders Company, 1994:26–42.
110. Kales A, Wilson T, Kales JD, et al. Measurements of all-night sleep in normal elderly persons, effects of aging. J Am Geriatr Soc 1967; 15(5):405–414.
111. Lariy BE, Cormordret M, Faure R, et al. Electroencephalographic study of sleep in the aged, normal and pathologic. Revue Neurologique (Paris) 1962; 107:188.

112. Passouant P, Bertrand L, Delange M, et al. Arteriosclerosis and sleep. Study of night sleep in the aged over 80 years old. Oto-Neuro-Ophtalmol (Paris) 1963; 35:1.
113. Roffwarg HP, Dement WC. Preliminary observations of the sleep-dream pattern in neonates, infants, children and adults. In: Harms E, ed. Problems of Sleep and Dreams in Children (Monograph on Child Psychiatry). New York: Pergamon Press, 1964:60–72.
114. Blois R, Feinberg I, Gaillard JM, et al. Sleep in normal and pathological aging. Experientia 1983; 39(6):551–558.
115. Bundlie SR. Sleep in aging. Geriatrics 1998; 53(suppl 1):S41–S43.
116. Floyd JA. Sleep and aging. Nurs Clin North Am 2002; 37(4):719–731.
117. Frank SA, Roland DC, Sturis J, et al. Effects of aging on glucose regulation during wakefulness and sleep. Am J Physiol 1995; 269(6 Pt 1):E1006–E1016.
118. Gigli GL, Placidi F, Diomedi M, et al. Sleep in healthy elderly subjects, a 24-hour ambulatory polysomnographic study. Int J Neurosci 1996; 85(3–4):263–271.
119. Huang YL, Liu RY, Wang QS, et al. Age-associated difference in circadian sleep–wake and rest–activity rhythms. Physiol Behav 2002; 76(4–5):597–603.
120. Landolt HP, Dijk DJ, Achermann P, et al. Effect of age on the sleep EEG, slow-wave activity and spindle frequency activity in young and middle-aged men. Brain Res 1996; 738(2):205–212.
121. Mourtazaev MS, Kemp B, Zwinderman AH, et al. Age and gender affect different characteristics of slow waves in the sleep EEG. Sleep 1995; 18(7):557–564.
122. Reynolds CF III, Kupfer DJ, Taska LS, et al. Slow wave sleep in elderly depressed, demented, and healthy subjects. Sleep 1985; 8(2):155–159.
123. Klerman EB, Davis JB, Duffy JF, et al. Older people awaken more frequently but fall back asleep at the same rate as younger people. Sleep 2004; 27(4):793–798.
124. Landolt HP, Borbely AA. Age-dependent changes in sleep EEG topography. Clin Neurophysiol 2001; 112(2):369–377.
125. Avidan AY. Sleep changes and disorders in the elderly patient. Curr Neurol Neurosci Rep 2002; 2(2):178–185.
126. Feinsilver SH. Sleep in the elderly. What is normal? Clin Geriatr Med 2003; 19(1):177–188, VIII.
127. Ficca G, Gori S, Ktonas P, et al. The organization of rapid eye movement activity during rapid eye movement sleep is impaired in the elderly. Neurosci Lett 1999; 275(3):219–221.
128. Weitzman ED, Moline ML, Czeisler CA, et al. Chronobiology of aging, temperature, sleep–wake rhythms and entrainment. Neurobiol Aging 1982; 3(4):299–309.
129. Dijk DJ, Czeisler CA. Contribution of the circadian pacemaker and the sleep homeostat to sleep propensity, sleep structure, electroencephalographic slow waves, and sleep spindle activity in humans. J Neurosci 1995; 15(5 Pt 1):3526–3538.
130. Carskadon MA, Dement WC. Sleep loss in elderly volunteers. Sleep 1985; 8(3):207–221.
131. Drapeau C, Carrier J. Fluctuation of waking electroencephalogram and subjective alertness during a 25-hour sleep-deprivation episode in young and middle-aged subjects. Sleep 2004; 27(1):55–60.
132. Murillo-Rodriguez E, Blanco-Centurion C, Gerashchenko D, et al. The diurnal rhythm of forebrain of young and adenosine levels in the basal old rats. Neuroscience 2004; 123(2):361–370.
133. Mackiewicz M, Nikonova EV, Zimmermann JE, et al. Age-related changes in adenosine metabolic enzymes in sleep/wake regulatory areas of the brain. Neurobiol Aging 2006; 27(2):351–360.
134. Meerlo P, Roman V, Farkas E, et al. Ageing-related decline in adenosine A1 receptor binding in the rat brain, an autoradiographic study. J Neurosci Res 2004; 78(5):742–748.
135. Meyer PT, Elmenhorst D, Boy C, et al. Effect of aging on cerebral A1 adenosine receptors, A [18f]Cpfpx pet study in humans. Neurobiol Aging 2007; 28(12):1914–1924.
136. Dijk DJ, Duffy JF. Circadian regulation of human sleep and age-related changes in its timing, consolidation and EEG characteristics. Ann Med 1999; 31(2):130–140.
137. Dijk D-J, Edgar DM. Circadian and homeostatic control of wakefulness and sleep. In: Turek FW, Zee PC, eds. Regulation of Sleep and Wakefulness. New York: Marcel Dekker, Inc., 1999:111–147.

138. Richardson GS. Circadian rhythms and aging. In: Schneider EL, Rowe JW, eds. Handbook of the Biology of Aging, 3rd edn. San Diego: Academic Press, Inc., 1990:275–305.
139. Zeitzer JM, Daniels JE, Duffy JF, et al. Do plasma melatonin concentrations decline with Age? Am J Med 1999; 107(5):432–436.
140. Duffy JF, Dijk DJ, Hall EF, et al. Relationship of endogenous circadian melatonin and temperature rhythms to self-reported preference for morning or evening activity in young and older people. J Investig Med 1999; 47(3):141–150.
141. Yoon IY, Kripke DF, Elliott JA, et al. Age-related changes of circadian rhythms and sleep–wake cycles. J Am Geriatr Soc 2003; 51(8):1085–1091.
142. Duffy JF, Dijk D-J, Klerman EB, et al. Later endogenous circadian temperature nadir relative to an earlier wake time in older people. Am J Physiol 1998; 275:R1478–R1487.
143. Duffy JF, Zeitzer JM, Rimmer DW, et al. Peak of circadian melatonin rhythm occurs later within the sleep of older subjects. Am J Physiol Endocrinol Metab 2002; 282(2):E297–E303.
144. Carrier J, Paquet J, Morettini J, et al. Phase advance of sleep and temperature circadian rhythms in the middle years of life in humans. Neurosci Lett 2002; 320(1–2):1–4.
145. Carrier J, Land S, Buysse DJ, et al. The effects of age and gender on sleep EEG power spectral density in the middle years of life (ages 20–60 years old). Psychophysiology 2001; 38(2):232–242.
146. Cajochen C, Brunner DP, Krauchi K, et al. Power density in theta/alpha frequencies of the waking EEG progressively increases during sustained wakefulness. Sleep 1995; 18(10):890–894.
147. Carrier J, Monk TH, Buysse DJ, et al. Amplitude reduction of the circadian temperature and sleep rhythms in the elderly. Chronobiol Int 1996; 13(5):373–386.
148. Monk TH, Buysse DJ, Reynolds CF, et al. Subjective alertness rhythms in elderly people. J Biol Rhythms 1996; 11(3):268–276.
149. Cajochen C, Munch M, Knoblauch V, et al. Age-related changes in the circadian and homeostatic regulation of human sleep. Chronobiol Int 2006; 23(1–2):461–474.
150. Wei HG, Riel E, Czeisler CA, et al. Attenuated amplitude of circadian and sleep-dependent modulation of electroencephalographic sleep spindle characteristics in elderly human subjects. Neurosci Lett 1999; 260(1):29–32.
151. Van Someren EJW. More than a marker, Interaction between the circadian regulation of temperature and sleep, age-related changes, and treatment possibilities. Chronobiol Int 2000; 17(3):313–354.
152. Hughes RJ, Sack RL, Lewy AJ. The role of melatonin and circadian phase in age-related sleep-maintenance insomnia, assessment in a clinical trial of melatonin replacement. Sleep 1998; 21(1):52–68.
153. Satinoff E, Li H, Tcheng TK, et al. Do the suprachiasmatic nuclei oscillate in old rats as they do in young ones? Am J Physiol 1993; 265(5 Pt 2):R1216–R1222.
154. Aujard F, Herzog ED, Block GD. Circadian rhythms in firing rate of individual suprachiasmatic nucleus neurons from adult and middle-aged mice. Neuroscience 2001; 106(2):255–261.
155. Nygard M, Hill RH, Wikstrom MA, et al. Age-related changes in electrophysiological properties of the mouse suprachiasmatic nucleus in vitro. Brain Res Bull 2005; 65(2):149–154.
156. Klerman EB, Duffy JF, Dijk DJ, et al. Circadian phase resetting in older people by ocular bright light exposure. J Investig Med 2001; 49(1):30–40.
157. Duffy JF, Zeitzer JM, Czeisler CA. Decreased sensitivity to phase-delaying effects of moderate intensity light in older subjects. Neurobiol Aging 2007; 28(5):799–807.
158. Benloucif S, Green K, L'hermite-Baleriaux M, et al. Responsiveness of the aging circadian clock to light. Neurobiol Aging 2006; 27(12):1870–1879.
159. Zeitzer JM, Dijk D-J, Kronauer RE, et al. Sensitivity of the human circadian pacemaker to nocturnal light, melatonin phase resetting and suppression. J Physiol (Lond) 2000; 526(3):695–702.
160. Charman WN. Age, lens transmittance, and the possible effects of light on melatonin suppression. Ophthal Physiol Opt 2003; 23(2):181–187.

161. Zhang Y, Brainard GC, Zee PC, et al. Effects of aging on lens transmittance and reti-nal input to the suprachiasmatic nucleus in golden hamsters. Neurosci Lett 1998; 258(3):167–170.

162. Zhang Y, Kornhauser JM, Zee PC, et al. Effects of aging on light-induced phase-shifting of circadian behavioral rhythms, FOS expression and CREB phosphorylation in the hamster suprachiasmatic nucleus. Neuroscience 1996; 70(4):951–961.

163. Von Gall C, Weaver DR. Loss of responsiveness to melatonin in the aging mouse suprachiasmatic nucleus. Neurobiol Aging 2006, Nov 22 [Epub ahead of print].

164. Benloucif S, Masana MI, Dubocovich ML. Light-induced phase shifts of circadian activ-ity rhythms and immediate early gene expression in the suprachiasmatic nucleus are attenuated in old C3 h/Hen mice. Brain Res 1997; 747(1):34–42.

165. Kolker DE, Fukuyama H, Huang DS, et al. Aging alters circadian and light-induced expression of clock genes in golden hamsters. J Biol Rhythms 2003; 18(2):159–169.

166. Davidson AJ, Yamazaki S, Arble DM, et al. Resetting of central and peripheral circadian oscillators in aged Rats. Neurobiol Aging 2006.

167. Yamazaki S, Straume M, Tei H, et al. Effects of aging on central and peripheral mam-malian clocks. Proc Natl Acad Sci U S A 2002; 99(16):10801–10806.

168. Monk TH. Sleep disorders in the elderly. Circadian rhythm. Clin Geriatr Med 1989; 5(2):331–346.

169. Porkka-Heiskanen T, Strecker RE, Thakkar M, et al. Adenosine, a mediator of the sleep-inducing effects of prolonged wakefulness. Science 1997; 276(5316):1265–1268.

170. Lavie P, Segal S. Twenty-four-hour structure of sleepiness in morning and evening per-sons investigated by ultrashort sleep–wake cycle. Sleep 1989; 12(6):522–528.

171. Achermann P, Borbely AA. Mathematical models of sleep regulation. Front Biosci 2003; 8:S683–S693.

172. Tobler I, Franken P, Trachsel L, et al. Models of sleep regulation in mammals. J Sleep Res 1992; 1(2):125–127.

173. Wright KP Jr., Hull JT, Czeisler CA. Relationship between alertness, performance, and body temperature in humans. Am J Physiol Regul Integr Comp Physiol 2002; 283(6):R1370–R1377.

174. Dijk DJ, Czeisler CA. Paradoxical timing of the circadian rhythm of sleep propensity serves to consolidate sleep and wakefulness in humans. Neurosci Lett 1994; 166(1):63–68.

175. Wyatt JK, Ritz-De Cecco A, Czeisler CA, et al. Circadian temperature and melatonin rhythms, sleep, and neurobehavioral function in humans living on a 20-h day. Am J Physiol 1999; 277:R1152–R1163.

176. Ohayon MM, Carskadon MA, Guilleminault C, et al. Meta-analysis of quantitative sleep parameters from childhood to old age in healthy individuals: developing normative sleep values across the human lifespan. Sleep 2004; 27:1255–1273.

2 Sleep and Medical Comorbidities

Steven R. Barczi

Department of Medicine, Section of Geriatrics, University of Wisconsin School of Medicine and Public Health, and The Madison V.A. Geriatric Research, Education and Clinical Center, William S. Middleton Veterans Administration Hospital, Madison, Wisconsin, U.S.A.

INTRODUCTION: THE INTERACTIONS OF SLEEP, MEDICAL ILLNESS, MEDICATIONS, AND AGING

Sleep is an essential human behavior and a tightly regulated biological rhythm. It is often considered a barometer of health and is susceptible to the disruptive effects of many endogenous and exogenous influences. This is especially evident in older persons with multiple medical comorbidities. Sleep complaints increase in prevalence with aging in a pattern that parallels the increase in medical conditions and medication use (1). Acknowledging the complex interaction between sleep, medical illness, medications, and age enables the clinician to more comprehensively and effectively address sleep difficulties in older adults.

Secondary insomnia is a term used to describe the sleep changes associated with medical or psychiatric diagnoses. It implies a causal relationship between the illness and the accompanying sleep disruption. Given the inconsistency of scientific evidence for many of these associations, expert consensus recommends a change in terminology. The 2005 National Institutes of Health (NIH) State-of-the-Science Conference on Insomnia proposed using the diagnosis of comorbid insomnia when an illness coexists with sleep changes but the details of cause and effect are not proven (2). Furthermore, medical and psychiatric diagnoses often necessitate complicated medication regimens that can further confound sleep architecture and daytime wakefulness. The International Classification of Sleep Disorders (ICSD), the nosological framework used by sleep clinicians, was recently revised with substantive changes made in areas relevant to insomnia (3). The new ICSD-2 includes two categories that encompass the breadth of comorbid insomnia: (1) Other Insomnia Due to Mental Disorder and (2) Other Insomnia Due to a Known Physiological Condition.

The Epidemiology of Sleep Changes with Medical Comorbidities

A number of studies have characterized the associated risks for sleep disturbance in individuals in mid and later life. Evidence supports that these sleep changes are more strongly associated with health and psychosocial factors rather than aging per se (1,4–6). These findings have important implications when one considers the disease prevalence in populations over age 60 and the frequency of coexisting medical and psychiatric conditions in this age group. Furthermore, these health problems appear to have additive effects when the likelihood of concomitant sleep complaints is considered. The 2003 "Sleep in America" survey conducted by the National Sleep Foundation found that 36% of people aged 55 years and older without chronic illness had sleep problems, 52% with one to three comorbidities had sleep disturbances, and 69% of those with four or more comorbidities had disturbed sleep (1). The self-perceived quality of these respondents' sleep was also inversely proportional to the number of comorbidities they possessed (1).

Chronic Health Conditions in Later Life

Chronic health problems increase in prevalence with age. In 1999, 82% of aged Medicare beneficiaries had one or more chronic conditions, and 65% had multiple chronic conditions (7). The simultaneous occurrence of several medical conditions in the same person constitutes the concept of multimorbidity. From an epidemiological perspective, the definition requires at least two coexisting chronic diseases. The prevalence of multimorbidity increases significantly with age in both men and women. Epidemiological studies in clinic-based samples demonstrate the mean number of chronic conditions to range from 5.2 to 6.5 in those aged 65 and older (8,9). The specific prevalence of individual conditions varies on the basis of the age strata, gender, and population sampled (e.g. community-based versus clinic cohort). The epidemiological literature supports that the most commonly defined chronic conditions in those 70 years or older include osteoarthritis, hypertension, heart disease, diabetes, obstructive lung disease, and cancer in an approximate descending order of frequency from 55% to 10% (10,11).

Medication Use in Older Persons

The use of prescription drugs and over-the-counter (OTC) drugs is common in older adults. Results of several population-based surveys suggest that between 89% and 94% of those over 65 years take prescription medication, with nearly 40% taking over 5 medications and 12% taking over 10 medications (12,13). Polypharmacy is frequently defined as taking over five medications and increases incrementally in relation to the number of coexisting age-associated diseases (13). Previously, polypharmacy implied inappropriate prescribing, but as the burden of medical illness increases, many or all of the prescribed drugs may have an appropriate indication. Furthermore, existing practice guidelines recommend use of multiple medications for certain chronic diseases (i.e., osteoporosis, congestive heart failure, and diabetes). The consequences of polypharmacy include adverse drug effects, drug–drug interactions, disease–drug interactions, nutraceutical –drug interactions, and medication cascade effects (13). The cascade effect refers to the use of medications to treat the side effects of other medications. This further adds to the risks and complexity of medication use in older adults.

About one-third of older persons taking at least five medications will experience an adverse drug event (ADE) each year, and about two-thirds of these patients will require medical attention (14). Multiple physicians treating one patient, increasing comorbidities, and an increase in the variety of drugs available contribute to the adverse effects of polypharmacy on the elderly patient. The adverse drug effects of sleepiness, insomnia, and nightmares occur with many OTC and prescription medications. Sleepiness or drowsiness is probably the most common ADE, with the 2000 Drug Interactions and Side Effect Index of the Physicians' Desk Reference® listing drowsiness as a side effect of 384 prescription or OTC preparations. DrugDex® lists 131 medications as producing insomnia as an adverse effect. Alternatively some medications or substances of abuse can exacerbate insomnia during periods of discontinuation or withdrawal.

MECHANISMS FOR SLEEP–WAKE DYSREGULATION WITH COEXISTING HEALTH ISSUES

The precise relationship between an illness and the neuropsychological, biochemical, and hormonal sequelae that contribute to sleep decay remains speculative in many cases. Frequently health conditions produce symptoms of discomfort or emotional distress that may lead to sympathetic response, hypothalamic-pituitary-adrenal activity, and ultimately activation of neural systems to produce arousal (15–17). Psychological factors of hyperarousal, stress response, predisposing personality traits, and maladaptive attitudes can perpetuate sleep changes seen during illness in later life (18). Acute pathophysiological changes such as hypoxemia, metabolic derangements, fever, or systemic inflammatory responses can also lead to delirium in frail, older patients with characteristic alterations in sleep–wake patterns (19).

Poor Sleep Hygiene Associated with Illness

Sleep habits or behaviors are commonly referred to as sleep hygiene. Abnormalities in sleep hygiene are pervasive across the general population and commonly co-occur in older persons with concomitant health problems (20). In the setting of acute illness, it is common to see a shift in the sleep–wake cycle, an increase in time napping in bed and a greater degree of overnight sleep fragmentation. These secondary changes can be perpetuated well beyond the initial acute episode and propagate ongoing maladaptive sleep hygiene. While the underlying factors for sleep difficulty or insomnia are being addressed, teaching good sleep hygiene may decrease the likelihood of development of persistent, chronic insomnia. Sleep hygiene practices are typically used in combinations with restriction of time spent in bed and regularization of the sleep schedule, since they may not be as efficacious alone for improving sleep (21). The specifics of sleep hygiene education are described elsewhere, but they focus on maintaining a stable bedtime and wakeup times, reducing daytime napping, increasing physical activity in the afternoon, and avoiding caffeine, alcohol, and nicotine near bedtime (22).

Physical Symptoms Associated with Illnesses that Contribute to Awakenings

Many chronic diseases have been associated with nocturnal awakenings. In a sample of 8937 community-dwelling adults, the prevalence of nightly awakenings significantly increased with age, reaching 34.6% in the group of subjects aged 65 years or older (23). Furthermore, the prevalence for nocturnal awakenings that occurred every night varied from 27% to 41% in a number of common chronic illnesses, as reflected in Table 1. When nocturnal awakenings occur, nearly half of the people had difficulty resuming sleep and 59% had at least two awakenings during the night. In those over 65 years, the most common symptoms that contribute to awakenings include pain, nocturia, thirst, dyspnea, and gastrointestinal acid reflux (23).

It is intuitive that many of these symptoms can interfere with sleep; however, the means by which this happens is poorly defined. Although many potential physiological mechanisms exist, it is plausible that any final common pathway would include activation of specific brain centers involved in wakefulness and shifts in neurotransmitter profiles. The high amount of overlap in brain areas as well as neurotransmitters involved in sleep, stress, and mood disorders further supports this idea. Neuropeptides such as corticotrophin-releasing factor (CRF) may interrupt

TABLE 1 Insomnia and Awakenings in Common Chronic Diseases

Chronic illness	Insomnia prevalence (%)	Nightly awakenings (%)
Heart disease	44	38
Cancer	41	Not available
Obstructive lung disease	59	Not available
Diabetes	47	Not available
Hypertension	44	35
Chronic pain	48	27

Source: From Refs. 10,23.

both rapid eye movement (REM) and non-REM sleep, with subsequent arousals. Physiological stress is associated with insomnia and activation of the hypothalamic-pituitary-adrenal axis with increased CRH and cortisol (17). These neurotransmitters tend to inhibit sleep and increase alertness (24). Sleep continuity disturbances are associated with biological correlates of heightened arousal, including increased cortical activity and increased sympathetic activation.

Pain is felt to be one of the more common mechanisms for comorbid insomnia. Studies suggest that 25% to 50% of community-dwelling older persons have significant pain problems (25). In a general population of adults aged 55 to 84, 19% reported that pain disrupted their sleep at least a few nights per week and 12% reported almost nightly sleep fragmentation due to pain (1). Among referral populations of patients with chronic pain, prevalence rates of insomnia can range between 50% and 70%(26). Painful conditions are frequently associated with reduced total sleep time, reduced REM sleep, frequent brief arousals, and increased wakefulness after sleep onset (20,27). There is a paucity of data reviewing pain and objective sleep parameters in older adults. The relationship between pain and sleep is complex; pain can disrupt sleep, and poor sleep may increase perceived pain intensity(28).

The Relationship Between Common Medical Conditions and Concurrent Primary Sleep Disorders

A number of chronic medical conditions coexist or increase the likelihood for an older adult to manifest a primary sleep disorder. Although the spectrum of these associations is extensive, it is essential that the clinician or scientist acknowledge some of the more common relationships as another means by which chronic illness can impact sleep. Table 2 is a composite of a number of published epidemiological studies that highlight how certain chronic medical conditions increase the risk for co-occurrence of two common primary sleep conditions of later life. These associations support the position that comorbid insomnia in medically complex, older persons is frequently a multifactorial process and numerous explanations should be sought to optimally address the older individual's insomnia complaints.

Medications that Affect Sleep Architecture

Many OTC and prescription medications are known to influence the sleep–wake cycle and produce comorbid insomnia. Their adverse effects are different but can be broadly categorized as those that produce drowsiness or daytime somnolence, those that are stimulating to the brain, those that interfere with sleep by indirect mechanisms, those that may directly exacerbate primary sleep disorders, and those that

TABLE 2   Selected Associations between Chronic Illness
and Primary Sleep Disorders

Primary sleep disorder	Associated chronic illness
Sleep apnea	Obesity
	Congestive heart failure
	Diabetes mellitus
	Chronic kidney disease
	Cerebrovascular accident
Restless legs syndrome	Anemia with ferritin < 50
	Diabetes mellitus
	Spinal cord disease
	Peripheral neuropathy
	Chronic kidney disease
	Rheumatoid arthritis

influence sleep architecture via other means. The practitioner should be sensitized to consider how adverse side effects and drug–drug or drug–disease interactions are more likely to occur in older adults and can include central nervous system depressing or excitatory sequelae.

Certain medications disturb sleep via excitation or activation of the central nervous system. Sleep quality may be affected if these agents are taken prior to the patient's bedtime or have a sustained half-life that extends into the typical sleep period. Commonly prescribed OTC therapies for cold and flu containing pseudoephedrine, ephedrine, or other symphathomimetics can do so. OTC analgesics with caffeine used for headache therapy are also a concern. Agents used to manage chronic lung disease such as beta-agonist inhalants or oral formulations, corticosteroids, and theophylline can all contribute to sleep disruption. Activating antidepressants can sometimes adversely affect sleep initiation and maintenance. These can include desipramine, bupropion, venlafaxine, reboxetine, and most selective serotonin receptor inhibitors (SSRIs). Insomnia has been reported as a frequent side effect with SSRI use, with a prevalence of 16.4% with sertraline, 15% with fluoxetine, and 14% with paroxetine (29). While individuals may appreciate an improvement in subjective sleep quality with SSRIs, objective sleep often worsens (30). Other activating medications such as methylphenidate, selegiline, and modafinil are often seen on geriatric medication lists. Accordingly it would be reasonable for such medications, if needed, to be taken far from the desired sleep period when possible, and stopped if not needed.

Medications can sometimes interfere with sleep by worsening an underlying medical or psychiatric condition that then affects sleep. Medications that worsen heart failure, such as nonsteroidal anti-inflammatory drugs, calcium channel blockers, or sodium-complexed antibiotics, have the potential to cause central sleep apnea, nocturia, or other sleep problems seen in this condition. Medications including nitrates and calcium channel blockers can decrease lower esophageal sphincter tone with resultant nocturnal gastroesophageal reflux. Amitriptyline and other anticholinergic medications, while potentially helpful with sleep due to sedation, can also contribute to confusion as well as urinary retention, with subsequent arousals from delirium or nocturia. Late-afternoon or evening diuretic treatment may cause nocturia and sleep fragmentation. Many antipsychotic medications, while being used for various symptoms in older adults have the potential to produce parkinsonian features, with sleep difficulties commonly associated with these conditions. Quetiapine may be one of the least common offenders in this category of medications. Hypoglycemic agents, if they produce nocturnal hypoglycemia, can increase nocturnal arousals.

A number of medications have been reported to exacerbate primary sleep disorders. Nocturnal movement disorders such as restless legs syndrome (RLS) and periodic limb movements of sleep (PLMS) can worsen in the setting of a number of antidepressant medications. In looking at 274 consecutive patients on antidepressants, and 69 control subjects not on antidepressants, those taking SSRIs or venlafaxine had an odds ratio over 5 that they would have the PLM index greater than 20, compared with the control group (31). Bupropion was similar to controls. Tricyclic antidepressants and lithium are also associated with a greater prevalence of nocturnal movement disorders. Caffeine, antihistamines, alcohol, and benzodiazepine withdrawal can all worsen RLS. Antipsychotic therapies are associated with greater PLMS prevalence.

On the basis of a series of small studies and case reports, opiate analgesia use, especially sustained release or long half-life formulations, is associated with increased central apneas, sustained hypoxemia, and prolonged duration of the abnormal breathing events (32). These changes occur in the context of the well-established acute respiratory depressant effects. Hypnotics such as benzodiazepines may also worsen sleep-disordered breathing by lowering the arousal threshold.

Certain medications are associated with worsening of sleep architecture by other influences. Beta-blockers are frequently prescribed in older adults in the context of hypertension and heart disease. The more lipophilic agents such as propanolol and some of the newer-generation beta-blockers have been shown to suppress melatonin, increase sleep fragmentation, as well as increase nightmares in some people (33). Other agents such as lithium, benzodiazepine receptor agonists, and gaba-hydroxy-butyrate, in addition to benzodiazepine withdrawal, are associated with a worsening of disorders of non-REM parasomnias. Tricyclic antidepressants, monoamine oxidase inhibitors, venlafaxine, and mirtazapine have all been documented to induce REM sleep behavior disorder, a parasomnia very specific to older adults.

Drowsiness is a common effect of medications. Excessive daytime sleepiness is a frequent sleep complaint in older adults, with a baseline tendency for older adults to have shorter sleep latency during the day (34). Many medications have the capacity to interfere with acetylcholine or histamine, both regulatory neurotransmitters for wakefulness. These anticholinergic agents are known to have somnogenic effects, waking drowsiness, as well as negative cognitive, affective, and quality-of-life outcomes in older adults (35). Antihistaminergic drugs appear to have variable central nervous system penetration and binding, with H1-antagonists like diphenhydramine having a much greater likelihood for sedation and cognitive impairment than do tertiary antihistamines (36). General classes of agents with these effects include antihistamines, antispasmodics, antipsychotics, antiemetics, and antiparkinsonian drugs. Notable specific examples include tricyclic antidepressants such as amitriptyline, doxepin, imipramine; cimetidine, mirtazapine, and oxybutynin. A comprehensive review of all of these agents is published elsewhere (37).

Medications can also produce sleepiness via other mechanisms. In individuals taking levodopa or dopamine agonists, there is an increased prevalence of excessive daytime sleepiness and sleep attacks (38). Anticonvulsant agents such as gabapentin, lamotrigine, tiagabine, and levetiracetam frequently produce sleepiness in older adults. Opiate analgesics can contribute to daytime somnolence and decreased alertness as well as disrupt overnight sleep efficiency and architecture.

The consumption of caffeine in coffee, tea, sodas, as well as medications is common in the older adult and may contribute to sleep disruption. Caffeine has stimulatory effects on the cerebral cortex and medullary centers, with blood levels peaking 15 to 45 minutes after intake and a half-life of 3 to 7.5 hours. In adult populations, daytime sleepiness and insomnia are associated with high daily caffeine consumption (39,40). Intake shortly prior to sleep time has been shown to disrupt sleep in adults on objective and subjective measures (41,42). Adults over 67 years old on caffeine-containing medications report significantly more trouble falling asleep after controlling for multiple factors (43). Hospital-dwelling older adults with a higher serum caffeine concentration reported sleep problems more than those with lower levels (44).

Nicotine is a frequently abused drug. Although the prevalence of smoking among older adults is lower than among younger persons, nearly 11% of Americans aged 65 and older smoke. (45). Several studies have suggested that insomnia and sleep apnea are more common in smokers, but establishing a causal relationship has been difficult (46). Nicotine enhances acetylcholine neurotransmission in the basal forebrain and dopamine release, potentially influencing sleep–wake control mechanisms toward wakefulness (47). A dose-dependent reduction in REM and slow-wave sleep, along with an increase in wakefulness and total sleep time, has been observed with nicotine (48). In persons 50 to 84 years old, smokers endorsed more difficulty with sleep onset and staying asleep as well as daytime sleep than nonsmokers.

SPECIFIC MEDICAL CONDITIONS
There are many examples of how medical illness negatively influences sleep quantity and quality. The list of medical conditions associated with disturbed sleep is extensive. Furthermore, an individual illness may have several mechanisms that interfere with sleep and it may have different effects on sleep architecture in its acute versus chronic state. The immediate physiological derangements or distress of an illness may produce transient sleep disruption. This sleep change can be perpetuated by maladaptive or learned responses to become a more protracted sleep difficulty that mirrors the profile of primary insomnia. Indirect support for this mechanism arises from recent randomized controlled trials demonstrating the efficacy for cognitive-behavioral therapies (CBTs) in the treatment of insomnia in a variety of medical illnesses (49). Chronic pain, cardiovascular disease, pulmonary disease, chronic kidney disease, gastrointestinal conditions, endocrine and genitourinary conditions have all been associated with poor sleep. Sleep disturbance may worsen symptoms in these disorders or even worsen the prognosis.

Heart Disease
Coronary artery disease is a leading cause of morbidity and mortality in older persons. Many interactions exist between ischemic heart disease and sleep. Nocturnal ischemia, nighttime arrhythmias, and sleep-disordered breathing are all linked

to altered sleep in underlying heart disease. A well-described circadian pattern of myocardial ischemia or infarction occurs early to mid-morning and is ascribed to the catecholamine surge that accompanies awakening and upright status. However, in a retrospective analysis of 3309 adults presenting with acute coronary syndrome (ACS), 26% of the individuals were awakened from sleep (50). On multivariate analysis only advanced age and lower left ventricular ejection fraction were independent predictors of a nocturnal episode of ACS in this cohort. Chronic problems with sleep initiation correlate with an increased risk of death from coronary artery disease in male patients (51). Finally, coronary artery bypass surgery is associated with protracted sleep disturbance up to two years following the procedure (52). The mechanism for this is unclear with occult heart failure, secondary mood issues, or brain microvascular ischemic changes as possibilities.

With increasing life span and improvements in the management of acute coronary ischemia, it is projected that the occurrence of congestive heart failure (CHF) will continue to rise. The classic sleep maintenance disturbance associated with CHF includes orthopnea, paroxysmal nocturnal dyspnea, nocturia, and sleep-disordered breathing. Increasingly concomitant depression is also identified as a factor that contributes to sleep disturbance in older adults with CHF (53). More than 50% of patients with moderate to severe CHF experience a form of periodic breathing called Cheynes–Stokes respiration. This may lead to increased sleep fragmentation and an increase in daytime sleepiness (54,55). When reviewing risk factors for central sleep apnea (CSA) and obstructive sleep apnea (OSA) in men and women with CHF, age over 60 years is an independent predictor for OSA in both genders and for CSA in women (56). More severe nighttime periodic breathing occurring in heart failure correlates with worse prognosis and increased cardiac death (55). It is also suggested that sleep apnea subjects the failing heart to adverse adrenergic and hemodynamic loads, which may further worsen heart failure. Small trials that treat OSA with continuous positive airway pressure have shown improvement in blood pressure and left ventricular systolic function in those with clinical heart failure (57).

Cancer
Cancer is principally a disease of older adults insofar that 60% of all cancers are diagnosed after age 65 (58). The prevalence of sleep problems in individuals with cancer is difficult to determine with wide variance dependent upon type and stage of cancer. Large epidemiological studies suggest that sleep problems are very common involving 55% to 87% of patients (59,60). Persons with cancer may have a baseline history of insomnia or a primary sleep disorder; or they may have sleep effects as a consequence of the cancer, its treatment or the psychological response to the diagnosis (60). Most published studies have focused on sleep changes in early stage cancer (61). Cancer-related fatigue is a well-known symptom, but its relationship to impaired sleep continues to be elucidated. As in other populations, it can be difficult for patients to distinguish fatigue from daytime sleepiness.

Forty-four percent of hospitalized cancer patients are prescribed hypnotic therapy (62). Nevertheless, the suspicion is high that ongoing sleep difficulties may be undertreated in persons with cancer due to underreporting, underdiagnosis, minimization of importance in the context of the cancer diagnosis, concerns about drug–drug interactions, or reluctance to take more medication (63). Controlled hypnotic trials have not been conducted to date in this population. Although limited in number and size, trials using CBT in patients with cancer suggest significant improvements in their sleep (59).

Lung Disease
Chronic lung disease in the form of chronic obstructive pulmonary disease (COPD) contributes to poor sleep continuity, as well as increased daytime sleepiness (64). Approximately 25% of patients with COPD complain of excessive sleepiness. The mean age of subjects in these studies was typically greater than 60 years, consistent with the prevalence of COPD in older adults. Hypoxemia, which is common in COPD during REM sleep, correlates with an increase in arousal and excessive daytime sleepiness. While the use of oxygen therapy frequently corrects the underlying hypoxemia, it does not appear to improve sleep quality (65). This suggests that other mechanisms, such as cough, impaired airflow, excessive respiratory secretions, or dyspnea, may be contributing to the observed sleep disruption. The use of inhaled ipratropium bromide improves sleep quality and duration presumably via improved airflow (66). A small observational study of lung volume reduction surgery in older adults, mean age 63 years, also demonstrates improved polysomnographic sleep quality and nocturnal oxygenation (67).

Coexistent OSA and COPD is termed overlap syndrome. By retrospective analysis, the prevalence of overlap syndrome in COPD was 12%, and 41% in OSA patients in an older VA population (68). There is some concern that treatment of OSA with CPAP therapy may lead to greater declines in lung function tests in patients with overlap syndrome (68). Consideration of longer-acting bronchodilator therapy at night may help manage this issue.

Diabetes Mellitus
Type 2 diabetes mellitus is an age-associated condition with a rising global prevalence of 10% at age 60 and 15% at age 80 (69). Worldwide estimates for adults 65 and older with diabetes include nearly 30 million adults in 2000 and 50 million in 2030. Thirty percent of diabetic patients demonstrate sleep maintenance disturbances, with the severity of disruption correlating with the degree of hyperglycemia (70,71). One-third of patients with diabetes have problems with sleep fragmentation. Causes for this include nocturia, neuropathic leg pain, and leg cramps. Likewise, patients with diabetes have an increased prevalence of both RLS and PLMS (72). A growing body of epidemiological and experimental evidence links sleep apnea and disorders of glucose metabolism; however, the cause and effect relationship remains to be determined (73). Recent work has demonstrated an independent association between sleep-disordered breathing and insulin resistance, but treatment of sleep apnea has produced mixed results on insulin sensitivity and glycemic control (73,74).

Menopause
In menopause, an estimated 40% to 50% of women report sleep difficulties following cessation of menstruation. While some of this is transient during the time of acute hormonal changes, others have persisting symptoms for years later. Hormone replacement therapy has been shown to improve subjective but not objective sleep measures (75). The relationships between gender, hormonal status, and sleep–wake

patterns are complex and addressed more completely in the chapter by Drs. Misra and Malow in this book.

Rheumatic Disease

Arthritis affects an estimated 43 million Americans (8). The prevalence of arthritis increases with advancing age with nearly 45% of those over 80 manifesting knee osteooarthritis (76). Evidence suggests that as many as 60% of those with arthritis experience pain during the night. Adults over age 65 with knee arthritis have been observed to have problems initiating sleep (31%), problems maintaining sleep (81%), and a tendency to awaken early in the morning (51%) (77). Patients with rheumatoid arthritis have a high prevalence of RLS (25%) (78). Poor sleep in patients with osteoarthritis correlates with increased perceived pain, decreased self-rated health, poor functional status, and depression (77). Furthermore, individuals with self-reported arthritis-related sleep disruption are more likely then those without sleep disturbance to pursue multiple sources of self-care and medical care (79). A recent randomized clinical trial involving older adults with arthritis and comorbid insomnia demonstrated efficacy for cognitive-behavioral approaches in improving self-reported measures of sleep (80).

Gastrointestinal Conditions

Gastroesophageal reflux disease (GERD) is common, with over 44% of the general population having monthly symptoms and 7% having daily symptoms (81). These symptoms increase with aging, with a prevalence of 10% for daily reflux symptoms for those older than 50 years (82). In population surveys, between 50% and 70% of individuals with GERD report nighttime symptoms and reduced sleep quality (83). The relationship between disturbed sleep and GERD is bidirectional: sleeping increases the likelihood of reflux, and reflux episodes often awaken the patient (84,85). Patients with nighttime acid reflux may underestimate the degree of sleep disruption that occurs when objective measurements of pH and electroencephalogram (EEG) arousal are compared to patient recollection the next morning (85). Reviewing the patient history for nocturnal cough or wheezing as a surrogate for reflux is also important, since not all patients with overnight reflux will experience classic chest pain, but their sleep may be disrupted nevertheless. Published evidence demonstrates that acid suppression therapy reduces nighttime heartburn symptoms, reduces GERD-associated sleep disturbances, and improves subjective sleep quality and next day's work performance (86).

Urological and Renal Conditions

Sleep disruption is common in urological and kidney diseases. Benign prostatic hyperplasia (BPH) and prostate cancer are typically diseases of the aging male, steeply increasing with age. Urinary obstructive symptoms, including nocturia, are hallmarks for these conditions. Overactive bladder is characterized by urinary urgency, frequency, nocturia, and sometimes incontinence. It increases markedly with advancing age in both men and women (87). Nocturia is a well-recognized etiology for sleep maintenance disturbance in later life, and nighttime urination is often associated with poor quality of sleep and increased fatigue during the daytime (88).

Chronic kidney disease and end-stage renal disease have a steady increase over age 60, with a striking rise in prevalence beyond age 75 (89). Overall prevalence of insomnia in hemodialysis (HD) patients ranges between 45% and 86% (90). Fifty-seven percent of patients with end-stage renal disease report sleep maintenance problems, and 55% report early morning awakening. There are marked abnormalities seen in the sleep EEGs of patients with chronic kidney disease, with overall reduction in total sleep time, decreased sleep efficiency due to wakefulness after sleep onset, and reduced total REM (91). This may reflect the impact of uremia and other metabolic derangements on brain function during sleep. Patients on HD have a higher prevalence of OSA (which improves following dialysis), RLS, periodic limb movements, early insomnia, and excessive daytime sleepiness (92–94). In a study involving HD patients with a mean age of 65 years, the treatment of anemia of kidney disease with erythropoietin improved sleep quality by polysomnographic and subjective measures (95). This appears to correspond to reduced numbers of periodic limb movements. Over 50% of HD patients endorse chronic pain, and this is felt to be significantly associated with insomnia and depression in this condition (96).

Selected Geriatric Syndromes
Falls and gait problems are a common and serious problem facing older adults. About one-third of those aged 65 and older living in the community fall at least once a year. This increases to one in two for those aged 80 and older (97). Falls are typically the result of multiple, interacting etiologies. It is well acknowledged that older persons with insomnia on hypnotic therapy have a higher risk for falls. Prevailing evidence suggests that this is due in part to the adverse effects of benzodiazepines and other hypnotics on balance, cognition, and reaction time, with withdrawal of these agents reducing the risk for future falls (98). There is some evidence that it may be the underlying insomnia with its neurocognitive consequences that predispose an older person to falls in selected populations such as in the nursing home (99). Consensus from expert panels advise a multifaceted approach to reduce future falls, including behavioral interventions for sleep, drug review, adjustment of psychotropic and hypnotic agents as possible, an exercise program, and evaluation and treatment other comorbid medical problems as appropriate.

Approximately 40% of community-dwelling older adults report sporadic or chronic urinary incontinence (100). Urine loss is considered a geriatric syndrome insofar that it leads to a spectrum of physical, psychological, and social consequences that can be a detriment to a person's function and quality of life. Cross-sectional epidemiological studies in the community show correlation between awakenings, nocturia, and incontinence. The effects of incontinence on sleep are best studied in the nursing home population, with both polysomnographic and actigraphy samples demonstrating sleep disruption with nocturnal wetting episodes. Interestingly, 51% of these episodes occurred during or within 60 seconds of an abnormal sleep breathing event (101). In those who are chronically incontinent, the relationship between urine loss and awakening are not as tightly linked (102).

THERAPEUTIC APPROACHES/ STRATEGIES
The viewpoint on the management of comorbid insomnia is evolving. Historically if a sleep problem was attributed to an associated mental or physical illness, then the primary focus was on optimizing treatment of that underlying health concern.

This placed an emphasis on correcting metabolic, neurochemical, and physiological derangement in illness with the hope that sleep would improve. The role for CBTs and hypnotics was de-emphasized in this situation because pathophysiological mechanisms were believed to be different than those seen in primary insomnia. Many sleep authorities feel that this lead to undertreatment of the accompanying insomnia. More recently, a series of controlled trials have demonstrated the efficacy of CBT in managing insomnia complaints in a variety of different illnesses. On these grounds, some argue that all comorbid or secondary insomnia should be treated the same as primary insomnia with CBT and, when indicated, adjunctive hypnotic therapy (103). Although the most efficacious approach remains to be determined, it seems prudent that a multifaceted intervention that equally emphasizes optimizing comorbid health issues, using CBT and hypnotics, is justified.

A good sleep history is of primary importance in the effective treatment of sleep disturbance in patients with comorbid illness. When clinicians recognize how common medical problems affect sleep, they may choose a very different first-line therapy. For best outcomes, the underlying medical problems should be optimally managed, and any sleep-disruptive medications that can be changed should be adjusted or replaced. Sometimes targeted medical therapies, such as an analgesic for pain or intervention for anemia, may serve to be the best sleep aides. In addition, adjunctive behavioral and pharmacological approaches that are applicable for others forms of insomnia should be considered if a sleep problem persists. It is essential to treat patients with comorbid insomnia with a holistic approach that addresses the underlying illness, as well as incorporates the standard of care for managing all insomnia.

Cognitive-Behavioral Therapies with Comorbid Insomnia
The NIH Conference on insomnia concluded that CBT is as effective as prescription medications for brief treatment of chronic insomnia, with subsequent research suggesting that this approach is also appropriate for managing comorbid insomnia. There are indications that beneficial effects of CBT, in contrast to those produced by medications, may last well beyond completion of treatment.

While psychological and behavioral therapies require more effort on the part of the patient and the health care provider, they are very effective and may be more appropriate for older adults who develop comorbid insomnia. In insomnia overall, the results of a meta-analysis of 59 trials enrolling over 2000 patients showed that nonpharmacological treatments result in consistent improvements in the time-to-sleep onset and the ability to maintain sleep. CBT is generally considered the treatment of choice for chronic insomnia. CBT involves challenging a patient's attitudes and misconceptions regarding sleep, eliminating sleep-incompatible behaviors as well as reducing the overall amount of time in bed to match the amount of time the individual sleeps using restriction.

Experience has shown that giving a patient a printed handout of sleep hygiene rules is much less effective than discussing these principles with the patient and making one or two individualized recommendations. Once specific issues have been identified, the clinician should describe the rationale for instituting the change, provide detailed instructions, and encourage the patient to adhere to the change for at least 2 or 3 weeks, since sleep patterns change slowly over time. For example, a patient with sleep maintenance problems may be instructed to eliminate his or her evening alcoholic beverage and to reduce exposure to bright light if she or he awakens during the night to urinate.

The overlap of nicotine dependence in people with medical and psychiatric conditions is an important issue. In clinic and community populations of depressed patients, 40% to 60% smoke, with even higher rates in other mental illness such as PTSD (104). Quit rates are also much less in people with psychiatric disorder. Nevertheless, smoking cessation may be a viable intervention to improve sleep quality in older adults. When offered the tools they need, older smokers quit smoking at rates comparable to those of younger smokers.

The Risks and Benefits of Pharmacotherapy with Medically Complex Patients

As with primary insomnia, there may be a role for adjunctive pharmacotherapy. Studies examining the relative advantages of CBT and pharmacotherapy have found that improvements may be achieved more quickly with drug treatment but are more sustained with CBT. An evidence-based approach is lacking, however, for pharmacotherapy since few, if any, hypnotic trials have selected a medically complex, older population as its target group for treatment. Additionally, studies using medication treatments for comorbid insomnia due to specific disease states are almost nonexistent, so therapeutic options must be generalized from other geriatric and nongeriatric trials. It is beyond the scope of this chapter to provide a comprehensive overview of all potential treatments, but this is addressed elsewhere in this book. Of special concern, however, is that many patients with multimorbidity have much higher attendant risks for ADEs due to polypharmacy, multiple prescribers, and coexistent cognitive and balance issues. This group is particularly appropriate for nonpharmacological approaches first. When combination medication and behavioral therapies are felt necessary, then the prescriber should avoid higher anticholinergic or older-generation agents (e.g., antihistamines, long-acting benzodiazepines), start at the lowest feasible dose, and coordinate close follow-up to track for ADEs such as confusion, imbalance, and falls.

SUMMARY

With advancing medical sophistication and technology, people are living longer with their comorbid medical, psychiatric conditions and disabilities. This higher burden of illness and the numbers of medications used to treat these conditions play an important role in the quality and quantity of sleep in older adults. In approaching sleep complaints in geriatric patients, it is essential that practitioners consider the multidimensional ways by which illness impacts sleep. An appropriate first assumption is that the etiology of the sleep complaint(s) is likely multifactorial, with contributions from chronic health issues as well as the associated changes in a person's lifestyle, sleep hygiene, and medication regimes that occur secondary to the illness. Furthermore, these health problems rarely exist in isolation and instead frequently coexist with psychiatric diagnoses, neurological diseases, and primary sleep pathology, as described elsewhere in this book.

An equally multifaceted management approach is in order when dealing with comorbid insomnia. This includes optimizing the underlying illness, adjusting potentially offending medications, using cognitive-behavioral approaches, and employing judicious hypnotic therapy, which seems justified based on the current evidence. It is with this multipronged approach that one might expect the best treatment response for comorbid insomnia as supported by both evidence and expert opinion.

REFERENCES

1. Foley D, Ancoli-Israel S, Britz P, et al. Sleep disturbances and chronic disease in older adults: results of the 2003 National Sleep Foundation Sleep in America Survey. J Psychosom Res 2004; 56(5):497–502.
2. Panel S-o-t-S. National Institutes of Health State of the Science Conference Statement: manifestations and management of chronic insomnia in adults, June 13–15. Sleep 2005(28):1049–1057.
3. Medicine AAoS. International Classification of Sleep Disorders: Diagnostic and Coding Manual. 2nd ed. Westchester, IL; 2005.
4. Foley DJ, Monjan AA, Brown SL, et al. Sleep complaints among elderly persons: an epidemiologic study of three communities. Sleep 1995; 18(6):425–432.
5. Roberts RE, Shema SJ, Kaplan GA. Prospective data on sleep complaints and associated risk factors in an older cohort. Psychosom Med 1999; 61(2):188–196.
6. Ohayon MM, Smirne S. Prevalence and consequences of insomnia disorders in the general population of Italy. Sleep Med 2002; 3(2):115–120.
7. Wolff JL, Starfield B, Anderson G. Prevalence, expenditures, and complications of multiple chronic conditions in the elderly. Arch Intern Med 2002; 162(20):2269–2276.
8. Metsemakers JF, Hoppener P, Knottnerus JA, et al. Computerized health information in The Netherlands: a registration network of family practices. Br J Gen Pract 1992; 42(356):102–106.
9. Fortin M, Bravo G, Hudon C, et al. Prevalence of multimorbidity among adults seen in family practice. Ann Fam Med 2005; 3(3):223–228.
10. Fillenbaum GG, Pieper CF, Cohen HJ, et al. Comorbidity of five chronic health conditions in elderly community residents: determinants and impact on mortality. J Gerontol A Biol Sci Med Sci 2000; 55(2):M84–M89.
11. Tooth L, Hockey R, Byles J, et al. Weighted multimorbidity indexes predicted mortality, health service use, and health-related quality of life in older women. J Clin Epidemiol 2008; 61(2):151–159.
12. Kaufman DW, Kelly JP, Rosenberg L, et al. Recent patterns of medication use in the ambulatory adult population of the United States: the Slone survey. JAMA 2002; 287(3):337–344.
13. Linjakumpu T, Hartikainen S, Klaukka T, et al. Use of medications and polypharmacy are increasing among the elderly. J Clin Epidemiol 2002; 55(8):809–817.
14. Hanlon JT SK, Koronkowski MJ, Weinberger M, et al. Adverse drug events in high risk older outpatients. J Am Geriatr Soc 1997(45):945–948.
15. Vgontzas AN, Tsigos C, Bixler EO, et al. Chronic insomnia and activity of the stress system: a preliminary study. J Psychosom Res 1998; 45(1 Spec No):21–31.
16. Rodenbeck A, Huether G, Ruther E, et al. Interactions between evening and nocturnal cortisol secretion and sleep parameters in patients with severe chronic primary insomnia. Neurosci Lett 2002; 324(2):159–163.
17. Vgontzas AN, Bixler EO, Lin HM, et al. Chronic insomnia is associated with nyctohemeral activation of the hypothalamic-pituitary-adrenal axis: clinical implications. J Clin Endocrinol Metab 2001; 86(8):3787–3794.
18. Alapin I, Libman E, Bailes S, et al. Role of nocturnal cognitive arousal in the complaint of insomnia among older adults. Behav Sleep Med 2003; 1(3):155–170.
19. Peter R, Peter T, Brigitta B, et al. From psychophysiological insomnia to organic sleep disturbances: a continuum in late onset insomnia – with special concerns relating to its treatment. Med Hypotheses 2005; 65(6):1165–1171.
20. Ellis J HS, Cropley M. Sleep hygiene compensatory sleep practices: an examination of behaviors affecting sleep in older adults. Psychology, Health, & Medicine 2002; 7(2):157–162.

21. Morgenthaler T, Kramer M, Alessi C, et al. Practice parameters for the psychological and behavioral treatment of insomnia: an update. An American Academy of Sleep Medicine report. Sleep 2006; 29(11):1415–1419.

22. Stepanski EJ, Wyatt JK. Use of sleep hygiene in the treatment of insomnia. Sleep Med Rev 2003; 7(3):215–225.

23. Ohayon MM. Nocturnal awakenings and comorbid disorders in the American general population. J Psychiatr Res 2008.

24. Tsuchiyama Y, Uchimura N, Sakamoto T, et al. Effects of hCRH on sleep and body temperature rhythms. Psychiatry Clin Neurosci 1995; 49(5–6):299–304.

25. Helme RD, Katz B, Gibson SJ, et al. Multidisciplinary pain clinics for older people. Do they have a role? Clin Geriatr Med 1996; 12(3):563–582.

26. Latham J, Davis BD. The socioeconomic impact of chronic pain. Disabil Rehabil 1994; 16(1):39–44.

27. Rosenberg-Adamsen S, Skarbye M, Wildschiodtz G, et al. Sleep after laparoscopic cholecystectomy. Br J Anaesth 1996; 77(5):572–575.

28. Johnson EO, Roehrs T, Roth T, et al. Epidemiology of alcohol and medication as aids to sleep in early adulthood. Sleep 1998; 21(2):178–186.

29. Grimsley SR, Jann MW. Paroxetine, sertraline, and fluvoxamine: new selective serotonin reuptake inhibitors. Clin Pharm 1992; 11(11):930–957.

30. Argyropoulos SV, Hicks JA, Nash JR, et al. Correlation of subjective and objective sleep measurements at different stages of the treatment of depression. Psychiatry Res 2003; 120(2):179–190.

31. Yang C, White DP, Winkelman JW. Antidepressants and periodic leg movements of sleep. Biol Psychiatry 2005; 58(6):510–514.

32. Wang D, Teichtahl H, Drummer O, et al. Central sleep apnea in stable methadone maintenance treatment patients. Chest 2005; 128(3):1348–1356.

33. Brzezinski A. Melatonin in humans. N Engl J Med 1997; 336(3):186–195.

34. Richardson GS, Carskadon MA, Orav EJ, et al. Circadian variation of sleep tendency in elderly and young adult subjects. Sleep 1982; 5(suppl 2):S82–S94.

35. Mintzer J, Burns A. Anticholinergic side-effects of drugs in elderly people. J R Soc Med 2000; 93(9):457–462.

36. Nicholson AN, Stone BM. Antihistamines: impaired performance and the tendency to sleep. Eur J Clin Pharmacol 1986; 30(1):27–32.

37. Rudd KM, Raehl CL, Bond CA, et al. Methods for assessing drug-related anticholinergic activity. Pharmacotherapy 2005; 25(11):1592–1601.

38. Larsen JP, Tandberg E. Sleep disorders in patients with Parkinson's disease: epidemiology and management. CNS Drugs 2001; 15(4):267–275.

39. Ohayon MM, Caulet M, Philip P,et al. How sleep and mental disorders are related to complaints of daytime sleepiness. Arch Intern Med 1997; 157(22):2645–2652.

40. Shirlow MJ, Mathers CD. A study of caffeine consumption and symptoms; indigestion, palpitations, tremor, headache and insomnia. Int J Epidemiol 1985; 14(2):239–248.

41. Curatolo PW, Robertson D. The health consequences of caffeine. Ann Intern Med 1983; 98(5 pt 1):641–653.

42. Landolt HP, Dijk DJ, Gaus SE, et al. Caffeine reduces low-frequency delta activity in the human sleep EEG. Neuropsychopharmacology 1995; 12(3):229–238.

43. Brown SL, Salive ME, Pahor M, et al. Occult caffeine as a source of sleep problems in an older population. J Am Geriatr Soc 1995; 43(8):860–864.

44. Curless R, French JM, James OF, et al. Is caffeine a factor in subjective insomnia of elderly people? Age Ageing 1993; 22(1):41–45.

45. LaCroix AZ, Lang J, Scherr P, et al. Smoking and mortality among older men and women in three communities. N Engl J Med 1991; 324(23):1619–1625.

46. Wetter DW, Young TB. The relation between cigarette smoking and sleep disturbance. Prev Med 1994; 23(3):328–334.

47. Boutrel B, Koob GF. What keeps us awake: the neuropharmacology of stimulants and wakefulness-promoting medications. Sleep 2004; 27(6):1181–1194.

48. Davila D, Hurt R, Offord K, et al. Acute effects of transdermal nicotine on sleep architecture, snoring, and sleep-disordered breathing in nonsmokers. Am J Respir Crit Care Med 1994; 150(2):469–474.

49. Lichstein KL, Wilson NM, Johnson CT. Psychological treatment of secondary insomnia. Psychol Aging 2000; 15(2):232–240.

50. Peters RW, Zoble RG, Brooks MM. Onset of acute myocardial infarction during sleep. Clin Cardiol 2002; 25(5):237–241.

51. Mallon L, Broman JE, Hetta J. Sleep complaints predict coronary artery disease mortality in males: a 12-year follow-up study of a middle-aged Swedish population. J Intern Med 2002; 251(3):207–216.

52. Chocron S, Tatou E, Schjoth B, et al. Perceived health status in patients over 70 before and after open-heart operations. Age Ageing 2000; 29(4):329–334.

53. Lesman-Leegte I, Jaarsma T, Sanderman R, et al. Depressive symptoms are prominent among elderly hospitalised heart failure patients. Eur J Heart Fail 2006; 8(6):634–640.

54. Ingbir M, Freimark D, Adler Y. [Cheyne-Stokes breathing disorder in patients with congestive heart failure: incidence, pathophysiology, treatment and prognosis]. Harefuah 2001; 140(12):1209–1212, 1227.

55. Lanfranchi PA, Braghiroli A, Bosimini E, et al. Prognostic value of nocturnal Cheyne-Stokes respiration in chronic heart failure. Circulation 1999; 99(11):1435–1440.

56. Sin DD, Fitzgerald F, Parker JD, et al. Risk factors for central and obstructive sleep apnea in 450 men and women with congestive heart failure. Am J Respir Crit Care Med 1999; 160(4):1101–1106.

57. Kaneko Y, Floras JS, Usui K, et al. Cardiovascular effects of continuous positive airway pressure in patients with heart failure and obstructive sleep apnea. N Engl J Med 2003; 348(13):1233–1241.

58. Ries L, Eisner M, Kosary C, et al. SEER Cancer Statistics Review, 1973–2002. In.

59. Davidson JR, Waisberg JL, Brundage MD, et al. Nonpharmacologic group treatment of insomnia: a preliminary study with cancer survivors. Psychooncology 2001; 10(5):389–397.

60. Savard J, Morin CM. Insomnia in the context of cancer: a review of a neglected problem. J Clin Oncol 2001; 19(3):895–908.

61. Davidson JR, MacLean AW, Brundage MD, et al. Sleep disturbance in cancer patients. Soc Sci Med 2002; 54(9):1309–1321.

62. Stiefel FC, Kornblith AB, Holland JC. Changes in the prescription patterns of psychotropic drugs for cancer patients during a 10-year period. Cancer 1990; 65(4):1048–1053.

63. Lee K, Cho M, Miaskowski C, et al. Impaired sleep and rhythms in persons with cancer. Sleep Med Rev 2004; 8(3):199–212.

64. Klink M, Quan SF. Prevalence of reported sleep disturbances in a general adult population and their relationship to obstructive airways diseases. Chest 1987; 91(4):540–546.

65. Fleetham J, West P, Mezon B, et al. Sleep, arousals, and oxygen desaturation in chronic obstructive pulmonary disease. The effect of oxygen therapy. Am Rev Respir Dis 1982; 126(3):429–433.

66. Martin RJ, Bartelson BL, Smith P, et al. Effect of ipratropium bromide treatment on oxygen saturation and sleep quality in COPD. Chest 1999; 115(5):1338–1345.

67. Krachman SL, Chatila W, Martin UJ, et al. Effects of lung volume reduction surgery on sleep quality and nocturnal gas exchange in patients with severe emphysema. Chest 2005; 128(5):3221–3228.

68. O'Brien A, Whitman K. Lack of benefit of continuous positive airway pressure on lung function in patients with overlap syndrome. Lung 2005; 183(6):389–404.

69. Wild S, Roglic G, Green A, et al. Global prevalence of diabetes: estimates for the year 2000 and projections for 2030. Diabetes Care 2004; 27(5):1047–1053.

70. Lamond N, Tiggemann M, Dawson D. Factors predicting sleep disruption in Type II diabetes. Sleep 2000; 23(3):415–416.

71. Sridhar GR, Madhu K. Prevalence of sleep disturbances in diabetes mellitus. Diabetes Res Clin Pract 1994; 23(3):183–186.

72. Rijsman RM, de Weerd AW. Secondary periodic limb movement disorder and restless legs syndrome. Sleep Med Rev 1999; 3(2):147–158.
73. Punjabi NM, Polotsky VY. Disorders of glucose metabolism in sleep apnea. J Appl Physiol 2005; 99(5):1998–2007.
74. Ip MS, Lam B, Ng MM,et al. Obstructive sleep apnea is independently associated with insulin resistance. Am J Respir Crit Care Med 2002; 165(5):670–676.
75. Purdie DW, Empson JA, Crichton C, et al. Hormone replacement therapy, sleep quality and psychological wellbeing. Br J Obstet Gynaecol 1995; 102(9):735–739.
76. Felson DT, Naimark A, Anderson J, et al. The prevalence of knee osteoarthritis in the elderly. The Framingham Osteoarthritis Study. Arthritis Rheum 1987; 30(8):914–918.
77. Wilcox S, Brenes GA, Levine D, et al. Factors related to sleep disturbance in older adults experiencing knee pain or knee pain with radiographic evidence of knee osteoarthritis. J Am Geriatr Soc 2000; 48(10):1241–1251.
78. Salih AM, Gray RE, Mills KR, et al. A clinical, serological and neurophysiological study of restless legs syndrome in rheumatoid arthritis. Br J Rheumatol 1994; 33(1):60–63.
79. Jordan JM, Bernard SL, Callahan LF, et al. Self-reported arthritis-related disruptions in sleep and daily life and the use of medical, complementary, and self-care strategies for arthritis: the National Survey of Self-care and Aging. Arch Fam Med 2000; 9(2):143–149.
80. Rybarczyk B, Stepanski E, Fogg L, et al. A placebo-controlled test of cognitive-behavioral therapy for comorbid insomnia in older adults. J Consult Clin Psychol 2005; 73(6):1164–1174.
81. Locke GR III, Talley NJ, Fett SL, et al. Prevalence and clinical spectrum of gastroesophageal reflux: a population-based study in Olmsted County, Minnesota. Gastroenterology 1997; 112(5):1448–1456.
82. Bretagne JF, Richard-Molard B, Honnorat C, et al. [Gastroesophageal reflux in the French general population: national survey of 8000 adults]. Presse Med 2006; 35(1 Pt 1):23–31.
83. Farup C, Kleinman L, Sloan S, et al. The impact of nocturnal symptoms associated with gastroesophageal reflux disease on health-related quality of life. Arch Intern Med 2001; 161(1):45–52.
84. Penzel T, Becker HF, Brandenburg U, et al. Arousal in patients with gastro-oesophageal reflux and sleep apnoea. Eur Respir J 1999; 14(6):1266–1270.
85. Orr WC. Sleep and gastroesophageal reflux disease: a wake-up call. Rev Gastroenterol Disord 2004; 4 Suppl 4:S25–S32.
86. Johnson DA, Orr WC, Crawley JA, et al. Effect of esomeprazole on nighttime heartburn and sleep quality in patients with GERD: a randomized, placebo-controlled trial. Am J Gastroenterol 2005; 100(9):1914–1922.
87. Milsom I, Abrams P, Cardozo L, et al. How widespread are the symptoms of an overactive bladder and how are they managed? A population-based prevalence study. BJU Int 2001; 87(9):760–766.
88. Donahue JL, Lowenthal DT. Nocturnal polyuria in the elderly person. Am J Med Sci 1997; 314(4):232–238.
89. Stolzmann KL, Camponeschi JL, Remington PL. The increasing incidence of end-stage renal disease in Wisconsin from 1982–2003: an analysis by age, race, and primary diagnosis. Wmj 2005; 104(8):66–71.
90. Sabbatini M, Minale B, Crispo A, et al. Insomnia in maintenance haemodialysis patients. Nephrol Dial Transplant 2002; 17(5):852–856.
91. Parker KP, Bliwise DL, Bailey JL, et al. Polysomnographic measures of nocturnal sleep in patients on chronic, intermittent daytime haemodialysis vs those with chronic kidney disease. Nephrol Dial Transplant 2005; 20(7):1422–1428.
92. Williams SW, Tell GS, Zheng B, et al. Correlates of sleep behavior among hemodialysis patients. The kidney outcomes prediction and evaluation (KOPE) study. Am J Nephrol 2002; 22(1):18–28.
93. Parker KP. Sleep disturbances in dialysis patients. Sleep Med Rev 2003; 7(2):131–143.
94. Hanly PJ, Pierratos A. Improvement of sleep apnea in patients with chronic renal failure who undergo nocturnal hemodialysis. N Engl J Med 2001; 344(2):102–107.

95. Benz RL, Pressman MR, Hovick ET, et al. A preliminary study of the effects of correction of anemia with recombinant human erythropoietin therapy on sleep, sleep disorders, and daytime sleepiness in hemodialysis patients (The SLEEPO study). Am J Kidney Dis 1999; 34(6):1089–1095.

96. Davison SN, Jhangri GS. The impact of chronic pain on depression, sleep, and the desire to withdraw from dialysis in hemodialysis patients. J Pain Symptom Manage 2005; 30(5):465–473.

97. O'Loughlin JL, Robitaille Y, Boivin JF, et al. Incidence of and risk factors for falls and injurious falls among the community-dwelling elderly. Am J Epidemiol 1993; 137(3):342–354.

98. Campbell AJ, Robertson MC, Gardner MM, et al. Psychotropic medication withdrawal and a home-based exercise program to prevent falls: a randomized, controlled trial. J Am Geriatr Soc 1999; 47(7):850–853.

99. Avidan AY, Fries BE, James ML, et al. Insomnia and hypnotic use, recorded in the minimum data set, as predictors of falls and hip fractures in Michigan nursing homes. J Am Geriatr Soc 2005; 53(6):955–962.

100. Chang CH, Gonzalez CM, Lau DT, et al. Urinary Incontinence and Self-Reported Health Among the U. S. Medicare Managed Care Beneficiaries. J Aging Health 2008; 20(4):405–419.

101. Bliwise DL, Adelman CL, Ouslander JG. Polysomnographic correlates of spontaneous nocturnal wetness episodes in incontinent geriatric patients. Sleep 2004; 27(1):153–157.

102. Ouslander JG, Buxton WG, Al-Samarrai NR, et al. Nighttime urinary incontinence and sleep disruption among nursing home residents. J Am Geriatr Soc 1998; 46(4):463–466.

103. Stepanski E, Rybarczyk B. Emerging research on the treatment and etiology of secondary or comorbid insomnia. Sleep Medicine Rev 2006; 10:7–18.

104. Kalman D, Morissette SB, George TP. Co-morbidity of smoking in patients with psychiatric and substance use disorders. Am J Addict 2005; 14(2):106–123.

Sleep and Psychiatric Illness

Wilfred R. Pigeon and Michael L. Perlis
Sleep and Neurophysiology Research Laboratory, Department of Psychiatry, University of Rochester School of Medicine and Dentistry, Rochester, New York, U.S.A.

INTRODUCTION

Both psychiatric disorders and sleep disorders are significant public health issues in the geriatric population. While the prevalence of sleep disorders such as insomnia, sleep apnea, and restless legs syndrome has a pronounced increase across the lifespan (1–3), the prevalence of psychiatric conditions such as mood and anxiety disorders remains somewhat constant from middle to old age (4). Sleep disturbance is a symptom criterion across a number of psychiatric illnesses, including many of the mood and anxiety disorders as delineated in the Diagnostic and Statistical Manual of Mental Disorders, 4th revision (DSM) (5). Most commonly, the sleep disturbance is in the form of an insomnia complaint and to a lesser extent it relates to hypersomnia and other common disorders of sleep such as sleep apnea. Alterations in sleep architecture are evidenced across a variety of mood and anxiety disorders when sleep is subjected to polysomnographic evaluation. It is also the case that a host of psychotropic medications either alter sleep architecture and/or contribute to subjective sleep complaints.

This chapter will review literature from older populations, although in some areas, the limited number of studies requires the extrapolation of findings from nonelder populations. It is also the case that sleep problems are not measured or defined in a consistent manner across studies. This is especially true for data drawn from epidemiologic and community samples, but is also found in studies in which depression status (and not sleep) was the primary outcome(s). Typically, such investigations report on single-item measures of sleep complaints either developed for the study or embedded within other instruments. For instance, the Hamilton Rating Scale for Depression (6) has three items related, respectively, to early, middle, and late night insomnia. Until recently, such an approach had not been validated, but Manber et al. (7) have now shown that, at least in a depressed sample, such approaches can be validated against the assessment of insomnia via daily sleep diaries traditionally used by sleep researchers. Thus, while the general term "sleep disturbance" has been used as a proxy for insomnia in the absence of measures required for diagnosis of insomnia, for this chapter, we have adopted a convention of using the term "insomnia" in such cases.

SLEEP DISTURBANCE IN MOOD DISORDERS AND BEREAVEMENT

Depression

By far, the largest body of evidence for a relationship between psychiatric illness and sleep disturbances exists for the association between depression and insomnia.

As would be expected, both disorders are highly prevalent and frequently co-occur in all age ranges and in older cohorts (8,9). Cross-sectional data also distinguish the relationship further by providing the prevalence of insomnia in depressed populations and of depression in insomnia populations. In a vast majority of these studies, both female gender and increased age are associated with higher prevalence rates. Longitudinal studies have been undertaken further elucidating this relationship over time. Finally, there is more limited data to draw from with respect to polysomnographic findings in the elderly.

Prevalence Estimates for Depression and Insomnia

A number of community and epidemiologic studies have been conducted to determine the prevalence of both depression and insomnia. While both disorders are variably defined across studies, in general, the prevalence of depression is approximately 9% and that of insomnia is approximately 17%. The estimates are lower in studies with more stringent criteria, approximately 5% and 10% for depression and insomnia, respectively. It is also interesting to assess the prevalence of depression in only those subjects deemed to have insomnia compared with the prevalence of insomnia in only those subjects deemed to be depressed.

For example, there are at least three large studies with stratified age samples. Baseline estimates from Ford and Kamerow's longitudinal study ($n = 7954$), derived from the National Institute of Mental Health Epidemiologic Catchment Area study, found prevalence rates of 10% for insomnia and 5% for depression. Among those subjects with insomnia, 23% were depressed, whereas among subjects with depression, 42% had insomnia (10). A cross-sectional study of the general population of France conducted via an automated telephone screening ($n = 5622$) found prevalence rates of 17% for insomnia and 6% for depression (11). Among the subjects with insomnia, 18% were depressed, whereas among subjects with depression, 57% had insomnia. Stewart et al. (12) applied more stringent diagnostic criteria than most prior studies and applied them to data from the Second National Survey of Psychiatric Morbidity conducted in the United Kingdom ($n = 8580$). They reported prevalence rates of 5% for insomnia and 3% for depression. Among those subjects with insomnia, 21% were depressed, whereas among subjects with depression, 40% had insomnia.

Two large scale studies have focused exclusively on older populations. Foley et al. (3) assessed data from 9282 elderly community dwellers with a mean age of 74 years and found prevalence rates of 28% for insomnia and 20% for depression. Among the subjects with insomnia, 34% were depressed, whereas among the subjects with depression, 49% had insomnia. In a longitudinal study of community residents aged 50 and over in Alameda County, California ($n = 2272$), baseline estimates for the prevalence of insomnia and depression were 24% and 9%, respectively (13). Among the subjects with insomnia, 19% were depressed, whereas among subjects with depression, 50% had insomnia. There have also been two studies assessing samples from primary care practice (14,15), which have found prevalence rates of 16% to 19% for insomnia and 7% to 8% for depression, with 18% to 31% of those with insomnia being depressed and 52% to 58% of those with depression having insomnia. Mahendran et al. (16) reported on 141 consecutive cases referred to an insomnia clinic in Singapore and found that 48% met DSM criteria for primary insomnia and 10% met criteria for major depression or dysthymia, suggesting that insomnia services may see a biased selection of patients compared with what the epidemiologic data report.

Table 1 summarizes data from studies that include, or exclusively sample, older populations and that have enough detail to calculate the above prevalence rates. Overall, the prevalence of insomnia is approximately twice that of depression. In addition, it appears that the likelihood of having depression in the context of insomnia is approximately twice that of having insomnia in the context of depression. Such data lead to a discussion of the relationship between the two disorders.

Historically, when it occurred with psychiatric illness, insomnia was viewed as a natural consequence of mood dysregulation, where sleep onset insomnia and early morning insomnia were considered the cardinal symptoms of anxiety and depression. Insomnia was thus viewed as a symptom that would resolve with amelioration of the parent disorder. Based in part on nosologies that identify insomnia as a primary or comorbid disorder (17–19) and in part on the accumulation of data from longitudinal studies and from clinical trails in depression, several authors have challenged this assumption (20,21).

Longitudinal Studies

A number of longitudinal studies provide some insight into the relationship between insomnia and depression. In a study, patients with recurrent, but remitted, major depressive disorders (MDDs) were followed for up to 42 weeks with the Beck Depression Inventory (22) and the sleep item from this instrument in order to identify those who experienced a recurrence of depression and compare them with matched controls with no recurrence (23). Time series data showed that the nonrecurrent group exhibited an elevated, but stable, level of insomnia, while the recurrent group exhibited an increased level of sleep disturbance that began 5 weeks prior to, and was of highest severity at, the week of recurrence. This suggests that insomnia may be a prodromal sign of a depressive episode.

Longitudinal studies in mixed-age populations have found that insomnia represents a risk factor for subsequent depression. Typically, these studies have assessed whether insomnia occurring at two time points predicts depression at the second time point. Three studies have evaluated the onset of new depression over a one-year time point. Two of these have found that insomnia posed an increased risk for the development of depression with odds ratios of 40 (CI,19.8–80) and 5.4 (2.6–11.3), respectively (10,24). Dryman and Eaton found an increased risk for depression (OR, 9.4 [4.3–20.3]) (odds ratio), but only in women (25). In a study that began with college-aged men who were reevaluated approximately 30 years later, insomnia in college conferred a relative risk of 2.0 (1.2–3.3) for developing depression at some point during the follow-up period (26).

In longitudinal studies performed in older cohorts, the findings are more mixed. In a study of 524 community-dwelling elderly persons, those with insomnia at baseline and 3 years later were more likely to have depression at 3 years than those with no insomnia or with insomnia at one time point (statistics were not provided) (27). Baseline insomnia was predictive of future depression, but only in the absence of baseline depression, calling into question the independence of insomnia as a predictor. In a reanalysis of this data set restricted to a sample that had activity limitations, but no psychiatric morbidity at baseline, baseline insomnia was not associated with depression 3 years later (28).

TABLE 1 Prevalence Rates of Depression and Insomnia in Study Samples with Older Age Cohorts

Study	Sample type (size)	Mean age	Sleep measures	Depressed (%)	Insomnia (%)	In depressed,% with insomnia	In insomnia,% with depression
Foley et al. (3)	Epid (9282)	74	5 sleep items	20	28	49	34
Weyerer and Dilling (144)	Comm (1536)	Mixed	6 sleep items	7	16	47	24
Bixler et al. (145)	Comm (1006)	Mixed	5–6 sleep items	15	32	43	19
Mellinger et al. (84)	Comm (3161)	Mixed	2 sleep items	5	17	71	21
Ohayon et al. (11)	Epid (5622)	Mixed	DSM criteria	6	17	57	18
Stewart et al. (12)	Epid (8580)	Mixed	Clinical interview	3	5.4	40	21
Taylor et al. (85)	Comm (772)	Mixed	Sleep diaries	10	20	41	20
Simon and Vonkorff (15)	PC (373)	39	6 Sleep Items	8	16	58	31
Ford and Kamerow (10)	Epid (7954)	Mixed	2 sleep items	5	10	42	23
Roberts et al. (13)	Epid (2272)	50+	1 sleep item	9	24	50	19
Hohagen et al. (14)	PC (2512)	Mixed	DSM criteria	7	19	52	18
Total number	43,070		Weighted averages	9	17	50%	27

Abbreviations: Epid, epidemiologic sample; Comm, community-based sample; PC, primary care sample.

Roberts et al. found that insomnia at baseline was associated with an increased risk of depression one year later (OR, 2.5[1.7–3.7]) and insomnia at both time points carried an eightfold risk, but that several other factors were more significant predictors (13). In older adults followed for 12 years (29), baseline insomnia was an independent predictor of depression at 12 years in women only (OR, 4.1 [2.3–7.2]). Brabbins determined that in a sample of 771 elders, only initial insomnia (and not middle-of-the-night or early-morning awakening) that occurred at both baseline and 3 years was associated with the development of new depression at 3 years (30). Finally, a meta-analysis of studies conducted in older adults found that sleep disturbance, with an odds ratio of 2.6, was second to recent bereavement (OR 3.3) as a risk factor for late-life depression (31). In summary, while there is a good body of evidence that suggests that both incident and persistent insomnia predict new onset depression, the findings are not unanimous, and insomnia is not the only significant risk factor.

One difficulty in interpreting this set of findings in a causal manner is that to best evaluate the prospective contribution of chronic insomnia to the development of depression via survey instruments, one must compare insomnia that is chronic (via instruments or structured interviews that can capture chronicity or via assessments that spans two time points) with depression status at a later time point. So, despite a set of findings suggesting that insomnia is more than a symptom of depression, it does not completely rule out the possibility. The desire to seek dualistic solutions to this complex issue is perhaps unrealistic. As Table 1 shows, insomnia and depression do not always co-occur, nor does one necessarily presage the other across all cases. It may be that for some individuals insomnia is simply a symptom that does follow the course of depression and for others insomnia represents a comorbid condition requiring targeted intervention, as will be discussed in the treatment section later.

Depression and Other Sleep Disorders
It is important to note that although insomnia represents the most commonly occurring sleep disorder in depression, two additional sleep disturbances have been investigated. Hypersomnia (or excessive daytime sleepiness) has not always been included in epidemiologic studies, but when included, it has been found to have a prevalence rate of 5% to 10% and to be associated with depression (10,13). In both epidemiologic and clinical studies, depression is also associated with obstructive sleep apnea. In a large sample of the general population, Ohayon reported that approximately 18% of subjects with sleep-related breathing disorders also met criteria for MDD, and similarly, approximately 18% of subjects with MDD also met criteria for a sleep-related breathing disorder (32). A recent review indicated that the prevalence of depression ranges from 20% to 60% in clinic patients with obstructive sleep apnea (OSA), with some evidence that depression increases with OSA severity (33). These data suggest that the presence of either OSA or MDD may be a clinical indication to assess for the other disorder.

Polysomnographic Findings in Depression
When sleep is measured with polysomnography (PSG), patients with depression reliably exhibit sleep continuity and sleep architectural abnormalities (8,34) In terms of sleep continuity, patients with depression tend to exhibit increased sleep latency, increased time awake, and decreased sleep efficiency. While this profile resembles

that of patients with primary insomnia, the magnitude of the problem tends to be smaller. In terms of sleep architecture, slow-wave sleep (SWS) deficits have been observed in patients with MDD (35–38), though not consistently so. More consistent in MDD have been the REM sleep findings, including short REM latencies (less than or equal to 65 minutes), increased REM density (number of rapid eye movements during REM sleep), and increased total time in REM sleep (20–30%) (35–37,39). By using power spectral analysis of EEG activity from PSG recordings, patients with depression have been shown to exhibit either reduced NREM delta power overall or abnormal distributions of delta activity across the sleep period (40–42). There are, however, studies that suggest that this finding is not replicable (43,44) at all or is so only in males (45) and/or is characteristic of depressed cohorts from past, but not present, generations (46).

Bereavement

Bereavement refers to the loss of a loved one by death, whereas grief refers to the emotional reaction to bereavement. Approximately 75% of all deaths occur in persons aged 65 years and older (47), so that bereavement is a condition whose incidence and prevalence increases across the life span. Bereavement is considered a diagnostic entity in the DSM Nosology and grouped with a plethora of heterogeneous conditions under "Other Conditions That May Be a Focus of Clinical Attention." In order to be the focus of treatment, bereavement must include a grief reaction that exceeds normal levels and that is distinct from a major depressive episode. Currently the list of abnormal reactions does not include sleep disturbance, although the suggestion has been made that sleep interference be included as one of seven symptom criteria for a proposed diagnostic entity for complicated grief disorder (48). Between 10% and 20% of persons experiencing bereavement have a complicated grief reaction (49). In a meta-analytic review of studies in community-dwelling elders, Cole and Dendukuri determined that recent bereavement was the biggest risk factor for depression (31).

Across a number of smaller studies, sleep disturbance in the form of difficulty sleeping and/or insomnia has been reported in one third to one-half of subjects with bereavement (48,5050–54), and the level of sleep disturbance was higher than in that of control groups without bereavement (52–54). In an epidemiologic study of 2121 subjects with insomnia, bereavement, along with stress and loneliness, was the most often cited precipitant of insomnia (55). Even when complicated grief is recognized as a possible therapeutic target, as in many comorbid conditions, sleep may not be adequately addressed. Indeed, some proposed diagnostic criteria for complicated grief disorder do not include sleep disturbance as a symptom (56), while recent treatment reviews and evidence-based guidelines do not include sleep as a direct therapeutic target (56,57). This represents an understandable, but considerable, oversight, which the sleep medicine community can address.

PSG findings in bereaved subjects, meanwhile, have not distinguished such subjects from other depressed populations (58).

Treatment of Mood Disorders and Sleep Disorders

While a variety of antidepressant medication therapies do improve sleep in a large number of patients, for some the successful resolution of psychiatric illness does not translate to resolution of insomnia, which remains a common residual symptom (59–63). For instance, in an 8-week trial of fluoxetine, disturbed sleep and fatigue were the most common residual symptom among depression remitters (62), present in 44% and 38% of remitters, respectively. In a trial of nortriptyline, depression remitters had significant decreases in mean sleep disturbance scores on the Pittsburgh Sleep Quality Index (PSQI) (64), but their mean global PSQI score remained higher than that of healthy controls and above the clinical cutoff for disturbed sleep (65).

At least for the selective serotonin reuptake inhibitors (SSRIs) class, residual insomnia may be related to the disruption of sleep (detailed in final section of this chapter) associated with these medications. Coadministration of a hypnotic drug such as zolpidem may help some patients avoid the sleep-disrupting adverse effects of some antidepressants. Selection of an antidepressant with sedating effects is another alternative that may be beneficial for some patients, although daytime somnolence may limit use in some cases. New SSRIs, such as escitalopram, which may be less disruptive, may be the preferred option for some patients.

Interestingly, the treatment of depression with targeted behavioral interventions mirrors some of the outcomes observed following pharmacotherapy for depression (66,67). A recent analysis of treatment responders in a randomized trial comparing cognitive-behavioral therapy (CBT) for depression to antidepressant medication over 20 weeks of treatment found residual insomnia to be evenly distributed between intervention groups and occurring in approximately 50% of those with remitted depression (68). Similar findings were observed in a trial comparing CBT with nefazadone (69). Finally, in a large cohort of acutely depressed elders presenting to primary care, those subjects with persistent insomnia were two to four times more likely to remain depressed at later time points than patients with no insomnia, despite either a treatment as usual approach to depression in primary care or an enhanced care for depression intervention that included both behavioral and pharmacologic approaches (70).

Taken together this set of findings suggests that for some individuals insomnia may linger despite a seeming resolution of depression and that when it is not targeted it may lead to increased morbidity. Given that residual symptoms in general represent a significant risk for relapse and that increasing numbers of depressive episodes increase morbidity even further, targeted approaches to common residual symptoms are required (71,72).

Some promising options have begun to emerge for the treatment of insomnia in depression in the comorbid phase (as opposed to waiting for the residual phase). A recent coadministration study found that eszopiclone with fluoxetine resulted in sustained sleep improvements as well as a faster and more robust antidepressant effects than fluoxetine alone (73). In a unique coadministration study highlighting the importance of behavioral interventions for sleep, the combined use of escitilopram and CBT for insomnia (CBT-I) resulted in larger improvements in both sleep and depression outcomes than escitilopram and a control therapy (74). Also, two uncontrolled studies have shown that patients presenting with insomnia and depression who completed only a course of CBT-I had improvements in both sleep and depression (75,76).

While there are currently no evidence-based guidelines for addressing insomnia in the context of depression, the above findings and clinical experience form the bases for some recommendations. First-line treatment should address insomnia complaints directly with CBT-I or an appropriate currently available hypnotic, such as a benzodiazepine receptor agonist or a melatonin receptor agonist (see Chapter 6 for a thorough review of these medications). Secondary considerations include the use of benzodiazepines in subjects with paradoxical insomnia (previously called sleep state misperception), low-dose sedating antidepressants as augmentation to SSRI therapy, and newer sedating antipsychotic medications in patients with psychotic features. Especially in the elderly these secondary treatment considerations should be considered with some caution given their far riskier side-effect profile. It is also important to note that regardless of the treatment approach, successful management of insomnia at the level of the individual patient requires regular symptom assessment. Ideally, this will occur at weekly intervals and can be accomplished minimally with the administration of a validated instrument such as the Insomnia Severity Index (77,78), though it is best achieved by having patients complete daily sleep diaries.

Treatment of sleep apnea with nasal administration of continuous positive airway pressure has been shown to reverse the depression associated with sleep apnea, though findings have been mixed (79–83). In general, there is a suggestion that continuous positive airway pressure (CPAP) treatment improves mood in patients with sleep apnea, but larger, well-controlled studies are needed to fully address this question.

Finally, as noted in the bereavement section, attention to the treatment of sleep disturbance in complicated grief is very much warranted and needed.

SLEEP DISTURBANCE IN ANXIETY DISORDERS

Sleep disturbances are even more prevalent in anxiety disorders than they are in mood disorders, but with the exception of posttraumatic stress disorder (PTSD), far less research has been conducted in these areas. The Ford and Kamerow study found that 24% of study respondents with insomnia also had an anxiety disorder and that those with insomnia were six times more likely to have an anxiety disorder than those without insomnia (10). Others have found anxiety orders to be equally or more prevalent than depression in their general population samples and among their respective insomnia subsamples (12,16,84,85).

Posttraumatic Stress Disorder

Sleep disturbances are a common feature of PTSD in both the general population (86) and in combat veterans (87). Nightmares in particular have historically been considered the hallmark of PTSD, and there are ample data suggesting a strong association between trauma exposure and nightmares as well as between PTSD and nightmares (88). Interestingly, insomnia is actually a more prevalent symptom in PTSD than are nightmares. This has been shown in an epidemiologic survey of the general population as well as in a clinical sample seeking treatment for insomnia (86,89). In an assessment of the National Vietnam Veterans Readjustment Study database (87), it was found that insomnia was more frequent than nightmares in both combat veterans with PTSD (90.7% vs. 52.4%) and combat veterans without PTSD (62.5% vs. 4.8%). While these findings speak to the specificity of nightmares for PTSD, they also underscore the extremely high prevalence of insomnia in trauma-exposed populations of 60% to 90%. On both counts, these prevalence rates make apparent the need for a sleep assessment in patients presenting with a trauma history.

PTSD-related insomnia is similar to primary insomnia on a number of dimensions, including the severity of the sleep disturbance and the association with a higher risk for other complications (90,91). Other factors are more specific to trauma/PTSD. For instance, perceived loss of control is believed to be a crucial factor in the etiology and maintenance of PTSD (92). Inability to initiate or maintain sleep can be perceived by patients as another indicator of a loss of control and trigger efforts to regain control of sleep, which tend to be counterproductive. Nightmares contribute to the problem in several ways (87,88,93). Anticipatory anxiety related to having distressing dreams can increase arousal, nightmares often cause repeated awakenings and reinforce the association between threat and the sleep environment, and alcohol and/or sleep deprivation may be used as avoidance strategies to escape nightmares. Finally, to the extent that trauma exposure occurred in the sleep environment or during sleep, both the bedroom and the very act of sleep may represent dangerous stimuli that such subjects seek to avoid and/or serve as cues for heightened vigilance and arousal. Thus, PTSD represents a complication to primary insomnia above and beyond the insomnia experienced in depression or generalized anxiety.

Polysomnographic Findings in PTSD

Sleep abnormalities observed during overnight sleep recordings are similar to those observed in insomnia, including increased sleep latency, wake after sleep onset (WSO), and awakenings with increased stage 1 sleep and decreased stage 2 and higher NREM sleep (94,95). Additional REM sleep abnormalities not typically noted in general insomnia (96) include fragmented REM sleep coupled with increased REM density. PTSD has also been associated with increased periodic limb movements and sleep-disordered breathing (97). Krakow et al. in particular have reported on the high prevalence of upper-airway resistance syndrome or mild obstructive sleep apnea in several PTSD populations, ranging from 50% to 80% of patients having a polysomnographically assessed sleep-disordered breathing (98–100). These findings further underscore the necessity of a thorough sleep interview in patients with PTSD.

Other Anxiety Disorders

The relative paucity of sleep data in generalized anxiety disorder (GAD) is surprising given that sleep disturbance is one of the six DSM symptom criteria for its diagnosis, two additional symptoms (irritability and fatigue) are often associated with insomnia, and both GAD and insomnia tend to present with features of hyperarousal (101–103). In a survey of referrals to an insomnia clinic ($n = 141$), GAD was the most common co-occurring psychiatric disorder (16).

Panic disorder, and especially the panic attacks that accompany it, has been the subject of some inquiry in terms of sleep. Approximately 20% of panic attacks occur during sleep, and 30% to 70% of patients with panic disorder report sleep-related panic (104). Nocturnal panic attacks have been recorded to occur following stage 2 or 3 sleep (105,106).

Treatment of Anxiety Disorders and Sleep Disorders

Evidence-based treatments for both depression and PTSD are available, utilized, and successful across a variety of trauma populations, although they do not specifically address insomnia (107). For some individuals, the successful treatment of

PTSD and/or trauma-related depression does, indeed, lead to a resolution of sleep disturbance. As in depression, in such cases, insomnia is perhaps best viewed as an epiphenomenon of the primary disorder, and more specifically as a hyperarousal symptom that ameliorates with the treatment of the primary disorder. In other cases, insomnia becomes a disorder in its own right, one that then confers significant risk for poorer outcomes. For example, in the context of trauma exposure without PTSD, following otherwise successful psychotherapy for depression, insomnia has been found to persist (108). Similarly, in the context of existing PTSD, following otherwise successful psychotherapy for PTSD, nightmares have been found to abate, but insomnia has been found to persist in approximately 50% of patients (87,89). Therefore, insomnia does not uniformly respond to standard CBT for depression or for PTSD.

Imagery rehearsal therapy (IRT), a brief form of exposure therapy to treat nightmares, has been used for both nightmares with and without PTSD in several trauma populations to successfully decrease the number of distressing dreams and their impact on sleep (109–111). In a case series, a five-session course of CBT-I alone, which was tailored to a PTSD population with residual insomnia following CBT for PTSD, resulted in dramatic decreases in insomnia severity (112). IRT has also been combined with a brief course of CBT-I to reduce both nightmares and insomnia severity in PTSD (113–115). None of these studies were carried out in subjects with combat exposure. Thus, it remains to be shown whether similar gains from trauma-specific CBT-I may be achieved in a combat trauma population, an important question for the management of PTSD in current veterans as well as in the large number of returning Iraq War and Operation Enduring Freedom personnel.

GAD has been successfully treated with both CBT focused on anxiety symptoms and a variety of anxiolytics (116–118). A CBT trial focusing on worry-related thoughts without addressing sleep nonetheless improved insomnia complaints (119). Given the high prevalence of GAD in the general population and its close association with insomnia, more intervention studies are clearly indicated in this area.

SLEEP DISTURBANCE IN SUBSTANCE ABUSE DISORDERS

The prevalence of both alcohol and substance dependence declines with age, so that 2% to 10% of older populations in epidemiologic cohorts report alcohol dependence and a smaller percentage report other drug dependencies (excluding nicotine addiction). In general, older adults are thought to diminish alcohol use with the onset of increased health problems. The use of prescription medications with abuse potential, on the other hand, tends to rise in older adults, as does the combined use of alcohol and sedating medications. Notwithstanding the decline in prevalence rates for substance dependence, one study found that 30% of drinkers began drinking after age 60 (120). Alcohol abuse and drug abuse are more common in those with complaints of insomnia or hypersomnia, and furthermore, persistent insomnia is associated with an increased risk of having an alcohol abuse disorder (10).

In patients with alcoholism, a number of sleep disorders may arise, including sleep apnea, periodic limb movement disorder (PLMD), insomnia, hypersomnia, circadian rhythm disorders, and parasomnias, though this has not been well established. The rate of insomnia comorbid with alcoholism has been estimated at approximately twice that of the general population (121). Insomnia is also the most likely concomitant sleep disorder with stimulant abuse, though alcohol abuse is arguably the more important substance abuse disorder with respect to older adults.

Polysomnographic Findings in Substance Abuse Disorders

Alcohol is often used as a hypnotic by nonabusing individuals, which can set the stage for dependence in some. More acutely, the effects of alcohol on a single night's sleep are at first sedating, but then associated with increased wakefulness, increased REM sleep, and overall sleep fragmentation (which worsens with repeated alcohol use). In addition, given its effect on ventilatory control, alcohol may also induce or worsen sleep apnea. This may be more prevalent in problematic in older patients given the increased incidence of apnea with aging.

PSG sleep in patients with alcoholism is characterized by increased sleep latencies, decreased total sleep time, poor sleep efficiency, and diminished SWS and REM sleep (122,123). Sleep abnormalities persist following cessation of drinking, with acute worsening of sleep disturbance, and return to baseline disturbance levels over 3 to 6 months.

As might be expected, stimulants such as amphetamines and cocaine, while counteracting daytime sleepiness, tend to prolong sleep latency and reduce total sleep time. They have also been found to be associated with decreased REM sleep and increased latency to REM, while withdrawal from stimulants is associated with increased difficulty initiating sleep (124). The effects of cocaine abstinence have been observed polysomnographically more often, though in only a handful of studies with small sample sizes. Findings include increases in REM variables with decreases in total sleep time, sleep efficiency and SWS (125), and that polysomnographic sleep disturbances get worse in the 2 weeks following acute abstinence (126).

In acute administration of cannabis, there have been mixed findings for sleep latency as well as for SWS changes, but consistent findings of decreases in REM sleep and REM density (127). In chronic cannabis users, where there are notably two studies with 30 and 32 subjects, respectively, any improvements in sleep latency, overall sleep, and increased SWS diminish over time, while the REM findings appear to persist (127).

Treatment of Substance Abuse Disorders and Sleep Disorders

Sleep disturbance, particularly in the form of insomnia, is associated with higher rates of relapse in recovering alcoholics (121,128); this has no been established in other substance abuse disorders. One open-label and two randomized controlled trials for treating insomnia comorbid with alcoholism have been undertaken. Arnedt et al. (129) treated seven recently abstinent patients with alcohol dependence with standard outpatient CBT for insomnia. They found significant improvements in all areas of sleep continuity and insomnia severity, and no relapses occurred during treatment, although no follow-up assessments were conducted in this pilot investigation. The first RCT compared progressive muscle relaxation with wait-list control, in which large effect sizes for improved sleep quality, but no other sleep measures, were reported (130). The second randomized clinical trial (RCT) compared standard outpatient CBT for insomnia with an insomnia self-help program with telephone support and with a wait-list condition in patients newly recovering from alcoholism (131). In this study both interventions were found to be associated with greater clinical improvement than the wait-list condition with more pronounced gains in the CBT-I condition. Rates of relapse did not differ between

TABLE 2 Typical Polysomnographic Changes Associated with Psychiatric Medications

Drug class/drug	Wake	TST	St 1	SWS	REM	Other
Antidepressants						
Buproprion				↓	↑	Insomnia, disturbing dreams
Citalopram						Insomnia
Fluoxetine	↑	↓	↑	↓	↓	PLMs
Fluvoxamine	↑	↑	↑		↓	Insomnia
MAOIs	↑	↓			↓↓	
Mitrazapine		↑	↓			
Nefazadone	↓	↑			↑	
Paroxetine	↑	↓	↑		↓	Insomnia
Sertraline		↓			↓	Insomnia
Trazadone	↓	↑			↓	
Tricyclics	↑	↓			↓↓	Insomnia
Venlafaxine	↑	↓			↓↓	Insomnia, PLMs
Antipsychotic agents	↑			↑	↑↓	
Antiparkinsonian agents				↑↓	↑↓	Insomnia (?)
Benzodiazepines				↓	↓	↑ Sleep spindles
Lithium				↑	↓	Improves sleep

Arrows indicate increase or decrease; double arrows indicate large changes; and up and down arrows indicate mixed findings.
Abbreviations: TST, total sleep time; St 1, stage 1 sleep; SWS, slow wave sleep; PLMs, periodic limb movements.

conditions, although the small sample size limits the generalizability of these findings. Particularly given the elevated risk of relapse associated with insomnia, more work is needed in this area with both CBT and pharmacologic approaches. It does not appear that any such work has been undertaken with respect to other substance abuse disorders, and no trials have been conducted in older populations of substance-abusing patients or those in early abstinence.

PSYCHIATRIC MEDICATIONS AND THEIR EFFECTS ON SLEEP

There are sleep effects for most psychotropic medications. This section will provide but a brief summary of those effects (see Table 2 for a summary). In general, if a medication has a sedative effect it can be expected to improve sleep continuity (reduce sleep latency, wake after sleep onset, and number of awakenings, while increasing total sleep time and sleep efficiency). Usually the effects can be seen on both objective (PSG) and subjective (sleep diaries) measures of sleep. Sleep architecture effects can be expected to include decreases in stage 1 and increases in stage 2 sleep, whereas effects on SWS and REM sleep tend to vary by medication.

SWS suppression is generally considered a negative as it parallels the effects of aging and may interfere with the putative-restorative functions of SWS. In contrast, SWS augmentation is generally considered useful, though empirical support of these benefits from SWS augmenting medications is lacking. To the extent that SWS augmentation results in nonnormally distributed SWS (i.e. SWS occurs later in the night than usual), it may produce better sleep continuity at the expense of having patients awaken from high levels of SWS; a scenario that may interfere with the perception of good sleep continuity and leave the individual with profound levels of sleep inertia and/or residual sedation. For a review of SWS findings in insomnia populations see Ref. 132.

The effects of medication-driven REM suppression are largely unknown in healthy subjects and patients with insomnia. To the extent that REM sleep is thought to subserve mood regulation and procedural memory, suppression of this stage may interfere with optimal functioning in these domains. The effects of REM suppression in patients with psychiatric illness (especially MDD) do not appear to be deleterious, but instead associated with good clinical outcomes, so much so that some have posited that REM suppression is a mechanism of actions for antidepressants (133). Adrien has proposed that insomnia initially occurs as a compensatory phenomenon in MDD to increase serotonergic tone, but that unlike its sleep deprivation counterpart, it cannot reach a level that exerts an antidepressant effect (134–136). On a very acute basis (single-night REM deprivation), sleep deprivation therapy produces marked, though temporary, improvements in the mood of depressed subjects (see, e.g., 137). In contrast, the effects of REM augmentation in healthy subjects or patients with primary or comorbid insomnia are unknown. One reason for pause is that increased REM time (percent and/or minutes) tends to be positively associated with the incidence and severity of mental illness.

Anxiolytics and Hypnotics
Sedative classes of medications tend to have the sedating effects on sleep noted earlier. In addition, the benzodiazepines suppress both REM sleep and SWS, while the benzodiazepine receptor agonists have little appreciable effect on REM or SWS. Chapter 6 thoroughly reviews the relevant classes of medications.

Antidepressants
SSRIs exhibit alerting effects during sleep and thus have the potential to be insomnogenic (138). They may also increase REM latency and decrease total time in REM sleep with little or no effect on SWS; and they may also induce bruxism and periodic limb movements in some patients (139). Trazodone is widely prescribed for its sedating qualities for patients with depression and insomnia, though this is based more on clinical and subjective report than empirical work (140). It may also decrease REM time (which is elevated in depressed patients) and increase SWS (138). Nefazadone has not been shown to diminish REM in depressed patients; $5HT_{2A}$ antagonists such as nefazadone appear to have sedating properties (141).

Other Psychiatric Medications
As alerting medications, stimulants can be expected to diminish sleep continuity, primarily by increasing sleep latency and the number of arousals and stage shifts. The antimania medication lithium increases REM latency, while decreasing total time in REM and increasing SWS, but is associated with worsening of restless leg syndrome (139). Atypical antipsychotic medications such as quetiapine have been found to improve sleep in bipolar patients (142) and generally have mixed effects on REM sleep and may augment SWS (143).

It is worth reiterating the statement that most psychotropics will have some effect on sleep and to further note that especially in treating elderly patients caution should be applied to any off-label use of medications despite trends to the contrary.

REFERENCES

1. Ancoli-Israel S, Kripke DF. Prevalent sleep problems in the aged. Biofeedback Self Regul 1991; 16(4):349–359.
2. Carskadon MA, Van Den Hoed J, Dement WC. Insomnia and sleep disturbances in the aged: sleep and daytime sleepiness in the elderly. J Geriatr Psychiatry 1980; 13:135–151.
3. Foley DJ, Monjan AA, Brown SL, et al. Sleep Complaints among elderly persons: an epidemiologic study of three communities. Sleep 1995; 18(6):425–432.
4. Lyness JM, Caine ED, King DA, et al. Depressive disorders and symptoms in older primary care patients: one-year outcomes. Am J Geriatr Psychiatry 2002; 10(3):275–282.
5. American Psychiatric Association. Diagnostic and Statistical Manual Of Mental Disorders, 4th edn., revised (DSM-IV-TR). Washington, DC: APA, 2000.
6. Hamilton M. Development of a rating scale for primary depressive illness. Br J Social Clin Psychol 1967; 6:278–296.
7. Manber R, Blasey C, Arnow B, et al. Assessing insomnia severity in depression: comparison of depression rating scales and sleep diaries. J Psychiatr Res 2005; 39(5):481–488.
8. Benca R. Mood disorders. In: Kryger M, Roth T, Dement W, eds. Principles and Practice of Sleep Disorders Medicine. Philadelphia, PA: W.B. Saunders Company, 2005:1311–1326.
9. Tsuno N, Besset A, Ritchie K. Sleep and depression. J Clin Psychiatry 2005; 66(10):1254–1269.
10. Ford DE, Kamerow DB. Epidemiologic study of sleep disturbances and psychiatric disorders. An opportunity for prevention? JAMA 1989; 262(11):1479–1484.
11. Ohayon MM, Caulet M, Lemoine P. Comorbidity of mental and insomnia disorders in the general population. Comp Psychiatry 1998; 39(4):185–197.
12. Stewart R, Besset A, Bebbington P, Brugha T, Lindesay J, Jenkins R Et Al. Insomnia Comorbidity And Impact And Hypnotic Use By Age Group In A National Survey Population Aged 16 To 74 Years. Sleep 2006; 29(11):1391–1397.
13. Roberts RE, Shema SJ, Kaplan GA, et al. Sleep complaints and depression in an aging cohort: a prospective perspective. Am J Psychiatry 2000; 157(1):81–88.
14. Hohagen F, Rink K, Kappler C, et al. Prevalence and treatment of insomnia in general practice: a longitudinal study. Eur Arch Psychiatry Clin Neurosci 1993; 242(6):329–336.
15. Simon GE, Vonkorff M. Prevalence, burden, and treatment of insomnia in primary care. Am J Psychiatry 1997; 154(10):1417–1423.
16. Mahendran R, Subramaniam M, Chan YM. Psychiatric morbidity of patients referred to an insomnia clinic. Singapore Med J 2007; 48(2):163–165.
17. American Sleep Disorders Association. The International Classification of Sleep Disorders: Diagnostic and Coding Manual – Revised. Rochester, MN: American Sleep Disorders Association, 1997.
18. Diagnostic and Statistical Manual of Mental Disorders, 4th edn. Washington, DC: American Psychiatric Association, 1994.
19. Edinger JD, Bonnet MH, Bootzin RR, et al. Derivation of research diagnostic criteria for insomnia: report of an American Academy of Sleep Medicine Work Group. Sleep 2004; 27(8):1567–1596.
20. Turek FW. Insomnia and depression: if it looks and walks like a duck. Sleep 2005; 28(11):1362–1363.
21. Pigeon WR, Perlis ML. Insomnia and depression: birds of a feather? Int J Sleep Disord 2007; 1(3):82–91.
22. Beck AT, Steer RA, Garbin MG. Psychometric properties of the Beck Depression Inventory – 25 years of evaluation. Clin Psychol Rev 1988; 8(1):77–100.
23. Perlis M, Smith LJ, Lyness JM, et al. Insomnia as a risk factor for onset of depression in the elderly. Behav Sleep Med 2006; 4(2):104–113.
24. Weissman MM, Greenwald S, Nino-Murcia G, Dement WC. The morbidity of insomnia uncomplicated by psychiatric disorders. Gen Hosp Psychiatry 1997; 19(4):245–250.

25. Dryman A, Eaton WW. Affective symptoms associated with the onset of major depression in the community: findings from the US National Institute of Mental Health Epidemiologic Catchment Area Program. Acta Psychiatr Scand 1991; 84(1):1–5.
26. Chang PP, Ford DE, Mead LA, et al. Insomnia in young men and subsequent depression. The Johns Hopkins Precursors Study. Am J Epidemiol 1997; 146(2):105–114.
27. Livingston G, Blizard B, Mann A. Does sleep disturbance predict depression in elderly people? A study in inner London. Br J Gen Pract 1993; 43(376):445–448.
28. Livingston G, Watkin V, Milne B, et al. Who becomes depressed? The Islington community study of older people. J Affect Disord 2000; 58(2):125–133.
29. Mallon L, Broman JE, Hetta J. Relationship between insomnia, depression, and mortality: a 12-year follow-up of older adults in the community. Int Psychogeriatr 2000; 12(3):295–306.
30. Brabbins CJ, Dewey ME, Copeland JR, et al. Insomnia in the elderly: prevalence, gender differences and relationships with morbidity and mortality. Int J Geriatr Psychiatry 1993; 8(6):473–480.
31. Cole MG, Dendukuri N. Risk factors for depression among elderly community subjects: a systematic review and meta-analysis. Am J Psychiatry 2003; 160(6):1147–1156.
32. Ohayon MM. The effects of breathing-related sleep disorders on mood disturbances in the general population. J Clin Psychiatry 2003; 64(10):1195–1200.
33. Schroder CM, O'hara R. Depression and obstructive sleep apnea (OSA). Ann Gen Psychiatry 2005; 4(13):1–8.
34. Mendlewicz J, Kerkhofs M. Sleep electroencephalography in depressive illness. a collaborative study by the World Health Organization. Br J Psychiatry 1991; 159:505–509.
35. Perlis ML, Buysse DJ, Thase ME, et al. Which depressive symptoms are related to which sleep EEG variables? Biol Psychiatry 1997; 42(10):904–913.
36. Buysse DJ, Jarrett DB, Miewald JM, et al. Minute-by-minute analysis of REM sleep timing in major depression. Biol Psychiatry 1990; 28(10):911–925.
37. Williams RL, Karacan I, Hursch CJ. Electoencephalography (EEG) of human sleep: clinical applications. New York: John Wiley and Sons, 1974.
38. Kupfer DJ, Frank E, Mceachran A, et al. Delta sleep ratio: a biological correlate of early recurrence in unipolar affective disorder. Arch Gen Psychiatry 1989; 47:1100–1105.
39. Giles DE, Roffwarg HP, Rush AJ, Guzick DS. Age-adjusted threshold values for reduced REM latency in unipolar depression using ROC analysis. Biol Psychiatry 1990; 27(8):841–853.
40. Borbely AA, Tobler I, Loepfe M, et al. All-night spectral analysis of the sleep EEG in untreated depressives and normal controls. Psychiatry Res 1984; 12:27–33.
41. Armitage R. Microarchitectural findings in sleep EEG in depression: diagnostic implications [see comments] [review]. Biol Psychiatry 1995; 37(2):72–84.
42. Kupfer DJ, Ulrich RF, Coble PA, et al. Application of automated REM and slow wave sleep analysis: II. Testing the assumptions of the two-process model of sleep regulation in normal and depressed subjects. Psychiatry Res 1984; 13(4):335–343.
43. Mendelson WB, Sack DA, James SP, et al. Frequency analysis of the sleep EEG in depression. Psychiatry Res 1987; 21(2):89–94.
44. Armitage R, Calhoun JS, Rush AJ, et al. Comparison of the delta EEG in the first and second non-REM periods in depressed adults and normal controls. Psychiatry Res 1992; 41(1):65–72.
45. Armitage R, Hoffmann R, Trivedi M, et al. Slow-wave activity in NREM sleep: sex and age effects in depressed outpatients and healthy controls. Psychiatry Res 2000; 95(3):201–213.
46. Landolt HP, Gillin JC. Similar sleep EEG topography in middle-aged depressed patients and healthy controls. Sleep 2005; 28(2):239–247.
47. Hamilton BE, Minino AM, Martin JA, et al. Annual summary of vital statistics: 2005. Pediatrics 2007; 119(2):345–360.
48. Horowitz MJ, Siegel B, Holen A, et al. Diagnostic criteria for complicated grief disorder. Am J Psychiatry 1997; 154(7):904–910.

49. Prigerson HG. When the path of adjustment leads to a dead-end. Bereavement Care 2004; 23:38–40.
50. Prigerson HG, Frank E, Kasl SV, et al. Complicated grief and bereavement-related depression as distinct disorders: preliminary empirical validation in elderly bereaved spouses. Am J Psychiatry 1995; 152(1):22–30.
51. Germain A, Caroff K, Buysse DJ, et al. Sleep quality in complicated grief. J Traum Stress 2005; 18(4):343–346.
52. Richardson SJ, Lund DA, Caserta MS, et al. Sleep patterns in older bereaved spouses. Omega – J Death Dying 2003; 47(4):361–383.
53. Valdimarsdottir U, Helgason AR, Furst CJ, et al. Long-term effects of widowhood after terminal cancer: a Swedish nationwide follow-up. Scand J Public Health 2003; 31(1):31–36.
54. Beem EE, Maes S, Cleiren M, et al. Psychological functioning of recently bereaved middle-aged women: the first 13 months. Psychol Rep 2000; 87(1):243–254.
55. Allaert FA, Urbinelli R. Sociodemographic profile of insomniac patients across national surveys. CNS Drugs 2004; 18:3–7.
56. Zhang BH, El Jawahri A, Prigerson HG. Update on bereavement research: evidence-based guidelines for the diagnosis and treatment of complicated bereavement. J Palliative Med 2006; 9(5):1188–1203.
57. Malkinson R. Cognitive-behavioral therapy of grief: a review and application. Res Social Work Pract 2001; 11(6):671–698.
58. Reynolds CF, Hoch CC, Buysse DJ, et al. Electroencephalographic sleep in spousal bereavement and bereavement-related depression of late life. Biol Psychiatry 1992; 31(1):69–82.
59. Hauri P, Chernik D, Hawkins D, et al. Sleep of depressed patients in remission. Arch Gen Psychiatry 1974; 31(3):386–391.
60. Karp JF, Buysse DJ, Houck PR, et al. Relationship of variability in residual symptoms with recurrence of major depressive disorder during maintenance treatment. Am J Psychiatry 2004; 161(10):1877–1884.
61. Opdyke KS, Reynolds CF III, Frank E, et al. Effect of continuation treatment on residual symptoms in late-life depression: how well is "well"? Depress Anxiety 1996; 4(6):312–319.
62. Nierenberg AA, Keefe BR, Leslie VC, et al. Residual symptoms in depressed patients who respond acutely to fluoxetine. J Clin Psychiatry 1999; 60(4):221–225.
63. Paykel ES, Ramana R, Cooper Z, et al. Residual symptoms after partial remission: an important outcome in depression. Psychol Med 1995; 25:1171–1180.
64. Buysse DJ, Reynolds CF, Monk TH, et al. The Pittsburgh Sleep Quality Index: a new instrument for psychiatric practice and research. Psychiatry Res 1989; 28(2):193–213.
65. Reynolds CF, Hoch CC, Buysse DJ, et al. Sleep in late-life recurrent depression. Changes during early continuation therapy with nortriptyline. Neuropsychopharmacology 1991; 5(2):85–96.
66. Simons AD, Murphy GE, Levine JL, et al. Cognitive therapy and pharmacotherapy for depression: sustained improvement over on year. Arch Gen Psychiatry 1986; 43:43–48.
67. Thase ME, Simons AD, Cahalane JF, et al. Cognitive behavior therapy of endogenous depression: I. An outpatient clinical replication series. Behav Ther 1991; 22(4):457–467.
68. Carney CE, Segal ZV, Edinger JD, et al. A comparison of rates of residual insomnia symptoms following pharmacotherapy or cognitive-behavioral therapy for major depressive disorder. J Clin Psychiatry 2007; 68(2):254–260.
69. Manber R, Rush J, Thase ME, et al. The effects of psychotherapy, nefazodone, and their combination on subjective assessment of disturbed sleep in chronic depression. Sleep 2003; 26(2):130–136.
70. Pigeon WR, Hegel MT, Unutzer J, et al. Is insomnia a perpetuating factor for late-life depression in the impact cohort? Sleep 2008; 31(4):481–488.
71. Fava GA, Fabbri S, Sonino N. Residual symptoms in depression: an emerging therapeutic target. Prog Neuropsychopharmacol Biol Psychiatry 2002; 26(6):1019–1027.

72. Fava GA. Long-term treatment with antidepressant drugs: the spectacular achievements of propaganda. Psychother Psychosomatics 2002; 71(3):127–132.
73. Fava M, Mccall WV, Krystal A, et al. Eszopiclone co-administered with fluoxetine in patients with insomnia coexisting with major depressive disorder. Biol Psychiatry 2006; 59(11):1052–1060.
74. Manber R, Edinger J, San Pedro M, et al. Combining escitalopram oxalate (ESCIT) and individual cognitive behavioral therapy for insomnia (CBTI) to improve depression outcome. Sleep 2007; 30(S):A232.
75. Morawetz D. Behavioral self-help treatment for insomnia: a controlled evaluation. Behav Ther 1989; 20:365–379.
76. Taylor DJ, Lichstein K, Weinstock J, et al. A pilot study of cognitive-behavioral therapy of insomnia in people with mild depression. Behav Ther 2007; 38:49–57.
77. Bastien CH, Vallieres A, Morin CM. Validation of the Insomnia Severity Index as an outcome measure for insomnia research. Sleep Med 2001; 2(4):297–307.
78. Morin CM. Insomnia, psychological assessment and management. New York, NY: Guilford Press, 1993.
79. Engleman HM, Cheshire KE, Deary IJ, et al. Daytime sleepiness, cognitive performance and mood after continuous positive airway pressure for the sleep apnoea/hypopnoea syndrome. Thorax 1993; 48(9):911–914.
80. Yu BH, Ancoli-Israel S, Dimsdale JE. Effect of CPAP treatment on mood states in patients with sleep apnea. J Psychiatr Res 1999; 33(5):427–432.
81. Cooke JR, Amador X, Lawton S, et al. Long-term CPAP may improve cognition, sleep, and mood in patients with Alzheimer's disease and SDB. Sleep 2006; 29:A103–A104.
82. Schwartz DJ, Kohler WC, Karatinos G. Symptoms of depression in individuals with obstructive sleep apnea may be amenable to treatment with continuous positive airway pressure. Chest 2005; 128(3):1304–1309.
83. Kawahara S, Akashiba T, Akahoshi T, et al. Nasal CPAP improves the quality of life and lessens the depressive symptoms in patients with obstructive sleep apnea syndrome. Intern Med 2005; 44(5):422–427.
84. Mellinger GD, Balter MB, Uhlenhuth EH. Insomnia and its treatment: prevalence and correlates. Arch Gen Psychiatry 1985; 42(3):225–232.
85. Taylor DJ, Lichstein KL, Durrence HH, et al. Epidemiology of insomnia, depression, and anxiety. Sleep 2005; 28(11):1457–1464.
86. Ohayon MM, Shapiro CM. Sleep disturbances and psychiatric disorders associated with posttraumatic stress disorder in the general population. Comp Psychiatry 2000; 41(6):469–478.
87. Neylan TC, Marmar CR, Metzler TJ, et al. Sleep disturbances in the Vietnam generation: findings from a nationally representative sample of male Vietnam veterans. Am J Psychiatry 1998; 155(7):929–933.
88. Mellman TA, Pigeon WR. Dreams and nightmares in posttraumatic stress disorder. In: Kryger M, Roth T, Dement WC, eds. Principles and Practice of Sleep Medicine. Philadelphia: Elsevier Saunders, 2005:573–578.
89. Zayfert C, Deviva JC. Residual insomnia following cognitive behavioral therapy for PTSD. J Traum Stress 2004; 17(1):69–73.
90. Nishith P, Resick PA, Mueser KT. Sleep difficulties and alcohol use motives in female rape victims with posttraumatic stress disorder. J Traum Stress 2001; 14(3):469–479.
91. Clum GA, Nishith P, Resick PA. Trauma-related sleep disturbance and self-reported physical health symptoms in treatment-seeking female rape victims. J Nervous Mental Dis 2001; 189(9):618–622.
92. Foa EB, Steketee G, Rothbaum BO. Behavioral/cognitive conceptualizations of posttraumatic stress disorder. Behav Ther 1989; 20:155–176.
93. Ross RJ, Ball WA, Sullivan KA, et al. Sleep disturbances as the hallmark of posttraumatic stress disorder. Am J Psychiatry 1989; 146(6):697–707.
94. Woodward SH, Bliwise DL, Friedman MJ, et al. Subjective versus objective sleep in Vietnam combat veterans hospitalized for PTSD. J Traum Stress 1996; 9(1):137–143.

95. Mellman TA, Kulick-Bell R, Ashlock LE, et al. Sleep events among veterans with combat-related posttraumatic stress disorder. Am J Psychiatry 1995; 152(1):110–115.
96. Mellman TA, Bustamante V, Fins AI, et al. REM sleep and the early development of posttraumatic stress disorder. Am J Psychiatry 2002; 159(10):1696–1701.
97. Lamarche LJ, De Koninck J. Sleep disturbance in adults with posttraumatic stress disorder: a review. J Clin Psychiatry 2007; 68(8):1257–1270.
98. Krakow B, Germain A, Tandberg D, et al. Sleep breathing and sleep movement disorders masquerading as insomnia in sexual-assault survivors. Comp Psychiatry 2000; 41(1):49–56.
99. Krakow B, Melendrez D, Pedersen B, et al. Complex insomnia: insomnia and sleep-disordered breathing in a consecutive series of crime victims with nightmares and PTSD. Biol Psychiatry 2001; 49(11):948–953.
100. Krakow B, Germain A, Warner TD, et al. The relationship of sleep quality and posttraumatic stress to potential sleep disorders in sexual assault survivors with nightmares, insomnia, and PTSD. J Traum Stress 2001; 14(4):647–665.
101. Saletu-Zyhlarz G, Saletu B, Anderer P, et al. Nonorganic insomnia in generalized anxiety disorder. 1. Controlled studies on sleep, awakening and daytime vigilance utilizing polysomnography and EEG mapping. Neuropsychobiology 1997; 36(3):117–129.
102. Saletu B, Anderer P, Brandstatter N, et al. Insomnia in generalized anxiety disorder: polysomnographic, psychometric and clinical investigations before, during, and after therapy with a long- versus a short-half-life benzodiazepine (quazepam versus triazolam). Neuropsychobiology 1994; 29:69–90.
103. Fuller KH, Waters WF, Binks PG, et al. Generalized anxiety and sleep architecture: a polysomnographic investigation. Sleep 1997; 20(5):370–376.
104. Mellman TA, Uhde TW. Sleep in panic and generalized anxiety disorders [references]. In: JCB, ed. Neurobiology of Panic Disorder. Frontiers of Clinical Neuroscience, Vol. 8. New York, NY, USA: Wiley-Liss, 1990:365–376.
105. Mellman TA, Uhde TW. Sleep panic attacks: new clinical findings and theoretical implications. Am J Psychiatry 1989; 146(9):1204–1207.
106. Mellman TA, Uhde TW. Electroencephalographic sleep in panic disorder. Arch Gen Psychiatry 1989; 46:178–184.
107. Effective Treatments for PTSD: Practice Guidelines from the International Society for Traumatic Stress Studies. Guildford Press, 2000.
108. Pigeon WR, Talbot NL, Perlis ML. The effect of interpersonal therapy for depression on insomnia symptoms in a cohort of women with sexual abuse histories. Sleep 2007; 30(S):A231.
109. Krakow B, Hollifield M, Johnston L, et al. Imagery rehearsal therapy for chronic nightmares in sexual assault survivors with posttraumatic stress disorder – a randomized controlled trial. JAMA – J Am Med Assoc 2001; 286(5):537–545.
110. Germain A, Nielsen TA. Polysomnographic changes in PTSD and idiopathic nightmare patients following imagery rehearsal treatment. Sleep 2002; 25(S):A249.
111. Forbes D, Phelps AJ, Mchugh AF, et al. Imagery rehearsal in the treatment of posttraumatic nightmares in Australian veterans with chronic combat-related PTSD: 12-month follow-up data. J Traum Stress 2003; 16(5):509–513.
112. Deviva JC, Zayfert C, Pigeon WR, et al. Treatment of residual insomnia after CBT for PTSD: case studies. J Traum Stress 2005; 18(2):155–159.
113. Krakow B, Johnston L, Melendrez D, et al. An open-label trial of evidence-based cognitive behavior therapy for nightmares and insomnia in crime victims with PTSD. Am J Psychiatry 2001; 158(12):2043–2047.
114. Germain A, Shear MK, Hall M, et al. Effects of a brief behavioral treatment for PTSD-related sleep disturbances: a pilot study. Behav Res Ther 2007; 45(3):627–632.
115. Krakow BJ, Melendrez DC, Johnston LG, et al. Sleep dynamic therapy for cerro grande fire evacuees with posttraumatic stress symptoms: a preliminary report. J Clin Psychiatry 2002; 63(8):673–684.
116. Zullino DF, Hattenschwiler J, Mattia M, et al. Pharmacotherapy of generalized anxiety disorder: state of the art. Schweiz Rundsch Med Prax 2003; 92(42):1775–1779.

117. Lydiard RB. An overview of generalized anxiety disorder: disease state-appropriate therapy. Clin Ther 2000; 22:A3–A19.
118. Casacalenda N, Boulenger JP. Pharmacologic treatments effective in both generalized anxiety disorder and major depressive disorder: clinical and theoretical implications. Can J Psychiatry – Revue Canadienne De Psychiatrie 1998; 43(7):722–730.
119. Belanger L, Morin CA, Langlois F, et al. Insomnia and generalized anxiety disorder: effects of cognitive behavior therapy for GAD on insomnia symptoms. J Anxiety Disord 2004; 18(4):561–571.
120. Crome IB. Alcohol problems in the older person. J R Soc Med 1997; 90:16–22.
121. Brower KJ, Aldrich MS, Robinson EAR, et al. Insomnia, self-medication, and relapse to alcoholism. Am J Psychiatry 2001; 158(3):399–404.
122. Irwin M, Miller C, Gillin JC, et al. Polysomnographic and spectral sleep EEG in primary alcoholics: an interaction between alcohol dependence and African-American ethnicity. Alcoholism – Clin Exp Res 2000; 24(9):1376–1384.
123. Clark CP, Gillin JC, Golshan S, et al. Polysomnography and depressive symptoms in primary alcoholics with and without a lifetime diagnosis of secondary depression and in patients with primary major depression. J Affect Disord 1999; 52(1–3):177–185.
124. Thompson PM, Gillin JC, Golshan S, et al. Polygraphic sleep measures differentiate alcoholics and stimulant abusers during short-term abstinence. Biol Psychiatry 1995; 38(12):831–836.
125. Valladares E, Irwin MR. Polysomnographic sleep dysregulation in cocaine dependence. Scientific World J 2007; 7(S2):213–216.
126. Pace-Schott EF, Stickgold R, Muzur A, et al. Sleep quality deteriorates over a simulated binge–abstinence cycle in chronic cocaine users: a combined nightcap and polysomnographic study. Sleep 2003; 26:A379–A380.
127. Schierenbeck T, Riemann D, Berger M, et al. Effect of illicit recreational drugs upon sleep: cocaine, ecstasy and marijuana. Sleep Med Rev 2008. (in press).
128. Brower KJ. Insomnia, alcoholism and relapse. Sleep Med Rev 2003; 7(6):523–539.
129. Arnedt JT, Conroy D, Rutt J, et al. An open trial of cognitive-behavioral treatment for insomnia comorbid with alcohol dependence. Sleep Med 2007; 8(2):176–180.
130. Greeff AP, Conradie WS. Use of progressive relaxation training for chronic alcoholics with insomnia. Psychol Rep 1998; 82(2):407–412.
131. Currie SR, Clark S, Hodgins DC, et al. Randomized controlled trial of brief cognitive-behavioural interventions for insomnia in recovering alcoholics. Addiction 2004; 99(9):1121–1132.
132. Pigeon WR, Perlis ML. Sleep homeostasis in primary insomnia. Sleep Med Rev 2006; 10(4):247–254.
133. Vogel GW. Evidence for REM sleep deprivation as the mechanism of action of antidepressant drugs. Prog Neuropsychopharmacol Biol Psychiatry 1983; 7(2–3):343–349.
134. Adrien J. Neurobiological bases for the relation between sleep and depression. Sleep Med Rev 2002; 6(5):341–351.
135. Adrien J. Reply to commentary. Sleep Med Rev 2002; 6(5):359.
136. Perlis M, Smith MT, Orff H. Invited commentary on: Joel Adrien's neurobiological bases for the relation between sleep and depression. Sleep Med Rev 2002; 6(5):353–357.
137. Giedke H, Schwarzler F. Therapeutic use of sleep deprivation in depression. Sleep Med Rev 2002; 6(5):361–377.
138. Sharpley AL, Cowen PJ. Effect of pharmacologic treatments on the sleep of depressed patients. Biol Psychiatry 1995; 37(2):85–98.
139. Walter T, Golish J. Psychotropic and neurologic medications. In: Lee-Chiong T, Sateia MJ, Carskadon MA, eds. Sleep Medicine. Philadelphia: Hanley & Belfus, Inc., 2002:587–599.
140. Montgomery I, Oswald I, Morgan K. Trazodone enhances sleep in subjective quality not in objective duration. Br J Clin Pharmacol 1983; 16:139–144.
141. Sharpley AL, Elliott JM, Attenburrow MJ, et al. Slow wave sleep in humans: role of 5-Ht2a and 5-Ht2c Receptors. Neuropharmacology 1994; 33(3–4):467–471.

142. Keating GM, Robinson DM. Quetiapine – a review of its use in the treatment of bipolar depression. Drugs 2007; 67(7):1077–1095.
143. Haffmans PMJ, Oolders HJ, Hoencamp E, et al. Sleep quality in schizophrenia and the effects of atypical antipsychotic medication. Acta Neuropsychiatr 2004; 16(6):281–289.
144. Weyerer S, Dilling H. Prevalence and treatment of insomnia in the community: results from the upper Bavarian field study. Sleep 1991; 14(5):392–398.
145. Bixler EO, Kales A, Soldatos CR, et al. Prevalence of sleep disorders in the Los Angeles metropolitan area. Am J Psychiatry 1979; 136:1257–1262.

4 Sleep and Neurologic Disorders in Older Adults

Alon Y. Avidan

Department of Neurology, David Geffen School of Medicine at UCLA, University of California, Los Angeles, California, U.S.A.

INTRODUCTION

Sleep disturbances are ubiquitous in geriatric patients with dementias and can cause hypersomnia, irritability, impaired motor and cognitive skills, psychiatric conditions such as depression, and fatigue (1). Sleep disturbances in patients with dementia may be related to both direct and indirect mechanisms (1,2). Direct mechanisms may be related to specific lesions in neuroanatomic regions involved in sleep physiology and neurochemistry. Structural alteration of the sleep–wake-generating neurons located in the suprachiasmatic nucleus (SCN) is one example of the direct mechanism, whereas insufficient light exposure or excessive noise at the patient's living quarter are examples of the indirect (external) mechanisms disturbing sleep. A summary of the predictable sleep-related changes in dementia is demonstrated in Figures 1 and 2.

SLEEP DISTURBANCES IN PATIENTS WITH NEURODEGENERATIVE DISEASES

Dementia may be defined as a syndrome that is characterized by progressive deterioration of neurocognitive function (3). Patients with dementia may also suffer from neuropsychiatric symptoms, such as apathy, agitation, and depression. The most important social consequence of progressive dementia is that with increasing loss of function, the patient is eventually robbed of his or her independence necessitating nursing home placement (3–5). Dementia affects about 6% of individuals over 65 years of age and has a strong age dependent prevalence (3). Alzheimer's disease (AD) is by far the most important and most common cause of dementia, accounting for approximately 70% of all cases of dementia (6), followed by dementia with Lewy bodies (DLB), which is the second most common irreversible cause of dementia, accounting for approximately 20% to 25% of cases.

Patients with dementia often present with a wide spectrum of sleep disturbances consisting of insomnia, hypersomnia, circadian rhythm disturbances, excessive motor activity at night [such as periodic leg movements and restless legs syndrome (RLS)], nocturnal agitation and wandering, and abnormal nocturnal behaviors such as rapid eye movement (REM) sleep behavior disorder commonly seen in synucleopathies (2).

Alzheimer's disease

In AD, degeneration of the neuroanatomic substrate of circadian physiology, the SCN, together with age-related macular degeneration, cataracts, decreased

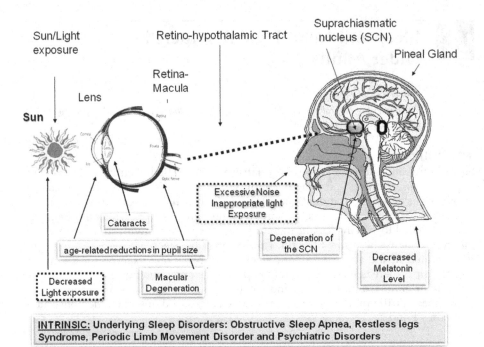

FIGURE 1 Pathophysiology of sleep disruption in patients with dementia: potential environmental and intrinsic factors (intrinsic factors are denoted by the broken line, whereas the slotted line denotes intrinsic or patient-related factors). *Source*: From Ref. 228.

melatonin levels, and environmental factors may be responsible for the circadian rhythm abnormalities (Fig. 1) (1,2). The severity of circadian rhythm disturbances correlates with the severity of dementia (7,8).

Degeneration of the cholinergic neurons in the nucleus basalis of Meynert, the pedunculopontine tegmental and laterodorsal tegmental nuclei, and noradrenergic neurons of the brainstem may induce reduction of REM sleep in AD (Fig. 2) (1,2). Degeneration of the brainstem respiratory neurons and the supramedullary respiratory pathways may place the patient at risk of sleep-disordered breathing (SDB) and other respiratory dysrhythmias in sleep in AD (Fig. 2) (1,2).

Indirect mechanisms may include medication-related side effects, underlying psychiatric diagnosis such as mood disorders, increasing incidence of periodic limb movements in older AD patients, and age-related alterations in sleep (Fig. 1). Other indirect mechanisms include general medical diseases affecting the cardiovascular and respiratory systems and environmental factors such as insufficient or dim light and environmental factors such as excessive noise and diminished light exposure in nursing homes or other long-term-care institutions (Fig. 1).

Sleep Architecture in Alzheimer's Disease

Sleep architectural changes in AD include reduction in sleep efficiency, increase in non-REM stage 1 sleep, increase in arousal and awakening frequency, decrease

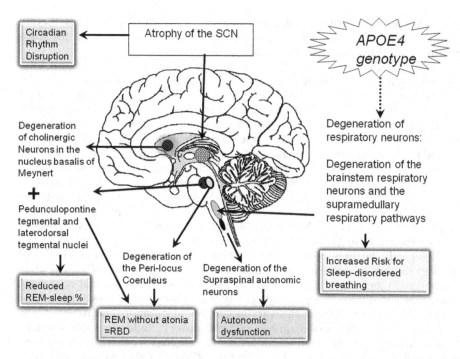

FIGURE 2 Pathophysiology of sleep disturbances in neurodegenerative disorders: direct mechanisms. *Abbreviations*: RBD, REM sleep behavior disorder; SCN, Suprachiasmatic nucleus, broken arrow demonstrates a hypothetical relationship. *Source*: From Ref. 228.

in total sleep time, and reduction in sleep spindles and K complexes. Predictable changes also consist of a profound disruption in sleep–wake rhythmicity primarily noted early in the onset of the disease. Sleep fragmentation subsequently leads to hypersomnia, insomnia, nocturnal wandering, increase in cognitive decline, increase in the number of daytime naps, increase in time in bed and time spent awake in bed, frequent nocturnal wandering, disorientation, and confusion (2,9–14).

As AD advances, patients typically experience more dramatic reduction of REM sleep, increased REM sleep latency, and a marked alteration of the circadian rhythm resulting in more significant daytime sleepiness (1). In fact, sleep and cognitive dysfunction are positively correlated in AD. Patients with AD are also susceptible to "sundowning," which is described as the nocturnal exacerbation of disruptive behavior or agitation in older people (15). It is frequently encountered in dementia and remains a common cause of institutionalization in patients with AD.

Circadian Rhythm Disturbances in Alzheimer's Disease

Circadian rhythm disturbances (CRD) are commonly seen in AD and older institutionalized patients (10,11,16). The symptoms of insomnia and hypersomnia can reflect a primary circadian dysrhythmias. In this clinical population setting, patients tend to sleep more during the day and be more active during the night. Significant caregiver distress stems from increased motor activity at night and the stress brought about due to this circadian misalignment.

Direct mechanisms thought to contribute to circadian rhythm abnormalities in patients with AD are thought to be related to degenerative changes at the level of SCN and due to decreased melatonin production in the pineal gland (Figs. 1 and 2) (17–20). Indirect mechanisms include comorbid medical conditions, psychiatric illness and are related to underlying medications prescribed for these patients that cause nocturnal confusion, or sundowning. Patients with AD are commonly affected by the irregular sleep–wake rhythm, which is characterized by the absence of discernable sleep–wake circadian rhythm. (This disorder is further described by Drs. Naylor and Zee in the chapter "Circadian Rhythm Sleep Disorders in Aging.") Sleep is fragmented into three or more periods during the 24-hour day, with the longest sleep period occurring between 2 and 6 AM. Patients may present with a complaint of insomnia and hypersomnia, depending on the timing of the sleep–wake episode. Although the total amount of sleep per day may be normal there should typically be three or more sleep episodes present at night. The lack of a clear circadian rhythm in sleep–wake is probably due to a disturbance of the circadian timing system and a reduced exposure to the most powerful external zeitgebers, light, as well as diminished physical activity that is often seen in institutionalized care (21–23). These sleep episodes vary in length and duration, and napping may be prevalent. The differential diagnosis of this disorder includes poor sleep hygiene and a voluntary irregular sleep schedule (24). The etiology for this disorder may be related to changes in the hypothalamus and the SCN (25). Other patients with associated neurologic disorders, and traumatic brain injury are also predisposed for this CRD (25,26).

Sleep-Disordered Breathing in Alzheimer's Disease

Sleep-related breathing disorders in the form of obstructive sleep apnea are very common in AD than when compared with controlled groups (27,28). One study demonstrated that the severity of AD is proportional to the severity of the underlying sleep apnea (29,30). Furthermore anecdotal reports of dementia-like symptoms associated with sleep apnea led to the speculation that there should be a causal relationship between SDB and AD (31). A significant number of patients with AD have an apnea index greater than 10 when compared with controls or patients with depression, and the predominant type of apnea is obstructive. In AD, however, sleep apnea occurs more frequently than in nondemented older subjects, and its severity is correlated with the degree of cognitive impairment.

In AD, sleep apnea could be a result of cell loss in the brainstem respiratory center. Conversely, neuronal degradation in AD could be accelerated by nightly insults of intermittent cerebral hypoxemia related to the underlying sleep apnea. One of the key genotypic markers for AD is the apolipoprotein E epsilon 4 (APOEε4) allele. A recent discovery that SDB is associated with the APOEε4 allele in the general population has sparked an interest in this topic, since obstructive sleep apnea is characterized by multiple genetic vulnerabilities (32,33). In individuals under age 65, the APOEε4 allele was associated with increased risk of OSA (34). However, other studies did not replicate the result in potentially owing to different genetic populations and different age cohorts (35,36). In another study examining 1775 participants aged 40 to 100 years and looking into the association between the APOEε4 and OSA, the prevalence of OSA was 19%. Even after adjustment for age, sex, and body mass index (BMI), the presence of any APOEε4 allele persisted to have an association with increased odds of OSA (37).

Treatment of Sleep Disturbances in Alzheimer's Disease

Current pharmacotherapy for cognitive loss in AD involves the use of cholinesterase inhibitors, which may increase REM sleep density, exacerbate insomnia, and induce vivid dreams (38). To date, there have been no randomized clinical trials of sedative-hypnotic medications specifically targeted at AD patients with sleep problems (38). SDB is related to agitation in AD, and treatment of the underlying SDB may improve agitation, lessen the burden of caregiving, and delay institutionalization (39). Neuropsychologic analyses have revealed that in patients with OSA, cognitive flexibility, attention, vigilance, and memory all improve with continuous positive airway pressure, CPAP therapy (40–44). Compliance with CPAP was also associated with greater improvements in attention, psychomotor speed, executive functioning, and nonverbal delayed recall (40).

Recent studies showed that melatonin, a neurohormone secreted by the pineal gland, may play a significant role in aging and AD as an antioxidant and neuroprotector. Melatonin levels diminish with aging, and patients with AD have a more profound reduction in this hormone (45). Data from clinical trials indicate that melatonin supplementation improves sleep and slows down the progression of cognitive impairment in AD (45). Melatonin protects neuronal cells via antioxidant and anti-amyloid-mediated activity properties, arrests the formation of amyloid fibrils, attenuates Alzheimer-like tau hyperphosphorylation, and protects cholinergic neurons (46,47). A misleading labeling of the hormone melatonin as a "food supplement" and the consistent lack of quality control over melatonin preparations on the market unfortunately continue to be a concern, and heath care providers should use caution when prescribing it to elderly patients with dementia, especially in the absence of large scale safety data (48).

Bright light therapy is being looked at as a possible treatment of circadian rhythm disturbances, as noted earlier, and of agitation in the nursing home setting (49). Given the decreased light exposure in the nursing home facilities and the potential impact on sleep disturbances, Ancoli-Israel et al. (52) examined the effect of light on sleep and circadian activity rhythms in patients with probable or possible AD. The results of their study showed that both morning and evening bright light resulted in more consolidated sleep at night, as measured with wrist actigraphy (50). It is therefore suggested that nursing homes increase ambient light in activity rooms, where patients the majority of their days (50).

Treatment for Circadian Rhythm Disturbances in Alzheimer's Disease

Treatments for circadian rhythm sleep disorders including the irregular sleep–wake type are aimed at consolidating the sleep–wake cycle with the potential use of melatonin and phototherapy. Melatonin, when given at bedtime, may improve sleep continuity and increase total sleep time in dementia. For institutionalized patients, increased daytime social interactions and light exposure have been shown to help consolidate and improve nighttime sleep (51,52). Other strategies aimed at consolidating sleep include scheduled physical activity and minimizing nighttime light and noise (53,54). Combination therapy of vitamin B12, bright light, chronotherapy, and hypnotics produced a 45% success rate in one cohort of patients suffering from

AD (55). Treatment with melatonin failed to improve sleep in one large multicenter study in Alzheimer's disease based on actigraphy-derived measurement of sleep time (56).

A recent multicenter, randomized, double-blind, placebo-controlled clinical trial funded by the National Institutes of Health at 31 AD centers in the United States demonstrated no beneficial effects of melatonin 2.5 or 10.0 mg on sleep disturbance in a well-characterized, large AD population ($n = 157$) (38,56). The data relied on actigraphically derived measures of sleep and are considered the definitive test of this hormone at this time. Light therapy or phototherapy has proven efficacy in the management of CRD in patients with dementia. However, the optimal timing and duration of phototherapy and illumination intensity have not yet been determined (57,58).

A practical approach to the management of irregular sleep–wake rhythms in AD is to begin with behavioral and environmental strategies. These include bright light exposure (Fig. 3) and structured social and physical activities and avoidance of naps during the day. During the sleep period, the environment should be conducive to sleep and consist of minimal noise, a darkened room, and a comfortable room temperature. The use of hypnotic or sedating psychoactive medications should be used with caution in elderly patients with dementia. Time exposure to bright light in the morning may be helpful in some patients. Evening bright light pulses may ameliorate sleep–wake cycle disturbances in some patients with AD (58). Ancoli-Israel et al. (52) reported that when light exposure is increased throughout the day and evening, it produced a beneficial effect on sleep and on circadian rhythms in patients with dementia. It would behoove nursing homes, therefore, to consider increasing ambient light in multipurpose rooms where patients often spend much of their days to help improve sleep quality (50). Another observation from the same group, evaluating the effect of bright light therapy on agitated behavior in a large sample of patients with severe AD, revealed that light was associated with improved caregivers' ratings but had little effect on observational ratings of agitation (59). It is believed that while the SCN of patients with severe AD is more likely to be degenerated and the circadian activity rhythms deteriorate as AD progresses, it is still possible that patients with more intact SCNs, that is, patients with mild to moderate AD, might benefit from light treatment even more than those with severe AD (59).

Sundowning Syndrome
Sundowning refers to agitation in dementia patients that has specific temporal exacerbation during the early evening or nocturnal hours (60,61). The "sundowning syndrome" describes a combination of nocturnal confusion, hyperactivity, delirium, disorganized thinking, wandering, restlessness, impaired attention, agitation, insomnia, hypersomnia, hallucinations, anger, delusions, anxiety, and illusions (14,61). Sundowning implies a predilection for the abnormal behavior to evolve or occur during the evening or night. Although caregivers and nursing home staff describe the escalation of symptoms toward the late afternoon or evening, there are actually little data to support that this indeed occurs (62). Sundowning may very likely have several different underling pathophysiologic mechanisms. It is suggested that rather than using the term sundowning, health care providers should use more descriptive terms when communicating among themselves and when approaching family members. Examples may include phrases such as the patient showed "agitation and physically aggressive behavior" or "wandering and

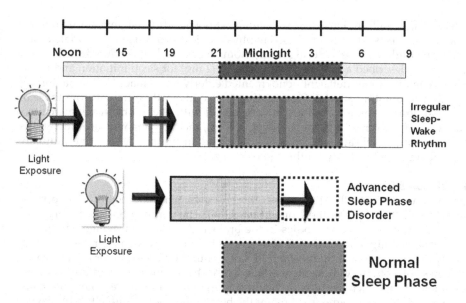

FIGURE 3 Light therapy for the treatment of the circadian rhythm disorders in dementia. Evening bright light pulse (→) may improve sleep–wake cycle disturbances in some patients with the Irregular sleep–wake rhythm. As light exposure is increased throughout the day, it produced a beneficial effect on sleep and on circadian rhythms in patients with dementia. The treatment for the Advanced Sleep Phase Disorder (ASPS), a circadian disorder characterized by evening sleepiness, early morning awakenings, and difficulties reinitiating sleep is early evening light exposure to 2500 lux in an attempt to delay sleep onset . In both conditions, a major limitation of bright light therapy in the older adult is the potential ineffectiveness from attenuated light transmission due to age-related reductions in pupil size and cataracts. *Source*: From Ref. 229.

pacing." When poorly controlled, sundowning may lead to eventual institutional-ization of the patient and thus it is critical to make an early diagnosis and prescribe appropriate management (5,63). Unfortunately, the use of the term sundowning is often used loosely and ambiguous describing nocturnal agitation without specifi-cally connoting a precise pathophysiology mechanism or diagnosis.

Specific therapy for sundowning is targeted at uncovering the underlying causes. Often, the clinical history and diagnostic testing do not provide a clear answer and therapy may take the approach of treating by trial and error approach. When specific pharmacologic therapy is contemplated, it is suggested "start low and go slow." The integration of psychosocial support, including education, and respite care can be very helpful. Several modalities have been suggested to ame-liorate various features of the sundowning syndrome. Data evaluating the use of antipsychotic agents and benzodiazepines have demonstrated improvements in sleep or nocturnal behavior but lacked real-time behavioral observations as relevant outcomes (60). Agents such as the antipsychotics often have adverse effects such as sedation, confusion, orthostatic hypotension, and parkinsonism, which are often clinically significant in elderly patients with dementia (60). The "high potency" antipsychotics are associated with an increased risk of producing extrapyramidal side effects, whereas the "low potency" agents have more sedating, anticholiner-gic, and orthostatic hypotensive properties (60). Clozapine is a unique antipsychotic agent in that it is specific to the dopamine D4 receptor and thus may improve the psychiatric manifestations of sundowning without causing significant extrapyramidal side effects. Melatonin, if used in physiologic doses and at appropriate times, can be helpful for those suffering from insomnia or circadian rhythm disorders(48). One study described a role for oral melatonin (2 mg) for sleep initiation and maintenance in melatonin-deficient nondemented elderly insomniacs (64). Behaviorally, the sleep-promoting effects of melatonin are also distinctly different from those of the traditional hypnotics and are not associated with alterations in sleep architecture (65). However, at high doses (over 0.3 mg), melatonin may cause side effects and disrupt the delicate mechanism of the circadian system, dissociating mutually dependent circadian body rhythms (48).

Parkinson's Disease

Parkinson's disease (PD), the most common movement disorder, affects approximately 500,000 people in the United States (66). The neuropathologic hallmark of PD is the finding of Lewy bodies in the brainstem nuclei and depigmentation of the substantia nigra. PD is a clinical diagnosis based on the signs of resting tremor, bradykinesia, cogwheel rigidity, and loss of postural reflexes (67). Bradykinesia, or slowness of voluntary movements, may cause disturbances in common yet simple motor tasks, such as dressing or turning in bed. Falls can become quite common as the disease progresses. Among the behavioral and cognitive troubles experienced in PD, depression and dementia affect approximately one-third of patients (68,69). Sleep disorders are encountered in a majority of patients with PD, adversely affecting their quality of life (70). Pathologic daytime sleepiness and fatigue are common in patients with PD and is most disabling features (71). As with patients with AD, sleep problems in PD patients also correlate with increased severity of disease.

The frequency of sleep complaints in patients with PD is estimated to be between 60% and 90%, and a variety of other mechanisms that are either disease related or secondary may come into play, including prescribed therapy for PD utilizing dopaminergic treatment. (72) Patients with PD may experience a number of sleep disorders, including insomnia, parasomnia, and daytime somnolence (including excessive daytime sleepiness and sleep attacks) (1). Excessive nocturia can disturbs sleep, particularly in the severe disease group, and may be related to the natural evolution of dysautonomia in PD (73) Typical sleep abnormalities include fragmented sleep with increased number of arousals and awakenings, and PD-specific motor phenomena such as nocturnal immobility, rest tremor, eye blinking, dyskinesias, and other phenomena such as periodic limb movements in sleep, RLS, fragmentary myoclonus, and respiratory dysfunction in sleep (72).

The underlying biologic basis of sleep disruption in PD is possibly related to the alteration of dopaminergic, noradrenergic, serotonergic, and cholinergic neurons in the brainstem (74). Typical polysomnographic features in PD include reduction of sleep efficiency, increased wake after sleep onset (WASO), increased sleep fragmentation, reduction of slow-wave sleep (SWS) and REM sleep, disruption of non-REM to REM cyclicity, loss of muscle atonia, and increased EMG activity, which is the basis for REM sleep behavior disorder RBD (75). Close to 90% of these patients often have sleep maintenance insomnia associated with frequent awakenings (2,76)

Patients with PD often have difficulties and the inability to ambulate or turn over during the night and get out of bed. This is most likely secondary to bradykinesia. Leg cramps and leg jerks are also very common as well as dystonic spasms of the limbs, face, and back. One community-based survey evaluating 245 patients with PD demonstrated that nearly two-thirds of patients reported sleep disorders, significantly more than among patients with diabetes (46%) and healthy control subjects (33%) (77). About a third of the patients with PD rated their overall night-time problem as moderate to severe (77). The most commonly reported sleep disorders included frequent awakening (sleep fragmentation) and early awakening (77). The study found a strong correlation between depression and sleep disorders in patients with PD, underlining the importance of identifying and treating both conditions in these patients (77).

Sleep maintenance problems and difficulties with sleep initiation are the earliest and most frequent sleep disorders observed in these patients (74). Sleep fragmentation and spontaneous daytime dozing occurred much more frequently in PD patients than in controls (78). Sleep fragmentation in PD may be due to an increased skeletal muscle activity, disturbed breathing, and REM-to-non-REM variations of the dopaminergic receptor sensitivity (74). In patients with PD who developed motor fluctuations (on-off phenomenon, wearing off) during the day, other common sleep-related motor complaints, including nocturnal akinesia, dystonia, and painful cramps, are observed (74). Chronic release formulation of levodopa/carbidopa (Sinemet CR) has been demonstrated to improve nocturnal akinesia and increase sleep efficiency of patients with PD with underlying sleep-related motor disturbances (74).

Motor abnormalities in PD during sleep include the parkinsonism tremor and REM onset blepherospasm, which disappears during REM sleep. Patients have rapid blinking at sleep onset and REM intrusion into non-REM sleep. REM-sleep behavior disorder is very common in patients PD (2,79) and may also precede the onset of PD (80). One-third of patients with PD are found to have periodic limb movement disorder (PLMD) of sleep based on a nocturnal polysomnogram. Patients with PD who have posture reflex abnormalities and autonomic impairment are at an increased risk for sleep-related breathing disorder in the form of central sleep apnea, obstructive sleep apnea, and alveolar hypoventilation syndrome (81). Parkinson's disease may lead to a restrictive pulmonary disease. Patients with PD are also found to have circadian rhythm abnormalities and depression (82). Circadian rhythm disturbances in PD, although probably less severe than in AD, may be related to mesocorticolimbic dopaminergic abnormalities and mesostriatal system abnormalities (74). Abnormalities of dopaminergic neurons in the ventral tegmentum area often lead to EEG desynchronization and abnormal sleep–wake schedule disorder (83).

Factors that are often responsible for sleep disruption in Parkinson's disease are probably due to tremors, dystonia, rigidity, dyskenesia, RBD, periodic leg movements of sleep, REM onset blinking, and increased awakening (70). These patients often have difficulty in changing position and the inability to initiate movement. Patients with PD who are already on medications may have additional sleep difficulties. Low-dose dopominergic agonists are often sedating. On the other hand, high-dose dopominergic agonists may lead to increased hallucinations, nightmares, and increased arousals. Levadopa is often associated with increased sleep latency but an increased sleep continuity (84,85). Attempts to explain the sleep–wake disruption in Parkinson's disease have been linked to reduction in serotonergic neurons of the dorsal raphe, noradrenergic neurons of the locus coeruleus, and cholinergic neurons of the pedunculopontine nucleus (74).

Treatment of sleep disorders in patients with PD deserves special consideration. Patients with PD who suffer from insomnia are often treated by improving sleep hygiene abnormalities. Pharmacologic treatment with small-dose dopaminergic preparation (i.e. levodopa/carbidopa 25/100) and small doses of sedating tricylic antidepressants (TCAs) may be tried. Problems with bradykinesia and nocturia are often improved by providing patients with a portable bedside commode. For patients with RLS symptoms, an evening and nocturnal dose of dopaminergic agonist such as carbidopa/levodopa or a dopamine (D3) agonist are useful(86,87). Patients with RBD are often treated with clonazepam (0.5 mg QHS) (88). Patients with OSA are often improved with CPAP. Patients who are diagnosed with OSA in addition to autonomic dysfunction can be treated effectively with CPAP. However, a definitive treatment (with tracheostomy) is indicated and is often mandatory due to the increased risk of fatal cardiac arrhythmias.

REM Sleep Behavior Disorder

RBD is characterized by pathologic augmentation of skeletal muscle tone during REM sleep (Fig. 4). Patients present with unusual, complex, and intense motor activity during a dream sequence. The range of motor activities can vary from a simple limb movement to very complex quasi-purposeful movements suggestive of dream content enactment (89). The potential for self- and bed partner injury is high, especially during severe episodes (90). Current speculations suggest that the pontine tegmentum is the locus of muscle tone inhibitor system, which normally causes muscle atonia during REM sleep (Fig. 4) (91). The peril-locus coeruleus of the rostral tegmentum of the pons produces activation of the medullary inhibitory zone via tegmentoreticular tract. RBD is characterized by a loss of atonia during REM sleep, which facilitates the motor behaviors during dreaming (92–94). Figure 5 summarizes the possible neuroanatomic explanation for RBD.

RBD is a common sleep disorder seen in PD (95,96). Recent findings from various studies suggest that (*i*) a high percentage of patients with PD without sleep complaints may have subclinical or clinical RBD, and (*ii*) RBD can be the heralding manifestation of parkinsonism by many years in older male patients (72,96–102). In addition to its high prevalence in patients with PD, RBD is a common sleep disturbance in other neurodegenerative disorders such as multiple system atrophy and dementia with Lewy bodies (102–104).

The majority of cases occur with advancing age; approximately 60% are idiopathic, while the remaining 40% may have an underlying neuropathology. RBD typically manifests itself in the sixth or seventh decade. This disorder has a particular predilection to occur in a number of synucleinopathies and other neurodegenerative disorders such as PD, DLB, olivopontocerebellar atrophy OPCA, Shy-Drager syndrome, and multiple system atrophy (90,105–110). Secondary causes or RBD include diseases that disrupt brainstem centers involved in REM-generated muscle atonia, such as multiple sclerosis, cerebral vascular accidents, and brainstem neoplasm. Twenty-five percent of patients may have a prodrome of subclinical behavioral release during sleep. The acute onset of RBD is related to drugs such as TCAs, monamine oxidase inhibitors (MAOIs), selective serotonin-reuptake inhibitors (SSRIs), and acute withdrawal of alcohol and barbiturates. Caffeine use has also been recently implicated in causing RBD (106,107,109).

In many cases, the diagnosis is suspected clinically by confirming the presence of recurrent dream-enacting behaviors with the help of the bed partner. The

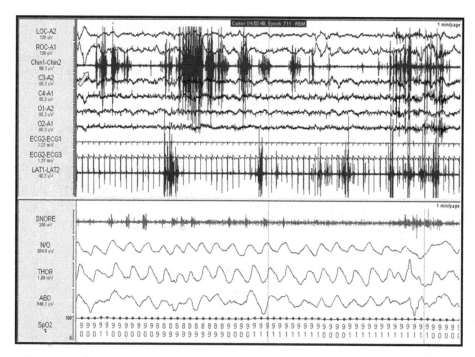

FIGURE 4 Polysomnographic Example of REM sleep behavior Disorder. A 60-second epoch from a diagnostic polysomnogram of an 80-year-old man with Parkinson's disease who was referred to the sleep disorders clinic for evaluation of recurrent violent nighttime awakenings. Illustrated in this figure is a typical spell that this patient was experiencing during the night. He was noted to yell, jump from bed, and have complex body movements. The figure shows abnormal augmentation REM-muscle atonia in the left anterior tibialis muscle and chin-EMG channel. The patient was diagnosed with REM sleep behavior disorder (RBD) and was treated successfully with 0.25 mg of Clonazepam. Channels are as follows: electro-oculogram (*left:* LOC-A2, *right:* ROC-A1), chin electromyogram (EMG), electroencephalogram (left central, right central, left occipital, right occipital), two ECG channels, limb EMG (LAT), snore channel, nasal-oral airflow, respiratory effort (thoracic, abdominal), and oxygen saturation (SaO$_2$).

diagnosis is confirmed by polysomnography (PSG) utilizing multiple-limb EMG leads with simultaneous continuous video monitoring demonstrating evidence of increased electromyographic bursts of chin EMG or limb electrodes during REM sleep. The sleep study may also capture the actual spells during which the abnormal spell is demonstrated (limb jerk, complex, vigorous, violent behaviors). If there is evidence of an abnormal neurologic examination, a full neurologic workup including a brain MRI may be also be needed (88,107).

The differential diagnosis of RBD includes sleepwalking, nocturnal seizures, posttraumatic stress disorder (PTSD), sleep terrors, nocturnal panic disorders, delirium, sleep-related gastroesophageal reflux, periodic limb movement disorder of sleep, psychogenic dissociative state, and confusional arousals with sleep apnea. Distinguishing RBD form nocturnal seizures may sometimes be difficult. However, unlike nocturnal seizures, the typical RBD spell is usually not stereotyped and is often variable (90,107,109,111). Additional laboratory studies may be needed

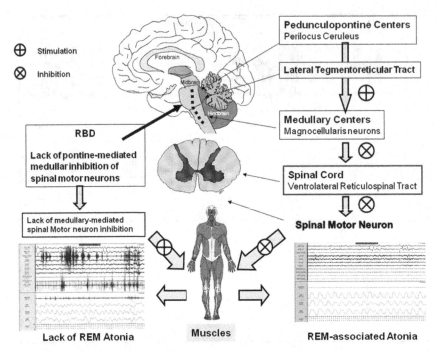

FIGURE 5 Pathophysiology of REM sleep behavior disorder. Muscle atonia during REM sleep results from pontine-mediated perilocus ceruleus inhibition of motor activity. This pontine activity exerts an excitatory influence on medullary centers (magnocellularis neurons) via the lateral tegmentoreticular tract (   ). These neuronal groups, in turn, hyperpolarize the spinal motor neuron postsynaptic membranes via the ventrolateral reticulospinal tract. In REM sleep Behavior Disorder (RBD), the brainstem mechanisms generating muscle become disrupted. The pathophysiology of RBD in humans is based on the cat model. In the cat model, bilateral pontine lesions result in a persistent absence of REM atonia associated with prominent motor activity during REM sleep, similar to that observed in RBD in humans. The pathophysiology of the idiopathic form of RBD in humans is still not very well understood but may be related to reduction of striatal presynaptic dopamine transporters. *Source*: From Ref. 229.

especially if the clinical history remains vague or ambiguous. When the possibility of nocturnal seizures cannot be reliably excluded, additional sleep testing may be warranted.

Environmental safety is crucial in every patient with likely RBD. This may include protecting and sleeping environment by removing sharp objects and padding the bed area. Suggested pharmacotherapy for RBD may be in the form of clonazepam (0.25 mg to 1 mg p.o. QHS), which is effective in 90% of cases (107). There is little evidence of tolerance or abuse with this form of treatment. Caution should be exercised when using it in patients with chronic respiratory diseases or impaired renal function, and it is contraindicated in patients with documented hypersensitivity, severe liver disease, or acute narrow-angle glaucoma. Abrupt discontinuation of clonazepam can precipitate withdrawal symptoms (107). Other agents that can be helpful include imipramine (25 mg p.o. QHS), carbamazepine (100 mg p.o. TID), and levodopa, in cases where RBD is associated with PD. Recent studies have also demonstrated improvement with the use of melatonin, which is believed to exert its therapeutic effect by restoring REM sleep atonia. One study reported that melatonin was effective in 87% of patients taking 3 to 9 mg at bedtime (112), whereas a later study reported resolution in those taking 6 to 12 mg of melatonin at bedtime (113). As stated earlier in this chapter, the reader is reminded that melatonin, a food supplement, is not approved by the Food and Drug Administration and has poor regulation in terms of pharmacologic preparation. Its use, especially in elderly patients, should be done with great care as its safety profile has not been widely studied. Tacrine, Donepezil, and Serzone, drugs used in AD and other dementing disorders may exacerbate RBD. Some antidepressant may potentially increase total REM sleep, which may worsen RBD.

Diffuse Lewy Body Dementia

Diffuse Lewy body disease (DLBD) is a neurodegenerative disorder characterized by parkinsonism, dementia, fluctuations in mental status, and hallucinations. REM sleep behavior disorder is now recognized as a feature of DLBD (114–116). Awareness of the presence of this symptom in patients with DLBD is important and treatment with low-dose clonazepam or levodopa may help (117). Nightmares without atonia may be an early symptom, and very often the initial manifestation, of DLBD (115,118).

Multiple-System Atrophy

Multiple-system atrophy (MSA) is characterized clinically by any combination of autonomic, extrapyramidal, or cerebellar signs and symptoms. Patients with MSA experience degeneration of the pontine tegmentum, nucleus tractus solitarius, nucleus ambiguous, hypoglossal nucleus, reticular formation of the brainstem, and at times the cervical and thoracic spinal cord. Therefore, the diffuse neurodegenerative process that encompasses these key structures involved in the regulation of the sleep–wake transition and respiratory function in MSA may account for the most frequent sleep disturbances in MSA, SDB, and RBD (119,120).

Patients with MSA are commonly affected with RBD, which represents the most common clinical sleep manifestation and polysomnographic findings in patients with MSA. In a large study involving MSA patients, RBD was diagnosed by PSG monitoring in 90%, dream-enacting behaviors were reported in 69%, and RBD preceded the clinical presentation of MSA in 44% patients (103). RBD can frequently herald the appearance of other MSA symptoms by years; therefore, expanded polysomnographic montage consisting of multiple limbs and video monitoring is recommended in patients MSA when these spells are suspected (88,108). Increasing evidence points to the role of basal ganglia dysfunction in the underlying pathophysiology of RBD in MSA; in fact, a recent study from our center has revealed that decreased nigrostriatal dopaminergic projections may contribute to RBD in MSA (121).

Patients with MSA frequently manifest a variety of sleep-related respiratory disturbances, some of which are life threatening. Above all, a common and serious complication is upper-airway OSA associated with stridor, which is caused by vocal cord abductor paralysis (VCAP) and may lead to sudden death during sleep (122). For this reason, nocturnal stridor in MSA has been considered a poor prognostic feature (123). For the early diagnosis of VCAP, it is critical to perform laryngoscopy during sleep, because VCAP does not appear during wakefulness in the early stage of MSA (124). PSG study should be obtained to assess the severity of respiratory disturbances, and tracheostomy is the most reliable treatment for respiratory disturbances due to VCAP, while CPAP may be a useful treatment for some patients. Absolute compliance is mandatory. Tracheostomy is probably the only effective measure for emergency treatment of severe respiratory dysfunction and hypoxia in patients with marked laryngeal stridor, as can be seen in laryngeal abductor paralysis in patients with MSA (123,124).

Olivopontocerebellar Degeneration

Patients with olivopontocerebellar degeneration (OPCD) present with parkinsonism, atrophy of the pontine nuclei and cerebellar cortex, and degeneration of the olivopontocerebellar region. The sleep problems encountered in this condition include central, obstructive, and mixed sleep apnea probably caused by bulbar muscle weakness (1). Patients may also have nocturnal stridor as well as RBD (125,126). Patients, unaware of their nocturnal sleep disturbance, complained only of the resulting daytime tiredness and sleepiness (126). Patients may also have nocturnal stridor as well as RBD. Nocturnal polyuria has also been reported in OPCA, possibly related to a disturbance in the circadian rhythm for arginine vasopressin secretion due to degeneration of SCN and marked increase in the secretion of atrial natriuretic peptide due to abnormal diurnal variation in blood pressure (127).

Shy-Drager Syndrome

Progressive autonomic failure and progressive somatic neurologic manifestations characterize patients with Shy-Drager syndrome (SDS). Neuropathologic findings include striatonigral degeneration, OPCA, and autonomic neuronal degeneration (2). The neuropathologic hallmark of this disease includes argyrophilic oligodendroglionic cytoplasmic inclusions in the cortical motor, premotor, and supplementary motor association regions; extrapyramidal, corticocerebellar, brainstem; and reticular formation, and the supraspinal autonomic system.

Patients with SDS most commonly present with sleep-related respiratory dysregulation with frequent arousals and hypoxemia (128). Apneas encountered in this syndrome include obstructive, mixed, and central apneas. Cheyne-Stokes respiratory dysfunction, apneustic breathing, and inspiratory gasping are commonly seen. The hypersomnia seen in these patients is probably secondary to the dramatic sleep disruption. Patients may be at risk of dying from sudden cardiac death related to the underlying sleep-related breathing disorder. RBD and insomnia are also common in this disease.

The mechanism of sleep disruption in this condition is probably due to pathology in the brainstem structures regulating sleep–wake transition. Patients with SDS are at increased risk for developing brainstem ischemia secondary to nocturnal hypotensive episodes, which may subsequently potentiate the tendency to develop RBD (129). Sleep studies in patients with SDS demonstrate reduced SWS, reduced REM sleep, reduced total sleep time, increased sleep latency, increase in the frequency of awakenings, absence of atonia in REM sleep, and an increase respiratory dysrhythmias (1,130).

Progressive Supranuclear Palsy

Patients with progressive supranuclear palsy (PSP) often present with dementia, axial rigidity, dystonia, gait disturbances, and supranuclear eye movement abnormalities leading to impairment of vertical eye gaze. Other features include pseudobulbar paresis, axial rigidity, gait disturbances, and subcortical dementia. Neuropathologic hallmarks of progressive supranuclear palsy (PSP) include neuronal loss and gliosis in brainstem nuclei and the locus coeruleus. Sleep disturbance is universal in PSP (1,131). Insomnia is probably the most severe sleep problem noted by decreased total sleep time and significant sleep disruption without a specific clinical complaint (1). Insomnia in PSP is worse than insomnia in PD or AD. This is probably secondary to the apathy of patients inflicted with this disease. Other sleep disturbances may be related to the well-documented immobility in bed and difficulty with transfers, depression, dysphagia, and frequent nocturia seen in PSP. RBD and SDB are not common features in PSP (1,131).

The polysomnographic features of PSP are unique. When one evaluates the eye leads of the recording, it is interesting to note the absence of vertical eye movement during REM sleep. Horizontal eye movements are present but are slower and reduced in amplitude. During REM sleep, PSG may show increased phasic twitching and increased fast activity with by alpha intrusion. The minority of patients with PSP may have periodic leg movements of sleep and obstructive sleep apnea. Sleep architecture profile consist of increased sleep latency, increased arousal and awakening frequency, decreased stage 2 non-REM, reduced REM sleep, and reduced REM latency (1,130)

Epilepsy

Consideration of epilepsy and epileptic-like spells in the elderly is important. These are a frequent problem in elderly patients referred to epilepsy centers. In a recent study from the Cleveland Clinic Foundation, looking at the frequency of nonepileptic seizures in elderly patients referred for epilepsy monitoring, 43% were found to have a diagnosis other than epilepsy, which included transient ischemic attacks, syncope, movement disorders, and sleep disorders (132). Although most of the patients did not have any evidence of epilepsy, more than two-thirds of these patients had been placed on anticonvulsive drugs (132). Sleep and epilepsy have a reciprocal relationship. Sleep can affect the frequency and distribution of epileptiform discharges, while epileptic discharges can change sleep regulation and induce sleep disruption. Patients with epilepsy complain of symptoms such as hypersomnia, insomnia, and even greater breakthrough seizures attributed to sleep disruptions. Sleep disturbances in epilepsy patients probably indicate the presence of an underlying sleep disorder rather than the effect of epilepsy or medication on sleep. Physicians must be able to identify and differentiate between potential underlying sleep disorders and sleep dysfunction related to epilepsy and direct therapy to improve the patient's symptoms (133).

Sleep deprivation was noted to increase interictal discharges in patients with generalized epilepsy (134). The sleep state can promote interictal activity in as many as a third of patients with epilepsy and up to 90% of patients with sleep state dependent epilepsy (133,135). Up to one-third of patients with medically refractory epilepsy had evidence of OSA, and treatment of the underlying sleep apnea with CPAP can improve seizure frequency (136–138).

Nocturnal seizures and certain types of parasomnias can have similar clinical semiologies and can become a diagnostic dilemma. Common sleep disorders and manifestations such as cataplexy, sleep attacks in the setting of narcolepsy, night terrors, and RBD may be confused with epilepsy (139). Some epilepsy syndromes such as benign rolandic and nocturnal frontal lobe epilepsies occur predominantly or exclusively during sleep.

Antiepileptic drugs (AEDs) also affect sleep architecture (140). Phenytoin increases the amount of non-REM sleep, decreases sleep efficiency, and reduces sleep latency (141). Carbamazepine increases the number of sleep-stage shifts and decreases REM sleep (142). Benzodiazepines decrease sleep latency and reduce SWS (140,143). Gabapentin has been shown to improve sleep efficiency, improve SWS, and increase REM sleep (144,145). In clinical practice, understanding the unique effects of these AEDs may offer the clinician an opportunity to improve sleep and wakefulness; medications that improve sleep disorders may require tailored dosing schedules to maximize their benefit (133).

Multiple Sclerosis
Multiple Sclerosis (MS) is the most common nontraumatic cause of neurologic disability in young adults (146). With improved therapy, many patients survive to older age. Sleep disturbance in multiple sclerosis are common but poorly recognized, and almost half of all patients demonstrate sleep disturbances due to leg spasms, pain, immobility, nocturia, or medication (147). Common sleep disorders in patients with MS include insomnia, RLS, narcolepsy, and RBD. Sleep disruption in MS may result in hypersomnolence, increased fatigue, and a lowered pain threshold. An increased clinical awareness of sleep-related problems is therefore warranted in this patient population because they are extremely common and have the potential to negatively impact overall health and quality of life (148).

Chronic Pain and Fibromyalgia
Pain is a common and major problem among nursing home residents. The prevalence of pain in elderly nursing home patients is 40% to 80%, showing that they are at great risk of experiencing pain (149). Sleep and pain, two important vital functions, interact in complex ways that ultimately impact the biologic and behavioral capacity of the individual (150). Sleep studies of patients experiencing acute pain during postoperative recovery demonstrate shortened and fragmented sleep with reduced amounts of SWS and REM sleep, and the recovery is accompanied by normalization of sleep (150). Chronic pain conditions such as arthritis frequently coexist with insomnia. Chronic pain produces a vicious cycle of inactivity and fatigue during the day and sleeplessness at night. Patients with chronic pain disorders, including fibromyalgia report significant more sleepiness, more fatigue, and less refreshing sleep (151,152). Thus, patients with chronic pain are a population at a high risk for sleep disturbances. Adequate management of chronic pain requires treatment of the pain itself and the associated comorbid mood disorders.

Sleep and Stroke
Stroke is the most common neurologic disease and the leading cause of adult disability in Western countries (153). The number of patients affected by stroke will increase by the effect of aging (153). Sleep and stoke interact in a number of fascinating and complex ways. Probably the most important of these interactions is the fact that patients with sleep apnea or nocturnal hypoxemia often present with cardiac arrhythmias, intellectual decline, and increased risk of stroke. Habitual snoring affects 4% to 24% of the adult population with a maximum prevalence around the age of 50 to 60 and is strongly associated with OSA (154). Habitual snoring may

have adverse effects on long-term stroke outcome. Snoring was found to adversely affects prognosis in stroke survivors (155). Hypersomnolence and prolonged sleep, which can be symptoms of SDB, may also represent independent risk factors for stroke (156,157). SDB breathing is common among stroke patients as defined by an apnea–hypopnea index (AHI) ≥10/hour (158–160).

Treatment of SDB has been recently shown to improve subjective well-being and mood in stroke patients with SDB (161,162). Based on blood pressure lowering effects of CPAP, treatment of SDB may lead to a stroke risk reduction of about 20% (163).Currently it remains to be establishes if SDB represents an independent risk factor for stroke. The relationship may be a genetically determined one due to the increased vascular risk associated with SDB.

Central sleep apnea (CSA) and sometimes Cheyne-Stokes breathing may be a latent phenomena after the stroke and may predominate in as many as 30% to 40% of patients (164,165). Subsequent to the stroke, patients may present with the coexistence of both OSA during REM sleep and Cheyne-Stokes breathing during light NREM sleep (164,166,167). Central hypoventilation syndrome and failure of automatic breathing (Ondine's curse) are more typically associated with brainstem strokes and are less common presentations (167).

Bilateral lacunar ischemic infarcts in the tegmentum of the pons, periventricular white matter damage can present as REM sleep without atonia, which leads to RBD (168,169). Patients with Binswanger's disease or subcortical leukoencephalopathy are at an increased risk for developing RBD primarily because white matter ischemia in the vicinity of the supratentorial system is often involved in modulating REM-related atonia. Brain MRI studies in patients with RBD with underlying strokes show ischemic lesions in the pontine tegmentum, which is the locus of muscle tone inhibitor system. Stroke can impair the regulation of sleep–wake and breathing control mechanisms. Secondary consequences from the stroke such as immobilization, pain, hypoxia, and depression can also impact sleep.

Amyotrophic Lateral Sclerosis

Amyotrophic lateral sclerosis (ALS) is a neurodegenerative disease of middle-aged and elderly patients. The incidence of the disease increases with age, with a peak occurrence between 55 and 75 years of age. Pathology shows degeneration of the lateral corticospinal tracts, loss of motor neurons and astrogliosis in the brain and brainstem, and neuronal inclusions. This produces both upper and lower motor neuron deficits (170). ALS has a relentless progression with no impairment of the mental function, or sensorium. Respiratory failure in this disorder occurs late in the course of the disease and may also be the presenting feature of this disease. It is not uncommon for physicians to encounter patients with breathing difficulties, bulbar weakness, and stridor in the emergency room, only to later diagnose ALS. The major sleep complaint of these patients includes excessive daytime sleepiness likely caused by sleep-related respiratory disturbances and insomnia (171–174).

The mechanism of respiratory disturbance in this disorder may be due to the weakness of the upper airways caused by bulbar weakness, diaphragmatic weakness (due to a phrenic nerve lesion), and intercostal muscle weakness (due to the degeneration of intercostal nerve nuclei). Degeneration of the central respiratory neurons accounts for both central and obstructive sleep apnea. Polysomnographic findings include apneas in the form of central, obstructive, and mixed apneas, increased awakenings, sleep fragmentation, and reduced nocturnal oxygen saturation (171,172,175–177)

Noninvasive positive pressure upper airway ventilation provides a long-lasting benefit on symptoms and quality of life indicators for ALS patients and should be offered to all patients with symptoms of SDB or inspiratory muscle dysfunction (178). Positive pressure therapy can also prolong tracheostomy-free survival (179).

Spinal Cord Diseases

Patients with spinal cord injury (SCI) often present with sleep disturbances related to respiratory dysfunction, particularly when the lesion occurs in the upper cervical spinal cord within the vicinity of the phrenic nerve nuclei (180). Patients with SCI have a greater difficulty in falling asleep, describe more frequent awakenings, are more likely to be prescribed sleeping pills, sleep more hours, take more frequent and longer naps, and are more likely to snore than controls (181). In particular, spasms, pain, paraesthesia, and voiding difficulties have a higher association with sleep problems (181).

The incidence of SDB in SCI is high in patients with tetraplegia, especially when the patient is elderly, has an increased large neck circumference, has a long duration of the disease, and is on cardiac medications (182). The increased use of cardiac medication in tetraplegics with SDB may implicate a link between SDB and cardiovascular morbidity, one of the leading causes of death in tetraplegia. Obstructive sleep apnea appears to be more common in older patients with SCI than in the general population and is related to ventilatory dysfunction secondary to spinal cord (183).

Neurologic conditions likely to damage and disrupt the phrenic and intercostal motor neurons in the spinal cord include poliomyelitis, ALS, spinal cord tumors, spinal trauma, spinal surgery (e.g., cervical cordotomy or anterior spinal surgery), and nonspecific or demyelinating myelitis (180). Patients with syringobulbia present with severe abnormalities in respiratory rhythm generation during sleep (184). The respiratory disturbances are not due to muscle weakness and are not correlated with the size of the cavity (184). Phrenic nerve damage may cause diaphragmatic paralysis, and while unilateral paralysis is asymptomatic, bilateral paralysis presents with orthopnea manifesting as difficulty on inspiration out of proportion to the cardiopulmonary status and may be life threatening (180).

Postpolio Syndrome

Postpolio syndrome (PPS) describes the late manifestations that occur in patients three to four decades after the occurrence of acute poliomyelitis (185). PPS is more common at the present time due to the large epidemics of poliomyelitis in the 1940s and 1950s. Neurologic manifestations of PPS consist of neurologic, musculoskeletal, and systemic symptoms and signs. The most prominent neurologic manifestation is a new progressive weakness, at times accompanied by atrophy referred to as postpolio progressive muscular atrophy (PPMA) when affecting the extremities. However, a new weakness can also affect respiratory and bulbar muscles, and it can be more serious, causing dysphagia, dysphonia, and respiratory failure (186,187). Respiratory failure in PPS may be treated with CPAP, Bi-level Positive Airway Pressure BiPAP, or tracheotomy and permanent ventilation, if necessary (188). Other sleep disturbances include random myoclonus, periodic movements in sleep with muscle contractions, ballistic movements of the legs, and RLS (189). Poliovirus-induced damage to the spinal cord and brain may be implicated as a possible cause of these abnormal movements in sleep (189). It is suggested that PSG be performed on PPS patients with excessive daytime sleepiness and respiratory complaints (190).

Huntington's Disease

Huntington's disease (HD) is a hereditary progressive, neurodegenerative condition characterized by significant motor dysfunction (typically appearing as involuntary and spasmodic movements), cognitive impairment, and psychiatric difficulties. It is caused by an expanded CAG nucleotide repeats in the gene-encoding huntingtin, a protein of unknown function. Sleep disturbances are common in HD and consist of disturbed sleep pattern with increased sleep onset latency, reduced sleep efficiency, increased arousals and sleep fragmentation, decreased SWS, frequent nocturnal awakenings, increased density of sleep spindles, increased time spent awake, and reduced sleep efficiency (191–193). Patients who have HD have also shown higher-density sleep spindles, in contrast with findings in other neurodegenerative dementia populations (192). These abnormalities correlated in part with duration of illness, severity of clinical symptoms, and degree of atrophy of the caudate nucleus (193).

On the basis of actigraphy data, patients with HD demonstrate significant activity and spent more time making high-acceleration movements compared with age-matched controls (194). No increase in sleep-related breathing disorders has been demonstrated in HD, also in contrast with findings in other neurodegenerative dementias (195). Circadian rhythm sleep disturbances, however, are an important pathologic feature of HD and may arise from a disruption of the expression of the circadian clock genes *mPer2* and *mBmal1* in the SCN, the principal circadian pacemaker in the brain (196).

Myotonic Dystrophy

Myotonic dystrophy or dystrophia myotonica (DM) is a multisystem disorder with myotonia, muscle weakness, cataracts, endocrine dysfunction, and intellectual impairment. This disorder is caused by a CTG triplet expansion of the DMPK gene on 19q13. Sleep abnormalities in patients with DM include hypersomnia, sharing with narcolepsy a short sleep latency and the presence of sleep-onset REM periods during the multiple sleep latency test (MSLT) (197). Hypersomnia is found in almost a third of patients with DM, and the severity of daytime sleepiness correlates with the severity of muscular impairment (198). Corpus callosum atrophy might occur in DM patients, and the size of the CC anterior area might be associated with the hypersomnia (199). Patients with DM patients report a longer sleep period, a less restorative sleep, difficulties with sleep initiation, and hypersomnia comparable with those found in idiopathic hypersomnia (198). In DM, hypersomnia may be aggravated by alveolar hypoventilation and SDB, but is not entirely reversed by satisfactory application of positive pressure airway ventilation, suggesting that hypersomnia is partially related to an intrinsic hypersomnia caused by central nervous system alteration (178).

A dysfunction of the hypothalamic hypocretin system has recently been found in patients with DM and may mediate the underlying hypersomnia (197). Modafinil, a wake-promoting agent, was recently found to reduce hypersomnolence and improve mood, quality-of-life measures of energy, and health change in patients with DM (200,201).

Patients with DM are found have increased risk of OSA, central sleep apnea, and excessive daytime sleepiness (178,202,203). These patients are also thought to have a centrally mediated impaired in breathing, probably related to brainstem respiratory center disorder rather than respiratory muscle weakness (204,205). Nonobstructive sleep apneas and alveolar hypoventilation may be related to an underlying central neurologic pathology in DM, and muscle weakness and myotonia may underlie the development of obstructive SDB (178).

Neuropathologic findings in patients with DM consist of severe neuronal loss and gliosis in the midbrain and pontine raphe, particularly in dorsal raphe nucleus and superior central nucleus, pontine and medullary reticular formation (206). Alveolar hypoventilation and hypersomnia in DM may be attributed to these morphologic abnormalities and would appear to be central in nature (206).

Narcolepsy

Narcolepsy is a syndrome of excessive daytime sleepiness, cataplexy, sleep paralysis, and hypnagogic hallucinations. The onset of narcolepsy is most common during the second decade of life; the onset of narcolepsy after age 50 is extremely rare. Early onset of REM sleep in the older person may be due to circadian rhythm abnormalities, medication-induced REM sleep suppression, sleep-related breathing disorder, and subsequent REM sleep disruption (207). In the elderly one may see a rare occasion of excessive daytime sleepiness or cataplexy that was previously undiagnosed. The polysomnographic characteristics of narcolepsy include a mean sleep latency less than five minutes and the presence of two or more sleep onset REM periods (208). However, recent data performed in well-defined narcolepsy–cataplexy patients suggest a progressive decrease in the number of sleep onset REM periods (SOREMP) and increase in the mean sleep latency on the MSLT as a function of age, indicating that the current criteria used for diagnosis may be too stringent in older patients (209). These results may reflect the progressive increase in sleep latency seen in normal aging and suggest that clinical improvement might be due to changes in the neural mechanisms responsible for SOREMP, which may weaken with age probably due to genetic factors, including the catechol-O-methyltransferase gene (209).

Fatal Familial Insomnia

Fatal Familial Insomnia (FFI) is a very rare autosomal dominant prion disease, which is clinically characterized by inattention, severe progressive insomnia, autonomic dysregulation such as orthostatic stability, increased salivation, increased body temperature, and daytime stupor alternating with wakefulness (210). Patients with FFI go on to develop preferential thalamic degeneration characterized by loss of neuroendocrine regulation and loss of vegetative circadian rhythmicity (211,212). In the final stage of the disease, patients may become very agitated, confused, and disorientated and eventually develop progressive stupor or coma, ultimately leading to death (211,212).

Positron emission tomography (PET) reveals thalamic hypometabolism and milder involvement of the cortex; neuropathology demonstrates severe neuronal loss in the thalamic nuclei variably affecting the caudate, gyrus cinguli, and frontotemporal cortices (210). The genotypic localization of patients with FFI is a mutation at codon 178 of the prion-protein (PrP) gene (213). Neuropathologic findings demonstrate severe degeneration and gliosis of the anterior and dorsomedial nucleus of the thalamus (214). FFI is an inherited disease caused by a mutation in the protein prion gene. Symptoms of FFI closely resemble those of familial Creutzfeldt-Jakob disease, making genetic testing and histologic examination of brain tissue the only means to determine a definitive diagnosis (215).

DIAGNOSITIC APPROACHES TO SLEEP DISTURBANCES IN DEMENTIA AND NEUROLOGIC DISORDERS

Clinical Assessment

The first and most important step in the workup of sleep disturbances of patients with dementia and neurologic disturbances is a detailed inventory of sleep complaints. The history should consist of present and past sleep history, family history, medication and substance use (such as caffeine, nicotine, and alcohol), and information about underlying medical or psychiatric pathologies. The history should also be specifically directed at possible respiratory disturbances during sleep. It is important to perform physical examination for the diagnosis of the primary condition or associated medical, including neurologic, disorders that may be responsible for the sleep disturbances.

Laboratory Assessment

Laboratory investigations should be undertaken to diagnose the nature of the sleep disturbance and the primary neurologic disorder. Overnight PSG and the MSLT are the two most important laboratory tests for the diagnosis of sleep disturbances. Sometimes, pulmonary-function tests are needed to address the question of sleep-related respiratory disturbances, specifically in the setting of underlying motor neuron disease or neuromuscular disorder as well as underlying respiratory pathologies. As detailed in the previous sections, more specific PSG montages (including multiple limb electrodes and EEG) may be helpful in the evaluation of potential parasomnias and nocturnal seizures.

SLEEP TESTS

Polysomnography

PSG should be performed in patients suspected of sleep-related respiratory disorders (41,42,216,217). Unfortunately, the diagnosis and treatment of sleep disturbances may be problematic in neurodegenerative diseases with severe functional impairment given the difficulties in ascertaining the clinical history from the patient. All-night PSG is critical in the assessment of the severity of the SDB and in documenting the consequences on the sleep architecture. Sleep itself may adversely affect breathing and primary neurologic disorders; conversely, primary neurologic disorders may adversely affect sleep. In addition to the typical montage obtained in patients without neurodegenerative disorders, in suspected cases of upper airway resistance syndrome (UARS), which can sometimes be encountered in extrapyramidal disorders, measurement of the esophageal pressure is important and can be accomplished by inserting an esophageal pressure manometry ((PES) (218).

Comprehensive EEG monitoring is also helpful in the context of neurodegenerative disorders to further characterize sleep architectural disturbances and when focal or diffuse cerebral lesions and epileptiform activities are suspected (219,220).

Multiple Sleep Latency Test
When patients with neurodegenerative diseases present with pathologic sleepiness, MSLT can be helpful in documenting the extent of sleepiness. A mean sleep latency of less than five minutes is consistent with pathologic excessive sleepiness. Sleep-onset REM periods in two or more of the four or five recordings during MSLT is suggestive of narcolepsy. Abnormalities of REM sleep regulatory mechanisms and circadian rhythm sleep disturbances may also lead to REM abnormalities during the MSLT.

Additional Laboratory Tests
As noted earlier, multichannel continuous-video PSG monitoring may be helpful when abnormal motor activities are encountered in patients with MSA, OPCA, PD, and AD. Actigraphy is a recently developed technique that uses a motion detector to record activities during sleep and waking and may be useful in the diagnosis of circadian rhythm sleep disorders in patients with neurodegenerative diseases. Neuroimaging is of particular help when patients present with a variety of complaints with unusual features such as dream enactment behavior (in a young female), severe hypersomnia (following head trauma), and apneic episodes (following a brainstem stroke).

TREATMENT OF SLEEP DISTURBANCES IN NEUROLOGIC AND NEURODEGENERATIVE DISORDERS
Treatment of the sleep disturbances in patients with underlying dementias should begin with the treatment of the primary underlying condition. The goal of therapy is to improve the quality of life. The general measures are directed at reducing the risk factors that may exacerbate sleep disruption. An attempt should be made to reduce or eliminate medications that could potentially disrupt. Associated conditions such as depression, anxiety, or pain need to be treated with appropriate medications. Patients should be encouraged to develop good sleep habits, maintain a regular sleep–wake cycle, and refrain from taking extensive daytime naps. Substances that may disrupt sleep, such as caffeine, alcohol, and nicotine, should be prohibited. Patients should be encouraged to exercise during the day, but not too close to the evening hours.

As in the case of AD, the treatment of sleep problems in other forms of dementia requires a combined multidisciplinary approach, including behavioral approach, pharmacotherapy, and in some cases light therapy (221). The specific sleep hygiene recommendations discussed elsewhere in this book are always a first step. Helpful practices include those aimed at reducing daytime sleep and improving the sleep environment and routine (222). Pharmacologic treatments may be useful for symptomatic treatment of insomnia and nighttime behavioral disturbances in dementia patients, but there have been few controlled trials demonstrating their efficacy or long-term safety. Clonazepam is highly effective for treating the nighttime behaviors associated with REM behavior disorder. For most dementia patients, however, the side-effect risks of prolonged use of sedating medications must be weighed against the potential benefits. Dementia patients should be evaluated for common primary sleep disorders that may contribute to nighttime behavioral disturbances and impact treatment decisions. Continuous positive airway pressure, the gold standard for treating obstructive sleep apnea, can be tolerated by mild to moderately demented individuals with support from supervising caregivers. Increased daily light exposure and physical activity may help normalize circadian rest–activity rhythms in some dementia patients, although the frequency and dose needed to maintain treatment effects is currently not known.

Therapy for Insomnia

Sleep changes in aging often compounds sleep changes related to the primary insomnia itself. Insomnia complaints may include difficulty in initiating and maintaining sleep and early-morning awakening. Untreated insomnia can cause an insufficient amount of sleep and poor sleep, resulting in hypersomnolence, irritability, disruption in concentration, and depression, sometimes mistaken for dementia itself (1,223). Insomnia may be complicated by agents prescribed for the specific management of underlying neurodegenerative diseases. The medications used to treat these disturbances can worsen SDB and daytime symptoms (224).

Specific pharmacotherapy for sleep disturbances in neurodegenerative diseases is not particularly effective. In patients with insomnia, a trial with short- to intermediate-acting benzodiazepines (e.g., Temazepam) or zolpidem (Ambien) may be tried for a short period. For nocturnal wanderings or agitation and sundowning, a trial with small doses (0.5–1 mg) of haloperidol may be instituted.

Therapy for Hypersomnia

Hypersomnia is a common problem in patients with dementia resulting from inadequate sleep, sleep fragmentation due to primary sleep disturbances such as obstructive sleep apnea and circadian rhythm disturbances. Patients with hypersomnia may fall asleep at inappropriate times and situations (42,225). These patients may also have additional complaints of daytime fatigue, lack of concentration, and impaired motor skills and cognition and may not show any improvement despite adequate sleep time. Some patients may be at additional risk for sleep-related respiratory disturbances and loud snoring during sleep, as well as periodic leg movements (2).

Unfortunately, data regarding the incidence and prevalence of hypersomnia in dementia are unknown. Data are available, however, in a cohort consisting of elderly patients residing in nursing homes in whom low-dose methylphenidate (≤ 5 mg) has been shown to improve alertness (226). Currently, the exact neurochemistry and neurophysiology of hypersomnia in dementing conditions remains a mystery.

CONCLUSION

Sleep changes dramatically with old age and even more dramatically with dementia. When encountering daytime sleepiness in an older patient with dementia or neurodegenerative disorders, it is crucial to first review the patient's medical history, psychiatric history, medications, underlying medical illnesses, and sleep–wake schedule pattern. The prevalence of SDB, PLM disorder of sleep, RLS, and RBD increases with aging and may lead to excessive daytime sleepiness or insomnia. Many sleep disorders are potentially reversible. A carefully thought-out clinical decision-making process can greatly benefit the patient and family. Sleep problems of the elderly contribute heavily to the decision to institutionalize an elder and thus to the social and economic cost of institutional care and appear to do this largely by interfering with the sleep of caregivers. The nature, prevalence, and treatability of the sleeping problems of both elders and their caregivers need further study (227).

REFERENCES

1. Bhatt MH, Podder N, Chokroverty S. Sleep and neurodegenerative diseases. *Semin Neurol* 2005; **25**(1): 39–51.
2. Chokroverty S. Sleep and degenerative neurologic disorders. *Neurol Clin* 1996; **14**(4): 807–26.
3. van der Flier WM, Scheltens P. Epidemiology and risk factors of dementia. *J Neurol Neurosurg Psychiatry* 2005; **76 Suppl 5**: v2–7.
4. Little JT, Satlin A, Sunderland T, Volicer L. Sundown syndrome in severely demented patients with probable Alzheimer's disease. *J Geriatr Psychiatry Neurol* 1995; **8**(2): 103–6.
5. Pollak CP, Perlick D, Linsner JP, Wenston J, Hsieh F. Sleep problems in the community elderly as predictors of death and nursing home placement. *J Community Health* 1990; **15**(2): 123–35.
6. Janssens JP PS, Hilleret H, and Michel J-P. Sleep disordered breathing in the elderly. *Aging Clin Exp Res* 2000; **12**: 417–429.
7. Ancoli-Israel S, Klauber MR, Jones DW, Kripke DF, Martin J, Mason W *et al.* Variations in circadian rhythms of activity, sleep, and light exposure related to dementia in nursing-home patients. *Sleep* 1997; **20**(1): 18–23.
8. Ancoli-Israel S, Klauber MR, Gillin JC, Campbell SS, Hofstetter CR. Sleep in non-institutionalized Alzheimer's disease patients. *Aging (Milano)* 1994; **6**(6): 451–8.
9. Bliwise DL, Tinklenberg J, Yesavage JA, Davies H, Pursley AM, Petta DE *et al.* REM latency in Alzheimer's disease. *Biol Psychiatry* 1989; **25**(3): 320–8.
10. Vitiello MV, Prinz PN, Williams DE, Frommlet MS, Ries RK. Sleep disturbances in patients with mild-stage Alzheimer's disease. *J Gerontol* 1990; **45**(4): M131–8.
11. Vitiello MV, Prinz PN. Alzheimer's disease. Sleep and sleep/wake patterns. *Clin Geriatr Med* 1989; **5**(2): 289–99.
12. Vitiello MV, Poceta JS, Prinz PN. Sleep in Alzheimer's disease and other dementing disorders. *Can J Psychol* 1991; **45**(2): 221–39.
13. Vitiello MV, Borson S. Sleep disturbances in patients with Alzheimer's disease: epidemiology, pathophysiology and treatment. *CNS Drugs* 2001; **15**(10): 777–96.
14. Vitiello MV, Bliwise DL, Prinz PN. Sleep in Alzheimer's disease and the sundown syndrome. *Neurology* 1992; **42**(7 Suppl 6): 83–93; discussion 93–4.
15. Taylor JL, Friedman L, Sheikh J, Yesavage JA. Assessment and Management of "Sundowning" Phenomena. *Semin Clin Neuropsychiatry* 1997; **2**(2): 113–122.
16. Volicer L, Harper DG, Manning BC, Goldstein R, Satlin A. Sundowning and circadian rhythms in Alzheimer's disease. *Am J Psychiatry* 2001; **158**(5): 704–11.
17. Stopa EG, Volicer L, Kuo-Leblanc V, Harper D, Lathi D, Tate B *et al.* Pathologic evaluation of the human suprachiasmatic nucleus in severe dementia. *J Neuropathol Exp Neurol* 1999; **58**(1): 29–39.
18. Czeisler C, Dumont M, Duffy JF. Association os sleep-wake habits in older people with changes in output of circadian pacemaker. *Lancet* 1992; **340**: 933–936.
19. Swaab DF, Fisser B, Kamphorst W, Troost D. The human suprachiasmatic nucleus; neuropeptide changes in senium and Alzheimer's disease. *Basic Appl Histochem* 1988; **32**(1): 43–54.
20. Swaab DF, Fliers E, Partiman TS. The suprachiasmatic nucleus of the human brain in relation to sex, age and senile dementia. *Brain Res* 1985; **342**(1): 37–44.
21. van Someren EJ, Hagebeuk EE, Lijzenga C, Scheltens P, de Rooij SE, Jonker C *et al.* Circadian rest-activity rhythm disturbances in Alzheimer's disease. *Biol Psychiatry* 1996; **40**(4): 259–70.
22. Pollak CP, Stokes PE. Circadian rest-activity rhythms in demented and nondemented older community residents and their caregivers. *J Am Geriatr Soc* 1997; **45**(4): 446–52.

23. Reid KJ, Chang AM, Zee PC. Circadian rhythm sleep disorders. *Med Clin North Am* 2004; **88**(3): 631–51, viii.
24. Diagnostic and Statistical Manual of Mental Disorders. In. Fourth Edition, Text Revision ed. Washington, DC: American Psychiatric Association, 2000.
25. Liu RY, Zhou JN, Hoogendijk WJ, van Heerikhuize J, Kamphorst W, Unmehopa UA *et al.* Decreased vasopressin gene expression in the biological clock of Alzheimer disease patients with and without depression. *J Neuropathol Exp Neurol* 2000; **59**(4): 314–22.
26. Witting W, Mirmiran M, Bos NP, Swaab DF. Effect of light intensity on diurnal sleep-wake distribution in young and old rats. *Brain Res Bull* 1993; **30**(1–2): 157–62.
27. Hoch CC RIC, Kupfer DJ, *et al.* Sleep disordered breathing in normal and pathological aging. *J Clin Psychiatry* 1986; **47**(10): 499–503.
28. Erkinjuntti T PM, Sulkava R, *et al.* Sleep apnea in multiinfarct dementia and Alzheimer's disease. *Sleep* 1987; **10**(5): 419–425.
29. Janssens JP, Pautex S, Hilleret H, Michel JP. Sleep disordered breathing in the elderly. *Aging (Milano)* 2000; **12**(6): 417–29.
30. Ancoli-Israel S, Klauber MR, Butters N, Parker L, Kripke DF. Dementia in institutionalized elderly: relation to sleep apnea. *J Am Geriatr Soc* 1991; **39**(3): 258–63.
31. Schletens P VF, Van Keimpema A, Lindebloom J, Taphoorn M, Wolters E. Sleep apnea syndrome presenting with cognitive impairment. *Neurology* 1991; **41**: 155–156.
32. Bliwise DL. Sleep apnea, APOE4 and Alzheimer's disease 20 years and counting? *J Psychosom Res* 2002; **53**(1): 539–46.
33. Kadotani H, Kadotani T, Young T, Peppard PE, Finn L, Colrain IM *et al.* Association between apolipoprotein E epsilon4 and sleep-disordered breathing in adults. *Jama* 2001; **285**(22): 2888–90.
34. Punjabi NM, Shahar E, Redline S, Gottlieb DJ, Givelber R, Resnick HE. Sleep-disordered breathing, glucose intolerance, and insulin resistance: the Sleep Heart Health Study. *Am J Epidemiol* 2004; **160**(6): 521–30.
35. Foley DJ, Masaki K, White L, Redline S. Relationship between apolipoprotein E epsilon4 and sleep-disordered breathing at different ages. *Jama* 2001; **286**(12): 1447–8.
36. Saarelainen S, Lehtimaki T, Kallonen E, Laasonen K, Poussa T, Nieminen MM. No relation between apolipoprotein E alleles and obstructive sleep apnea. *Clin Genet* 1998; **53**(2): 147–8.
37. Gottlieb DJ, DeStefano AL, Foley DJ, Mignot E, Redline S, Givelber RJ *et al.* APOE epsilon4 is associated with obstructive sleep apnea/hypopnea: the Sleep Heart Health Study. *Neurology* 2004; **63**(4): 664–8.
38. Bliwise DL. Sleep disorders in Alzheimer's disease and other dementias. *Clin Cornerstone* 2004; **6** Suppl 1 A: S16–28.
39. Gehrman PR, Martin JL, Shochat T, Nolan S, Corey-Bloom J, Ancoli-Israel S. Sleep-disordered breathing and agitation in institutionalized adults with Alzheimer disease. *Am J Geriatr Psychiatry* 2003; **11**(4): 426–33.
40. Aloia MS IN, Di Dio P, Perlis ML, Greenblatt DW, Giles DE. Neuropsychological changes and treatment compliance in older adults with sleep apnea. *Journal of Psychosomatic Research* 2003; **54**(1): 71–6.
41. Avidan AY. Sleep disorders in the older patient. *Prim Care* 2005; **32**(2): 563–86.
42. Avidan AY. Sleep in the geriatric patient population. *Semin Neurol* 2005; **25**(1): 52–63.
43. Mazza M, Della Marca G, De Risio S, Mennuni GF, Mazza S. Sleep disorders in the elderly. *Clin Ter* 2004; **155**(9): 391–4.
44. Cohen-Zion M, Stepnowsky C, Marler, Shochat T, Kripke DF, Ancoli-Israel S. Changes in cognitive function associated with sleep disordered breathing in older people. *J Am Geriatr Soc* 2001; **49**(12): 1622–7.
45. Wu YH, Swaab DF. The human pineal gland and melatonin in aging and Alzheimer's disease. *J Pineal Res* 2005; **38**(3): 145–52.
46. Olakowska E, Marcol W, Kotulska K, Lewin-Kowalik J. The role of melatonin in the neurodegenerative diseases. *Bratisl Lek Listy* 2005; **106**(4–5): 171–4.
47. Wang JZ, Wang ZF. Role of melatonin in Alzheimer-like neurodegeneration. *Acta Pharmacol Sin* 2006; **27**(1): 41–9.

48. Zhdanova IV, Tucci V. Melatonin, Circadian Rhythms, and Sleep. *Curr Treat Options Neurol* 2003; **5**(3): 225–229.
49. Lovell BB, Ancoli-Israel S, Gevirtz R. Effect of bright light treatment on agitated behavior in institutionalized elderly subjects. *Psychiatry Res* 1995; **57**(1): 7–12.
50. Ancoli-Israel S, Gehrman P, Martin JL, Shochat T, Marler M, Corey-Bloom J *et al.* Increased light exposure consolidates sleep and strengthens circadian rhythms in severe Alzheimer's disease patients. *Behav Sleep Med* 2003; **1**(1): 22–36.
51. Okawa M, Mishima K, Hishikawa Y, Hozumi S, Hori H, Takahashi K. Circadian rhythm disorders in sleep-waking and body temperature in elderly patients with dementia and their treatment. *Sleep* 1991; **14**(6): 478–85.
52. Ancoli-Israel S, Martin JL, Kripke DF, Marler M, Klauber MR. Effect of light treatment on sleep and circadian rhythms in demented nursing home patients. *J Am Geriatr Soc* 2002; **50**(2): 282–9.
53. Schnelle JF, Cruise PA, Alessi CA, Ludlow K, al-Samarrai NR, Ouslander JG. Sleep hygiene in physically dependent nursing home residents: behavioral and environmental intervention implications. *Sleep* 1998; **21**(5): 515–23.
54. Naylor E, Penev PD, Orbeta L, Janssen I, Ortiz R, Colecchia EF *et al.* Daily social and physical activity increases slow-wave sleep and daytime neuropsychological performance in the elderly. *Sleep* 2000; **23**(1): 87–95.
55. Asayama K, Yamadera H, Ito T, Suzuki H, Kudo Y, Endo S. Double blind study of melatonin effects on the sleep-wake rhythm, cognitive and non-cognitive functions in Alzheimer type dementia. *J Nippon Med Sch* 2003; **70**(4): 334–41.
56. Singer C, Tractenberg RE, Kaye J, Schafer K, Gamst A, Grundman M *et al.* A multicenter, placebo-controlled trial of melatonin for sleep disturbance in Alzheimer's disease. *Sleep* 2003; **26**(7): 893–901.
57. Lyketsos CG, Lindell Veiel L, Baker A, Steele C. A randomized, controlled trial of bright light therapy for agitated behaviors in dementia patients residing in long-term care. *Int J Geriatr Psychiatry* 1999; **14**(7): 520–5.
58. Satlin A, Volicer L, Ross V, Herz L, Campbell S. Bright light treatment of behavioral and sleep disturbances in patients with Alzheimer's disease. *Am J Psychiatry* 1992; **149**(8): 1028–32.
59. Ancoli-Israel S, Martin JL, Gehrman P, Shochat T, Corey-Bloom J, Marler M *et al.* Effect of light on agitation in institutionalized patients with severe Alzheimer disease. *Am J Geriatr Psychiatry* 2003; **11**(2): 194–203.
60. McGaffigan S, Bliwise DL. The treatment of sundowning. A selective review of pharmacological and nonpharmacological studies. *Drugs Aging* 1997; **10**(1): 10–7.
61. Bliwise DL. What is sundowning? *J Am Geriatr Soc* 1994; **42**(9): 1009–11.
62. Bliwise DL, Carroll JS, Lee KA, Nekich JC, Dement WC. Sleep and "sundowning" in nursing home patients with dementia. *Psychiatry Res* 1993; **48**(3): 277–92.
63. Pollak CP, Perlick D. Sleep problems and institutionalization of the elderly. *Journal of Geriatric Psychiatry and Neurology* 1991; **4**: 204–210.
64. Haimov I, Lavie P, Laudon M, Herer P, Vigder C, Zisapel N. Melatonin replacement therapy of elderly insomniacs. *Sleep* 1995; **18**(7): 598–603.
65. Zhdanova IV. Melatonin as a hypnotic: pro. *Sleep Med Rev* 2005; **9**(1): 51–65.
66. Tanner CM, Aston DA. Epidemiology of Parkinson's disease and akinetic syndromes. *Curr Opin Neurol* 2000; **13**(4): 427–30.
67. Sethi KD. Clinical aspects of Parkinson disease. *Curr Opin Neurol* 2002; **15**(4): 457–60.
68. McDonald WM, Richard IH, DeLong MR. Prevalence, etiology, and treatment of depression in Parkinson's disease. *Biol Psychiatry* 2003; **54**(3): 363–75.
69. Elmer L. Cognitive issues in Parkinson's disease. *Neurol Clin* 2004; **22**(3 Suppl): S91-S106.
70. Partinen M. Sleep disorder related to Parkinson's disease. *J Neurol* 1997; **244**(4 Suppl 1): S3–6.
71. Fabbrini G, Barbanti P, Aurilia C, Vanacore N, Pauletti C, Meco G. Excessive daytime sleepiness in de novo and treated Parkinson's disease. *Mov Disord* 2002; **17**(5): 1026–30.
72. Stocchi F, Barbato L, Nordera G, Berardelli A, Ruggieri S. Sleep disorders in Parkinson's disease. *Journal of Neurology.* 1998; **245 (Suppl 1):** S15–8.

73. Young A, Home M, Churchward T, Freezer N, Holmes P, Ho M. Comparison of sleep disturbance in mild versus severe Parkinson's disease. *Sleep* 2002; **25**(5): 573–7.
74. Stocchi F, Barbato L, Nordera G, Berardelli A, Ruggieri S. Sleep disorders in Parkinson's disease. *J Neurol* 1998; **245** Suppl 1: S15–8.
75. Schenck CH, Mahowald MW. REM parasomnias. *Neurology Clinics* 1996; **14**: 697–720.
76. Frucht S, Greene P, Fahn S. Sleep episodes in Parkinson's disease: A wake-up call. *Mov Disord* 2000; **15**: 601–603.
77. Tandberg E, Larsen JP, Karlsen K. A community-based study of sleep disorders in patients with Parkinson's disease. *Mov Disord* 1998; **13**(6): 895–9.
78. Factor SA, McAlarney T, Sanchez-Ramos JR, Weiner WJ. Sleep disorders and sleep effect in Parkinson's disease. *Mov Disord* 1990; **5**(4): 280–5.
79. Comella CL. Sleep disturbances in Parkinson's disease. *Curr Neurol Neurosci Rep* 2003; **3**(2): 173–80.
80. Tan A, Salgado M, Fahn S. Rapid eye movement sleep behavior disorder preceding Parkinson's disease with therapeutic response to levodopa. *Mov Disord* 1996; **11**(2): 214–6.
81. Apps MC, Sheaff PC, Ingram DA, Kennard C, Empey DWK. Respiration and sleep in Parkinson's disease. *Journal of Neurology, Neurosurgery & Psychiatry* 1985; **48**(12): 1240–5.
82. Trenkwalder C. Sleep dysfunction in Parkinson's disease. *Clin Neurosci* 1998; **5**(2): 107–14.
83. Eisensehr I, Linke R, Noachtar S, Schwartz J, Gildehaus FJ, Tatsch K. Reduced striatal dopamine transporters in idiopathic rapid eye movement sleep behavior disorder. Comparison with Parkinson's disease and controls. *Brain* 2000; **123**: 1155–1160.
84. Askenasy JJ, Yahr MD. Reversal of sleep disturbance in Parkinson's disease by antiparkinsonian therapy: a preliminary study. *Neurology.* 1985; **35**(4): 527–32.
85. Pappert EJ, Goetz CG, Niederman FG, Raman R, Leurgans S. Hallucinations, sleep fragmentation, and altered dream phenomena in Parkinson's disease. *Movement Disorders* 1999; **14**(1): 117–21.
86. Wetter TC, Winkelmann J, Eisensehr I. Current treatment options for restless legs syndrome. *Expert Opin Pharmacother* 2003; **4**(10): 1727–38.
87. Silber MH, Ehrenberg BL, Allen RP, Buchfuhrer MJ, Earley CJ, Hening WA *et al.* An algorithm for the management of restless legs syndrome. *Mayo Clin Proc* 2004; **79**(7): 916–22.
88. Schenck CH, Bundlie SR, Patterson AL, Mahowald MW. Rapid Eye Movement Sleep Behavior Disorder: A treatable parasomnia affecting older adults. *JAMA* 1987; **257**(13): 1786–1789.
89. Chokroverty S. Sleep and degenerative neurologic disorders. *Neurol Clin* 1996; **4**(4): 807–26.
90. Aldrich MS. *Sleep Medicine*, vol. 53. Oxford University Press, Inc., 1999.
91. Schenck CH, Bundlie SR, Patterson AL, Mahowald MD. Rapid Eye Movement Sleep Behavior Disorder: A treatable parasomnia affecting older adults. *JAMA* 1987; **257**(13): 1786–1789.
92. Schenck CH, Mahowald MW. REM sleep parasomnias. *Neurologic Clinics.* 1996; **14**(4): 697–720.
93. Morrison AR. The pathophysiology of REM-sleep behavior disorder. *Sleep* 1998; **21**(5): 446–9.
94. Parkes JD. The parasomnias. *The Lancet* 1986; **2**(8514): 1021–5.
95. Lowe AD. Sleep in Parkinson's disease. *J Psychosom Res* 1998; **44**(6): 613–7.
96. Gagnon JF, Bedard MA, Fantini ML, Petit D, Panisset M, Rompre S *et al.* REM sleep behavior disorder and REM sleep without atonia in Parkinson's disease. *Neurology* 2002; **59**(4): 585–9.
97. Wetter TC, Trenkwalder C, Gershanik O, Hogl B. Polysomnographic measures in Parkinson's disease: a comparison between patients with and without REM sleep disturbances. *Wien Klin Wochenschr* 2001; **113**(7–8): 249–53.
98. Poryazova RG, Zachariev ZI. REM sleep behavior disorder in patients with Parkinson's disease. *Folia Med (Plovdiv)* 2005; **47**(1): 5–10.

99. Larsen JP, Tandberg E. Sleep disorders in patients with Parkinson's disease: epidemiology and management. *CNS Drugs* 2001; **15**(4): 267–75.
100. Boeve BF, Silber MH, Ferman TJ, Lucas JA, Parisi JE. Association of REM sleep behavior disorder and neurodegenerative disease may reflect an underlying synucleinopathy. *Mov Disord* 2001; **16**(4): 622–30.
101. Boeve BF, Silber MH, Ferman TJ. REM sleep behavior disorder in Parkinson's disease and dementia with Lewy bodies. *J Geriatr Psychiatry Neurol* 2004; **17**(3): 146–57.
102. Abad VC, Guilleminault C. Review of rapid eye movement behavior sleep disorders. *Curr Neurol Neurosci Rep* 2004; **4**(2): 157–63.
103. Plazzi G, Corsini R, Provini F, Pierangeli G, Martinelli P, Montagna P *et al*. REM sleep behavior disorders in multiple system atrophy. *Neurology* 1997; **48**(4): 1094–7.
104. Iranzo A, Santamaria J, Rye DB, Valldeoriola F, Marti MJ, Munoz E *et al*. Characteristics of idiopathic REM sleep behavior disorder and that associated with MSA and PD. *Neurology* 2005; **65**(2): 247–52.
105. Boeve BF, Silber MH, Ferman T. REM sleep behavior disorder and degenerative dementia: an association likely reflecting Lewy body disease. *Neurology* 1998; **51**: 363–70.
106. Ferini-Strambi L, Zucconi M. REM sleep behavior disorder. *Clin Neurophysiol* 2000; **111**(Suppl 2): sS136–40.
107. Mahowald MW, Schenck CH. *REM sleep behavior disorder*, WB Saunders: Philadelphia, 1994, 574–588pp.
108. Plazzi G, Corsinin R, Provini F. REM sleep behavior disorders in multiple sytem atrophy. *Neurology* 1997; **48**: 1094–7.
109. Schenck CH, Mahowald MW. REM sleep parasomnias. *Neurol Clin* 1996; **14**(4): 697–720.
110. Schenck CH, Bundlie SR, Mahowald MW. Delayed emergence of a parkinsonian disoderin 38% of 29 older men initially diagnosed with idiopathic rapid eye movement sleep behavior disorder. *Neurology* 1996; **46**: 388–93.
111. Kowey PR, Mainchak RA, *et al*. Things that go bang in the night. *N Engl J Med* 1992; **327**: 1884.
112. Takeuchi N, Uchimura N, Hashizume Y, Mukai M, Etoh Y, Yamamoto K *et al*. Melatonin therapy for REM sleep behavior disorder. *Psychiatry Clin Neurosci* 2001; **55**(3): 267–9.
113. Boeve B. Melatonin for treatment of REM sleep behavior disorder: response in 8 patients. *Sleep* 2001; **24(suppl)**: A35.
114. Zesiewicz TA, Baker MJ, Dunne PB, Hauser RA. Diffuse Lewy Body Disease. *Curr Treat Options Neurol* 2001; **3**(6): 507–518.
115. Boeve BF, Silber MH, Ferman TJ, Kokmen E, Smith GE, Ivnik RJ *et al*. REM sleep behavior disorder and degenerative dementia: an association likely reflecting Lewy body disease. *Neurology* 1998; **51**(2): 363–70.
116. Turner RS, Chervin RD, Frey KA, Minoshima S, Kuhl DE. Probable diffuse Lewy body disease presenting as REM sleep behavior disorde. *Neurology* 1997; **49**(2): 523.
117. Yamauchi K, Takehisa M, Tsuno M, Kaneda Y, Taniguchi T, Ohno H *et al*. Levodopa improved rapid eye movement sleep behavior disorder with diffuse Lewy body disease. *Gen Hosp Psychiatry* 2003; **25**(2): 140–2.
118. de Brito-Marques PR, de Mello RV, Montenegro L. Nightmares without atonia as an early symptom of diffuse Lewy bodies disease. *Arq Neuropsiquiatr* 2003; **61**(4): 936–41.
119. Ghorayeb I, Bioulac B, Tison F. Sleep disorders in multiple system atrophy. *J Neural Transm* 2005; **112**(12): 1669–1675.
120. Chokroverty S, Sharp JT, Barron KD. Periodic respiration in erect posture in Shy-Drager syndrome. *J Neurol Neurosurg Psychiatry* 1978; **41**(11): 980–6.
121. Gilman S, Koeppe RA, Chervin RD, Consens FB, Little R, An H *et al*. REM sleep behavior disorder is related to striatal monoaminergic deficit in MSA. *Neurology* 2003; **61**(1): 29–34.
122. Munschauer FE, Mador J, Ahuja A, Jacobs L. Selective paralysis of voluntary but not limbically influenced automatic respiration. *Archives of Neurology* 1991; **48**: 1190–1192.
123. Olson EJ, Boeve BF, Silber MH. Rapid eye movement sleep behaviour disorder: demographic, clinical and laboratory findings in 93 cases. *Brain* 2000; **123 (Pt 2)**: 331–9.
124. Sakakibara R, Odaka T, Uchiyama T, Asahina M, Yamaguchi K, Yamaguchi T *et al*. Colonic transit time and rectoanal videomanometry in Parkinson's disease. *J Neurol Neurosurg Psychiatry* 2003; **74**(2): 268–72.

125. Hughes RJ, Sack RL, Lewy AJ. The role of melatonin and circadian phase in age-related sleep-maintenance insomnia: assessment in a clinical trial of melatonin replacement. *Sleep* 1998; **21**(1): 52–68.
126. Salva MA, Guilleminault C. Olivopontocerebellar degeneration, abnormal sleep, and REM sleep without atonia. *Neurology* 1986; **36**(4): 576–7.
127. Miyamoto T, Miyamoto M, Yokota N, Hirata K, Katayama S. A case of nocturnal polyuria in olivopontocerebellar atrophy. *Psychiatry Clin Neurosci* 1999; **53**(2): 279–81.
128. Briskin JG, Lehrman KL, C. G. *Shy-Drager syndrome and sleep apnea.*, Liss: New York, 1978, 317–22pp.
129. Pauletto G, Belgrado E, Marinig R, Bergonzi P. Sleep disorders and extrapyramidal diseases: an historical review. *Sleep Med* 2004; **5**(2): 163–7.
130. Chokroverty S. Sleep and degnerative neurologi discoders. *Neurol Clin* 1996; **14**(4): 807–26.
131. Gross RA, Spehlmann R, Daniels JC. Sleep disturbances in progressive supranuclear palsy. *Electroencephalogr Clin Neurophysiol* 1978; **45**(1): 16–25.
132. Kellinghaus C, Loddenkemper T, Dinner DS, Lachhwani D, Luders HO. Non-epileptic seizures of the elderly. *J Neurol* 2004; **251**(6): 704–9.
133. Vaughn BV, D'Cruz OF. Sleep and epilepsy. *Semin Neurol* 2004; **24**(3): 301–13.
134. Degen R, Degen HE. Sleep and sleep deprivation in epileptology. *Epilepsy Res Suppl* 1991; **2**: 235–60.
135. Dinner DS. Effect of sleep on epilepsy. *J Clin Neurophysiol* 2002; **19**(6): 504–13.
136. Malow BA, Bowes RJ, Lin X. Predictors of sleepiness in epilepsy patients. *Sleep* 1997; **20**(12): 1105–10.
137. Vaughn BV, D'Cruz OF, Beach R, Messenheimer JA. Improvement of epileptic seizure control with treatment of obstructive sleep apnoea. *Seizure* 1996; **5**(1): 73–8.
138. Devinsky O, Ehrenberg B, Barthlen GM, Abramson HS, Luciano D. Epilepsy and sleep apnea syndrome. *Neurology* 1994; **44**(11): 2060–4.
139. Bazil CW. Nocturnal seizures. *Semin Neurol* 2004; **24**(3): 293–300.
140. Sammaritano M, Sherwin A. Effect of anticonvulsants on sleep. *Neurology* 2000; **54**(5 Suppl 1): S16–24.
141. Wolf P, Roder-Wanner UU, Brede M. Influence of therapeutic phenobarbital and phenytoin medication on the polygraphic sleep of patients with epilepsy. *Epilepsia* 1984; **25**(4): 467–75.
142. Gigli GL, Placidi F, Diomedi M, Maschio M, Silvestri G, Scalise A *et al*. Nocturnal sleep and daytime somnolence in untreated patients with temporal lobe epilepsy: changes after treatment with controlled-release carbamazepine. *Epilepsia* 1997; **38**(6): 696–701.
143. Copinschi G, Van Onderbergen A, L'Hermite-Baleriaux M, Szyper M, Caufriez A, Bosson D *et al*. Effects of the short-acting benzodiazepine triazolam, taken at bedtime, on circadian and sleep-related hormonal profiles in normal men. *Sleep* 1990; **13**(3): 232–44.
144. Placidi F, Diomedi M, Scalise A, Marciani MG, Romigi A, Gigli GL. Effect of anticonvulsants on nocturnal sleep in epilepsy. *Neurology* 2000; **54**(5 Suppl 1): S25–32.
145. Foldvary-Schaefer N, De Leon Sanchez I, Karafa M, Mascha E, Dinner D, Morris HH. Gabapentin increases slow-wave sleep in normal adults. *Epilepsia* 2002; **43**(12): 1493–7.
146. Johnson RT. Current therapy in neurologic disease. In. Philadelphia Saint Louis: B. C. Decker; C. V. Mosby Co. [distributor], 1985. p v.
147. Tachibana N, Howard RS, Hirsch NP, Miller DH, Moseley IF, Fish D. Sleep problems in multiple sclerosis. *Eur Neurol* 1994; **34**(6): 320–3.
148. Fleming WE, Pollak CP. Sleep disorders in multiple sclerosis. *Semin Neurol* 2005; **25**(1): 64–8.
149. Zwakhalen SM, Hamers JP, Huijer Abu-Saad H, Berger MP. Pain in elderly people with severe dementia: A systematic review of behavioural pain assessment tools. *BMC Geriatr* 2006; **6**(1): 3.
150. Roehrs T, Roth T. Sleep and pain: interaction of two vital functions. *Semin Neurol* 2005; **25**(1): 106–16.
151. Cote KA, Moldofsky H. Sleep, daytime symptoms, and cognitive performance in patients with fibromyalgia. *J Rheumatol* 1997; **24**(10): 2014–23.

152. Mahowald ML, Mahowald MW. Nighttime sleep and daytime functioning (sleepiness and fatigue) in less well-defined chronic rheumatic diseases with particular reference to the 'alpha-delta NREM sleep anomaly'. *Sleep Med* 2000; **1**(3): 195–207.

153. Carolei A, Sacco S, De Santis F, Marini C. Epidemiology of stroke. *Clin Exp Hypertens* 2002; **24**(7–8): 479–83.

154. Diehl M, Ragland DR. Habitual snoring as a risk factor for stroke: A meta-analysis. *Sleep* 2004; **(in press)**.

155. Spriggs DA, French JM, Murdy JM, Curless RH, Bates D, James OFW. Snoring increases the risk of stroke and adversely affects prognosis. *Quarterly Journal of Medicine* 1992; **303**: 555–562.

156. Qreshi AI, Giles WH, Croft JB, Bliwise DL. Habitual sleep patterns and risk for stroke and coronary disease: A 10-year follow-up from NHANES I. *Neurology* 1997; **48**: 904–910.

157. Davies DP, Rodgers H, Walshaw D, James OFW, Gibson GJ. Snoring, daytime sleepiness and stroke: a cse-control study of first-ever stroke. *J Sleep Res* 2003; **12**: 313–8.

158. Bassetti C, Aldrich M, Chervin R, Quint D. Sleep apnea in the acute phase of TIA and Stroke. *Neurology* 1996; **47**: 1167–1173.

159. Dyken ME, Somers VK, Yamada T, Ren Z, Zimmermann MB. Investigating the relationship between stroke and obstructive sleep apnea. *Stroke* 1996; **27**: 401–407.

160. Good DC, Henkle JQ, Gelber D, Weösh J, Verhulst S. Sleep-disordered breathing and poor functional outcome after stroke. *Stroke* 1996; **27**(2): 252–259.

161. Sandberg O, Franklin KA, Bucht G, Eriksson S, Gustafson Y. Nasal continuous positive airway pressure in stroke patients with sleep apnoea: A randomized treatment study. *Eur Respir J* 2001; **18**(4): 619–622.

162. Wessendorf TE, Wang YM, Thilmann AF, Sorgenfrei U, Konietzko N, Teschler H. Treatment of obstructive sleep apnoea with nasal continuous positive airway pressure. *Eur Respir J* 2001; **18**: 623–9.

163. Pepperell JCT, Ramdassingh-Dow S, Crosthwaite N, *et al.* Ambulatory blood pressure after therapeutic and subtherapeutic nasal continuous positive airway pressure for obstructive sleep apnoea: a randomized parallel trial. *Lancet* 2001; **359**: 204–210.

164. Parra O, Arboix A, Bechich S, *et al.* Time course of sleep-related breathing disorders in first-ever stroke or transient ischemic attack. *Am J Resp Crit Care Med* 2000; **161**: 375–80.

165. Iranzo A, Santamaria J, Berenguer J, Sanchez M, Chamorro A. Prevalence and clinical importance of sleep apnea in the first night after cerebral infarction. *Neurology* 2002; **58**: 911–6.

166. Power WR, Mosko SS, Sassin JF. Sleep-stage dependent Cheyne-Stokes respiration after cerebral infarct: a case study. *Neurology* 1982; **32**: 763–6.

167. Bassetti C, Aldrich MS, Quint D. Sleep-disordered breathing in patients with acute supra- and infratentorial stroke. *Stroke* 1997; **28**: 1765–1772.

168. Bahro M, Katzmann KJ, Guckel F, Sungurtekin I, Riemann D. [REM sleep parasomnia]. *Nervenarzt* 1994; **65**(8): 568–71.

169. Schenck CH, Mahowald MW. Injurious sleep behavior disorders (parasomnias) affecting patients on intensive care units. *Intensive Care Med* 1991; **17**(4): 219–24.

170. Gordon PH, Mitsumoto H, Hays AP. Amyotrophic lateral sclerosis. *Sci Aging Knowledge Environ* 2003; **2003**(35): dn2.

171. Ferguson KA, Strong MJ, Ahmad D, George CF. Sleep-disordered breathing in amyotrophic lateral sclerosis. *Chest* 1996; **110**(3): 664–9.

172. Ferguson KA, Strong MJ, Ahmad D, George CF. Sleep and breathing in amyotrophic lateral sclerosis. *Sleep* 1995; **18**(6): 514.

173. Arnulf I, Similowski T, Salachas F, Garma L, Mehiri S, Attali V *et al.* Sleep disorders and diaphragmatic function in patients with amyotrophic lateral sclerosis. *Am J Respir Crit Care Med* 2000; **161**(3 Pt 1): 849–56.

174. Arnulf I, Derenne JP. [Respiratory disorders during sleep in degenerative diseases of the brain stem]. *Rev Neurol (Paris)* 2001; **157**(11 Pt 2): S148–51.

175. Minz M, Autret A, Laffont F, Beillevaire T, Cathala HP, Castaigne P. A study on sleep in amyotrophic lateral sclerosis. *Biomedicine* 1979; **30**(1): 40–6.

176. Culebras A. Sleep and neuromuscular disorders. *Neurol Clin* 1996; **14**(4): 791–805.

177. Aboussouan LS, Lewis RA. Sleep, respiration and ALS. *J Neurol Sci* 1999; **164**(1): 1–2.
178. Culebras A. Sleep disorders and neuromuscular disease. *Semin Neurol* 2005; **25**(1): 33–8.
179. Butz M, Wollinsky KH, Wiedemuth-Catrinescu U, Sperfeld A, Winter S, Mehrkens HH *et al.* Longitudinal effects of noninvasive positive-pressure ventilation in patients with amyotrophic lateral sclerosis. *Am J Phys Med Rehabil* 2003; **82**(8): 597–604.
180. Culebras A. Sleep disorders associated with neuromuscular and spinal cord disorders. In: Gilamn S, (ed) *Neurology Medlink*. San Diego, 2006.
181. Biering-Sorensen F, Biering-Sorensen M. Sleep disturbances in the spinal cord injured: an epidemiological questionnaire investigation, including a normal population. *Spinal Cord* 2001; **39**(10): 505–13.
182. Stockhammer E, Tobon A, Michel F, Eser P, Scheuler W, Bauer W *et al.* Characteristics of sleep apnea syndrome in tetraplegic patients. *Spinal Cord* 2002; **40**(6): 286–94.
183. Short DJ, Stradling JR, Williams SJ. Prevalence of sleep apnoea in patients over 40 years of age with spinal cord lesions. *J Neurol Neurosurg Psychiatry* 1992; **55**(11): 1032–6.
184. Nogues M, Gene R, Benarroch E, Leiguarda R, Calderon C, Encabo H. Respiratory disturbances during sleep in syringomyelia and syringobulbia. *Neurology* 1999; **52**(9): 1777–83.
185. Jubelt B. Post-Polio Syndrome. *Curr Treat Options Neurol* 2004; **6**(2): 87–93.
186. Dalakas MC, Sever JL, Madden DL, Papadopoulos NM, Shekarchi IC, Albrecht P *et al.* Late postpoliomyelitis muscular atrophy: clinical, virologic, and immunologic studies. *Rev Infect Dis* 1984; **6 Suppl 2:** S562–7.
187. Jubelt B, Cashman NR. Neurological manifestations of the post-polio syndrome. *Crit Rev Neurobiol* 1987; **3**(3): 199–220.
188. Bach JR. Management of post-polio respiratory sequelae. *Ann N Y Acad Sci* 1995; **753:** 96–102.
189. Bruno RL. Abnormal movements in sleep as a post-polio sequelae. *Am J Phys Med Rehabil* 1998; **77**(4): 339–43.
190. Steljes DG, Kryger MH, Kirk BW, Millar TW. Sleep in postpolio syndrome. *Chest* 1990; **98**(1): 133–40.
191. Hansotia P, Wall R, Berendes J. Sleep disturbances and severity of Huntington's disease. *Neurology* 1985; **35**(11): 1672–4.
192. Emser W, Brenner M, Stober T, Schimrigk K. Changes in nocturnal sleep in Huntington's and Parkinson's disease. *J Neurol* 1988; **235**(3): 177–9.
193. Wiegand M, Moller AA, Lauer CJ, Stolz S, Schreiber W, Dose M *et al.* Nocturnal sleep in Huntington's disease. *J Neurol* 1991; **238**(4): 203–8.
194. Hurelbrink CB, Lewis SJ, Barker RA. The use of the Actiwatch-Neurologica system to objectively assess the involuntary movements and sleep-wake activity in patients with mild-moderate Huntington's disease. *J Neurol* 2005; **252**(6): 642–7.
195. Bollen EL, Den Heijer JC, Ponsioen C, Kramer C, Van Der Velde EA, Van Dijk JG *et al.* Respiration during sleep in Huntington's chorea. *J Neurol Sci* 1988; **84**(1): 63–8.
196. Morton AJ, Wood NI, Hastings MH, Hurelbrink C, Barker RA, Maywood ES. Disintegration of the sleep-wake cycle and circadian timing in Huntington's disease. *J Neurosci* 2005; **25**(1): 157–63.
197. Martinez-Rodriguez JE, Lin L, Iranzo A, Genis D, Marti MJ, Santamaria J *et al.* Decreased hypocretin-1 (Orexin-A) levels in the cerebrospinal fluid of patients with myotonic dystrophy and excessive daytime sleepiness. *Sleep* 2003; **26**(3): 287–90.
198. Laberge L, Begin P, Montplaisir J, Mathieu J. Sleep complaints in patients with myotonic dystrophy. *J Sleep Res* 2004; **13**(1): 95–100.
199. Giubilei F, Iannilli M, Vitale A, Pierallini A, Sacchetti ML, Antonini G *et al.* Sleep patterns in acute ischemic stroke. *Acta Neurol Scand* 1992; **86:** 567–571.
200. Damian MS, Gerlach A, Schmidt F, Lehmann E, Reichmann H. Modafinil for excessive daytime sleepiness in myotonic dystrophy. *Neurology* 2001; **56**(6): 794–6.
201. MacDonald JR, Hill JD, Tarnopolsky MA. Modafinil reduces excessive somnolence and enhances mood in patients with myotonic dystrophy. *Neurology* 2002; **59**(12): 1876–80.
202. Culebras A. Sleep and neuromuscular disorders. *Neurol Clin* 1996; **14**(4): 791–805.
203. Sivak ED, Shefner JM, Sexton J. Neuromuscular disease and hypoventilation. *Current Opinion in Pulmonary Medicine* 1999; **5**(6): 355–62.

204. Takasugi T, Ishihara T, Kawamura J, Kawashiro T. [Respiratory failure: respiratory disorder during sleep in patients with myotonic dystrophy]. *Rinsho Shinkeigaku* 1995; 35(12): 1486–8.
205. Ververs CC, Van der Meche FG, Verbraak AF, van der Sluys HC, Bogaard JM. Breathing pattern awake and asleep in myotonic dystrophy. *Respiration* 1996; 63(1): 1–7.
206. Ono S, Kurisaki H, Sakuma A, Nagao K. Myotonic dystrophy with alveolar hypoventilation and hypersomnia: a clinicopathological study. *J Neurol Sci* 1995; 128(2): 225–31.
207. Chervin RD, Aldrich MS. Sleep onset REM periods during multiple sleep latency tests in patients evaluated for sleep apnea. *Am J Respir Crit Care Med* 2000; 161(2 Pt 1): 426–31.
208. Aldrich MS, Chervin RD, Malow BA. Value of the multiple sleep latency test (MSLT) for the diagnosis of narcolepsy. *Sleep* 1997; 20(8): 620–9.
209. Dauvilliers Y, Gosselin A, Paquet J, Touchon J, Billiard M, Montplaisir J. Effect of age on MSLT results in patients with narcolepsy-cataplexy. *Neurology* 2004; 62(1): 46–50.
210. Montagna P. Fatal familial insomnia: a model disease in sleep physiopathology. *Sleep Med Rev* 2005; 9(5): 339–53.
211. Lugaresi E, Medori R, Montagna P, Baruzzi A, Cortelli P, Lugaresi A *et al*. Fatal familial insomnia and dysautonomia with selective degeneration of thalamic nuclei. *N Engl J Med* 1986; 315(16): 997–1003.
212. Cortelli P, Gambetti P, Montagna P, Lugaresi E. Fatal familial insomnia: clinical features and molecular genetics. *J Sleep Res* 1999; **8 Suppl 1:** 23–9.
213. Montagna P, Gambetti P, Cortelli P, Lugaresi E. Familial and sporadic fatal insomnia. *Lancet Neurol* 2003; 2(3): 167–76.
214. Cortelli P, Gambetti P, Montagna P, E. L. Fatal familial insomnia: clinical features and molecular genetics. *Journal of Sleep Research* 1999; 8(Suppl 1): 23–29.
215. Sundstrom DG, Dreher HM. A deadly prion disease: fatal familial insomnia. *J Neurosci Nurs* 2003; 35(6): 300–5.
216. Ancoli-Israel S. Sleep problems in older adults: putting myths to bed. *Geriatrics* 1997; 52(1): 20–30.
217. Phillips B A-IS. Sleep disorders in the elderly. *Sleep Medicine* 2001; 2: 99–114.
218. Guilleminault C, Stoohs R, Clerk A, Simmons J, Labanowski M. From obstructive sleep apnea syndrome to upper airway resistance syndrome: consistency of daytime sleepiness. *Sleep* 1992; 15(6 Suppl): S13–6.
219. Loewenstein RJ, Weingartner H, Gillin JC, Kaye W, Ebert M, Mendelson WB. Disturbances of sleep and cognitive functioning in patients with dementia. *Neurobiol Aging* 1982; 3(4): 371–7.
220. Montplaisir J, Petit D, Gauthier S, Gaudreau H, Decary A. Sleep disturbances and eeg slowing in alzheimer's disease. *Sleep Res Online* 1998; 1(4): 147–51.
221. McCurry SM, Logsdon RG, Vitiello MV, Teri L. Treatment of sleep and nighttime disturbances in Alzheimer's disease: a behavior management approach. *Sleep Med* 2004; 5(4): 373–7.
222. McCurry SM, Ancoli-Israel S. Sleep Dysfunction in Alzheimer's Disease and Other Dementias. *Curr Treat Options Neurol* 2003; 5(3): 261–272.
223. Chokroverty S, Jankovic J. Restless legs syndrome: a disease in search of identity. *Neurology* 1999; 52(5): 907–10.
224. Reynolds CF, 3rd, Kupfer DJ, Hoch CC, Sewitch DE. Sleeping pills for the elderly: are they ever justified? *J Clin Psychiatry* 1985; 46(2 Pt 2): 9–12.
225. Avidan AY. Sleep changes and disorders in the elderly patient. *Curr Neurol Neurosci Rep* 2002; 2(2): 178–85.
226. Gurian B, Rosowsky E. Low-dose methylphenidate in the very old. *J Geriatr Psychiatry Neurol* 1990; 3(3): 152–4.
227. Pollak CP, Perlick D. Sleep problems and institutionalization of the elderly. *J Geriatr Psychiatry Neurol* 1991; 4(4): 204–10.
228. Guilleminault C, Briskin JG, Greenfield MS, Silvestri R. The impact of autonomic nervous system dysfunction on breathing during sleep. *Sleep* 1981; 4(3): 263–78.

5 Insomnia in Aging

Octavio Choi and Michael R. Irwin

UCLA Semel Institute of Neuroscience, Los Angeles, California, U.S.A.

INTRODUCTION

Insomnia is a major public health problem that affects millions of individuals world-wide. In addition to reduced quality of life, chronic insomniacs suffer higher rates of medical and psychiatric morbidity and are higher utilizers of healthcare services (1). Estimates of direct and indirect costs of insomnia run in the tens of billions of dollars (2). How many people suffer from insomnia? What are the risk factors associated with it? How does aging affect sleep? How does insomnia affect our health?

This chapter will provide a broad overview of insomnia in aging, divided into three sections. The first section will review the epidemiologic literature as it relates to insomnia and aging. As we will discuss, older people suffer from higher rates of insomnia, and much of this increase appears to be related to the development of medical comorbidities that interfere with sleep. The second section will provide a conceptual approach to the diagnostic assessment of insomnia in the elderly. Many of the most common insomnia-related conditions in the aged population will be reviewed. As most cases of insomnia in this population are associated with comorbid psychiatric and medical illness, a thorough evaluation of insomnia in older adults requires a systematic consideration of related comorbidities. Finally, the third and last section will discuss the health and quality of life consequences of insomnia in the older adult. The presence of insomnia is thought to exacerbate numerous health conditions including psychiatric illness, obesity, and pain syndromes, which together emphasize the clinical importance of diagnostic ascertainment and treatment of insomnia in older adults.

EPIDEMIOLOGY AND CLASSIFICATION

Insomnia Prevalence in the General Population

Epidemiologic studies that attempt to ascertain the prevalence of insomnia in the general population have reported widely varying results that range from 6% to 48% (1). Much of this variation is due to the use of differing definitions of insomnia from study to study. In general, newer studies use more precise and stringent definitions of insomnia, which, as expected, result in lower prevalence rates. As proposed by Ohayon (1) in his 2002 review article, it is useful to conceptualize epidemiologic studies of insomnia as belonging to one of four different categories, which in a sense reflects the evolution of insomnia definitions over time:

1. studies that define insomnia by the presence of insomnia symptoms, such as difficulty initiating or maintaining sleep, which report prevalence rates of 30% to 48% in the general population;

2. studies that define insomnia by the presence of insomnia symptoms and daytime consequences, which report prevalence rates of 9% to 15%;
3. studies that define insomnia by subjective dissatisfaction with sleep quality, which report prevalence rates of 8% to 18%; and
4. studies that define insomnia by diagnosis using a formal classification system, such as the Diagnostic and Statistical Manual of Mental Disorders, fourth edition (DSM-IV), resulting in prevalence rates of 4.4% to 6.4%.

The first group encompasses older epidemiologic studies which detect insomnia simply by the presence of various symptoms, such as difficulty initiating sleep (DIS), difficulty in maintaining sleep (DMS), or early morning awakening (EMA). A representative study of this era is the 1979 study by Bixler et al. (3) of 1006 adults, which reported an insomnia prevalence rate of 32.2% in the general Los Angeles population. Subjects were simply asked whether they had trouble falling asleep, woke up during the night, or woke up too early in the morning. For this study, a positive response to any of these questions indicated the presence of insomnia. One limitation with this approach is that it may overestimate the prevalence of clinically significant insomnia, as it includes people who may suffer from insomnia only occasionally, or experience only mild symptoms. For example, subsequent studies attempted to further refine the notion of insomnia to include frequency and severity criteria. If insomnia is defined as insomnia symptoms (DIS, DMS, or EMA) occurring three or more times per week, prevalence rates drop to 16% to 21%. Similarly, if insomnia is defined as "great or very great difficulty" in initiating or maintaining sleep, prevalence rates drop to 10% to 28% (1).

The second group encompasses newer studies which further restrict the definition of insomnia to require the presence of insomnia symptoms (such as DIS, DMS, or EMA) as well as daytime functional impairment, such as daytime sleepiness, irritability, and trouble concentrating. These studies report prevalence rates ranging from 9% to 15% and averaging around 10% in the general population (1). As will be discussed in more detail later, the presence of clinically significant daytime impairment is a key criterion in establishing a diagnosis of insomnia in all modern sleep disorder classification systems.

The third group of studies has focused on an alternative definition of insomnia, requiring only the report of a subjective sense of dissatisfaction with sleep quality, with the consequence of feeling unrested upon awakening. These studies report prevalence rates similar to the second group, 8% to 18%. Note that this is a relatively recent definition, and there is still some controversy among sleep experts over whether individuals with this complaint share similar pathophysiologic mechanisms with insomniacs as defined in the first two groups (2). For example, patients with obstructive sleep apnea (OSA) may have severely disrupted sleep due to multiple apneic episodes throughout the night, but are often unaware of this, and thus tend to answer "no" when asked whether they have difficulty falling or staying asleep at night. These subjects would thus be categorized as noninsomniacs in the first two groups. However, they would tend to be included in the third group, as most patients suffering from this condition report waking up feeling unrested (4). Despite this controversy, however, there is a general consensus that a subjective sense of sleep dissatisfaction is a useful marker of insomnia, and it is included in the diagnostic criteria for insomnia under the DSM-IV classification system as the criterion of "nonrestorative sleep."

The fourth and last group of studies attempts to ascertain the prevalence of insomnia diagnoses using formal classification systems. The development of modern classification systems for insomnia reflects the evolving understanding that insomnia is a constellation of symptoms that may be part of a larger disease process or a diagnosis in its own right, according to specific inclusion and exclusion criteria. These systems recognize that insomnia symptoms frequently occur within the context of comorbid mental and physical illnesses, a point that will be discussed in more detail later in this chapter.

Because some patients with insomnia symptoms end up categorized with a noninsomnia diagnosis, studies that use classification systems report lower prevalence rates of insomnia diagnoses (4.4–6.4%), compared with studies that simply report prevalence of insomnia symptoms (1). This is beautifully illustrated in Ohayon's (5) 1997 epidemiologic study, which was the first study that attempted to estimate prevalence of insomnia diagnoses using a modern classification system, the DSM-IV. In this study, a representative sample of 5622 adults in the general population in France were each given an extensive structured interview. Interviewers were guided by a computer expert system that had been shown in previous studies to accurately diagnose DSM-IV disorders related to insomnia. In addition to insomnia symptoms, subjects were queried about the presence of medical conditions, substance use, breathing disorders, and mental disorders. If any of these conditions were present, further questions were asked, using a rule-based reasoning process similar to the differential diagnosis applied by a psychiatrist, and a final DSM-IV diagnosis reached.

For this study, an "insomnia complaint" was defined as the presence of insomnia symptoms and a subjective sense of dissatisfaction with sleep quality. Insomnia symptoms queried were DIS or DMS, EMA with inability to resume sleep, or a complaint of nonrestorative sleep in spite of normal sleep duration (NRS). By this definition, 18.6% of this population had an insomnia complaint. When duration of complaint was assessed, 15.3% of the sample experienced these symptoms for greater than one month. When daytime functional impairment was taken into account, the prevalence dropped further to 12.7%. Finally, when all relevant diagnostic information was applied, only 5.6% of the population met criteria for a formal insomnia diagnosis. The most common insomnia diagnoses were "insomnia related to a mental disorder" (2.9%), "primary insomnia" (1.3%), and insomnia related to a general medical condition (0.5%). Of the sample, 7.4% met criteria for an insomnia complaint with functional impairment, but did not end up with an insomnia diagnosis; instead, they were diagnosed with disorders that have insomnia as one of their core symptoms, such as major depression.

Risk Factors for Insomnia

Epidemiologic studies have uncovered numerous risk factors for insomnia, a few among them are female gender, advancing age, social isolation (divorced/widowed/separated), low socioeconomic status, unemployment, drug use (alcohol or illicit substances), medication use, and medical and psychiatric comorbidities. Many of these risk factors have been extensively reviewed elsewhere (1). However, several of these risk factors deserve further discussion in this chapter. First, the issue of medical and psychiatric risk factors will be discussed. As most cases of insomnia occur within the context of comorbid illnesses, it is essential for the clinician concerned with insomnia to be aware of these comorbidities so they can be diagnosed and treated, with consequent impacts on insomnia symptoms. Associated physical illness is especially prevalent in the elderly and is a major contributing factor to insomnia in this age group; this will also be discussed later in this chapter.

Insomnia Comorbidities

One of the most robust findings in the sleep literature is that the majority of those with insomnia suffer from comorbid physical and mental illnesses, which are presumed to contribute to insomnia (1,2,5). The 1979 study by Bixler et al. (3) revealed that 53% of respondents with insomnia symptoms reported suffering from a "recurring health problem," and 33% reported "needing help for emotional problems" in the previous year, both significantly higher than noninsomniacs. Subsequent studies have consistently reported that insomniacs suffer from physical and mental ailments at higher rates than persons without insomnia (6–8).

It should be noted that when discussing medical and psychiatric conditions contributing to insomnia, sleep specialists are moving away from the term "secondary," preferring instead the term "comorbid." This change reflects an appreciation for the fact that with most diseases associated with sleep disorders, especially mental illness, causality is unclear and complex. For example, insomnia may be an antecedent of major depressive disorder, or may develop after depressive symptoms (7,9). In addition, insomnia may persist after all other depressive symptoms remit, suggesting that once established, other factors, such as psychologic conditioning, may perpetuate it. In such cases, it would be inaccurate to label the insomnia as "secondary" to the major depression, and treatment of major depression alone (for example, with an antidepressant) would not be adequate for alleviation of insomnia. This is an important clinical issue, for the presence of insomnia alone is a major risk factor for future depressive relapse (9–12). Hence, among clinicians, the term "insomnia secondary to" may focus treatment efforts on the comorbid illness, which has the potential to lead ultimately to under-treatment of insomnia itself. Because of these concerns, as noted earlier, the emerging consensus among sleep experts is to move away from terms such as "secondary," to the more accurate term "comorbid" (2).

Insomnia and Psychiatric Illness

Cross-sectional surveys of insomnia and mental health symptoms have reported that 30% to 60% of those with insomnia symptoms have an associated mental disorder, compared with around 15% for persons without insomnia (5,6,7,9). The most frequently associated mental disorder is major depressive disorder, followed by generalized anxiety disorder. Viewed another way, over 80% of those with major depression, and over 90% of those with anxiety disorders suffer from insomnia (1). Surveys of individuals with chronic insomnia report that insomnia related to major depression is the most common single diagnosis (13). Multivariate logistical regression models indicate that the presence of depression is the strongest single factor predicting insomnia (6). In fact, this study revealed that insomnia is more strongly associated with major depression than with any other medical disorder, with relative risk two to three times greater than that for all other medical conditions surveyed.

Longitudinal studies have established that insomnia in the absence of psychiatric symptoms is a risk factor for the later development of major depression, in both young (11) and aged populations (10,12), with odds ratios ranging from 3 to 4. The risk for developing major depression is significantly higher when insomnia is chronic. Ford and Kamerow (9) reported that when insomnia was present for over one year, there was a 40-fold increased risk for developing a major depressive episode in that year. Interestingly, time sequence analyses have shown that insomnia symptoms precede the onset of depressive symptoms in the majority of cases (7).

From a pathophysiologic viewpoint, the mechanisms by which depression and insomnia influence each other remain unclear, but sleep-endocrine studies suggest that the hypothalamic–pituitary–adrenal (HPA) stress axis may be involved. In general, there is an emerging conceptual model of insomnia as a disorder of physiologic and emotional hyperarousal throughout the 24-hour sleep–wake cycle (14). Consistent with this model are studies that show that both insomniacs and depressed subjects have increased activity of the HPA axis as reflected by increased 24-hour circulating levels of the stress hormones ACTH and cortisol (15). Normal sleep-deprived subjects do not show this effect (16). As activation of the HPA axis is known to be arousing (17), this may be a unifying mechanism that links insomnia and depression. Similarly, patients with either depression or insomnia show an activation of sympathetic nervous system activity (18) and increases in sympathetic arousal mechanisms are implicated in insomnia onset and perpetuation (19). Further studies are needed to determine whether HPA axis and/or sympathetic activation are mechanisms that drive insomnia, or are simply state markers.

Taken as a whole, the data emphasize the clinical importance of ruling out psychiatric comorbidity in patients presenting with insomnia. Clinicians should be especially vigilant for depression, as older persons are subject to psychosocial factors that increase risk for depression, including retirement, social isolation, bereavement, and widowhood (8). Although not yet directly proven, these data also suggest that targeted treatment of insomnia, even in the absence of psychiatric symptoms, may reduce the risk of developing future depressive episodes. Sleep problems associated with mental illness are discussed in more detail in Chapter 3.

Insomnia and Medical Illness

Epidemiologic studies have consistently reported that insomniacs suffer from medical illnesses at higher rates than do persons without insomnia. As mentioned earlier, the 1979 survey by Bixler et al. (3) of the general population in Los Angeles revealed that about half of respondents with insomnia symptoms reported suffering from a "recurring health problem," significantly higher than those who do not have insomnia symptoms. In addition, compared with persons without insomnia, individuals with insomnia symptoms experienced more multiple health problems, were hospitalized more often, and for longer periods of time. A more recent study by Bixler et al. (6) of a general population in Pennsylvania replicated these findings and, using multivariate regression models, reported that colitis, hypertension, anemia, ulcers, and cancer were the medical conditions most highly associated with insomnia and/or sleep difficulties among the conditions the study surveyed. Ohayon's (5) 1997 study found that in those diagnosed with insomnia due to a general medical condition, the most frequent medical conditions were airway diseases such as asthma, and chronic pain conditions such as arthritis and back pain. A survey of older adults conducted by the National Sleep Foundation revealed a greater prevalence of insomnia in those suffering from hypertension, heart disease, arthritis, and lung disease (20). Other medical conditions associated with insomnia are heart failure, gastrointestinal disorders such as gastroesophageal reflux disease (GERD), neurodegenerative conditions such as dementia and Parkinson's disease, and stroke (2,20). Finally, it should be noted that there are a variety of physiologic disorders that frequently give rise to disordered sleep but are not considered "insomnia due to a general medical condition" under the DSM-IV classification system. These disorders are commonly collectively referred to as the *primary sleep disorders* and include breathing-related sleep disorders (OSA, central sleep apnea, hypoventilation syndrome), circadian rhythm sleep disorders, narcolepsy, restless legs syndrome (RLS), and periodic limb movement disorder (PLMD).

The strong cross-sectional association between insomnia and medical illness suggests that medical illness may play a role in the development or perpetuation of insomnia, although prospective data testing this hypothesized causal link are limited. What are the possible mechanisms by which medical disorders may affect sleep? For some disorders, the mechanisms appear straightforward. Obstruction of regular breathing due to airway disease, heart failure (resulting in pulmonary edema), or breathing-related sleep disorders can obviously interfere with a good night's rest. Hyperarousal due to pain/discomfort appears to be the unifying cause for insomnia in many diverse medical conditions, such as arthritis, gastrointestinal disease, RLS, and PLMD. In other disorders, the causal pathways, if present, are less clear. Hypertension may be a reflection of autonomic hyperarousal which would interfere with sleep (14). In cancer, insomnia may be the result of multiple factors, such as the anxiety engendered by a cancer diagnosis, and pain/discomfort engendered by both the cancer and the cancer treatments such as chemotherapy and radiation therapy (21). Disordered sleep due to neurologic conditions is often due to a complex variety of causes including degeneration of sleep-regulating brain centers, disordered respiration, drug treatment side effects, and the absence of a clear day/night light cues in institutionalized patients (20,22).

As will be further discussed in the next section, medical comorbidity is an especially prominent issue in the elderly. The increasing prevalence of medical illness with age is thought to account for much of the increasing prevalence of insomnia in the elderly.

Insomnia and Aging

Numerous studies have documented a positive correlation between insomnia symptoms and advancing age, with prevalence rates reaching close to 50% in elderly individuals (defined as >65 years old), depending on the definition of insomnia used (1). In a representative study, the 1979 survey Bixler et al. of 1006 adults in the Los Angeles area reported an increasing incidence of insomnia symptoms (difficulty falling asleep, staying asleep, or early morning awakening) with age: 23% for 18 to 30 year olds, 37% for 31 to 50 year olds, and 40% for those older than 51 years. The composite rate for all age groups was reported to be 32.2% (3).

Ohayon's (5) 1997 study of 5622 adults in the French population reported a similar relationship of insomnia with age, with prevalence rates starting at 12.5% for 15 to 24 year olds, and rising to 29.4% in those more than 65 years old, as shown in Figure 1. Ohayon's numbers are smaller than Bixler's due to a more stringent definition of insomnia which required presence of insomnia symptoms as well as a subjective sense of sleep dissatisfaction. Consistent with other studies (1), females

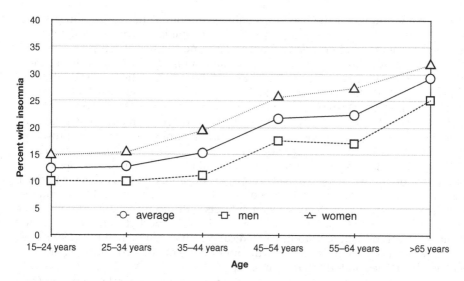

FIGURE 1 Increasing prevalence of insomnia with age. *Source*: Adapted from Table 1 and Ref. 5.

had higher prevalence rates of insomnia at all age points studied, with an average ratio of 1.4:1.

Although the prevalence of insomnia *symptoms* increases with advancing age, the relationship between age and insomnia *diagnoses* is less clear, with some studies reporting a stable prevalence with age and others reporting an increasing prevalence with age [reviewed in Ref. (1)]. Taken as a whole, the rate of insomnia diagnoses appears to be stable between age 15 and 45, increase from age 45 to 65, and remain stable after age 65 (1). Interestingly, this correlates well with sleep polysomnography studies, which indicate that sleep architecture in healthy subjects begins to change starting in early adulthood and becomes relatively constant after the age of 60. Age-related changes include decreases in sleep efficiency, decreases in percentage of slow-wave and rapid eye movement (REM) sleep, decreases in REM latency, and increases in percentage of stage 1 and stage 2 sleep (23).

What accounts for the discrepancy between insomnia symptoms and insomnia diagnoses in terms of prevalence rates with age? Although the reasons are not known, several factors should be considered. For example, older people often report more sleep complaints, such as nighttime awakenings, but these complaints are often not associated with daytime functional impairment, a necessary criterion for an insomnia diagnosis. Hence, many of these older adults receive a diagnosis of "dyssomnia not otherwise specified" rather than insomnia (5). Additionally, older adults often suffer from a higher prevalence of nocturia, which may result in multiple nighttime awakenings. However, without difficulty falling back asleep, daytime functional consequences are minimal (24). Finally, many elderly suffer from insomnia symptoms resulting from the so-called "primary sleep disorders" that are conceptualized as noninsomnia diagnoses within the DSM-IV classification system, such as circadian rhythm shift disorder, breathing-related sleep disorder, and limb movement disorders (5). The prevalence rates of all these conditions increases sharply with age (20).

What accounts for the rise in insomnia symptoms with age? It appears that most, if not all, of the increased prevalence of insomnia symptoms in the elderly is due to the increasing prevalence of medical comorbidities in this population. In 2004, Foley et al. (25) surveyed 1506 older adults (aged 55–84 years) in the general U.S. population as part of the National Sleep Foundation's 2003 "Sleep in America" poll. Participants were asked to report medical and psychiatric conditions, as well as a self-perceived quality of sleep. When comparing 55 to 64-year-old and >65-year-old groups, they found that the older group reported significantly more heart disease, hypertension, arthritis, cancer, stroke, and enlarged prostates. Whereas 25% of the 55 to 64 year olds reported no medical conditions, only 12.8% of those older than 65 years reported no medical conditions, a statistically significant difference between the two age groups. In addition, this study demonstrated a significant inverse relationship between the number of medical conditions and the self-perceived quality of sleep. Among subjects with no medical conditions, 54% reported an "excellent" quality of sleep, and only 10% reported "fair/poor" quality of sleep. For those with one to three medical conditions, 42% had excellent sleep, and 22% fair/poor sleep. For those with four or more medical conditions, only 32% had excellent sleep and 41% fair/poor sleep.

This work confirmed an earlier study in the elderly general population (24), which found a significant correlation between age and number of medical symptoms. Interestingly, using multivariable regression models, insomnia rates were not correlated with age among the elderly (those >65 years old), after controlling for health status. In other words, age was not a significant independent variable in predicting sleep complaints in the elderly; rather, declines in physical and mental health predicted insomnia.

Taken as a whole, the data indicate that the elderly suffer from higher rates of insomnia symptoms compared with younger subjects, and much of this appears to be due to increasing medical comorbidity with age. Indeed, despite the normal age-related changes in sleep architecture mentioned earlier, healthy elderly appear to sleep as well as young adults. The prevalence of primary insomnia diagnoses (that is, insomnia without medical, psychiatric, or neurologic comorbidities) is the same in elderly and young adults (5). Thus, when insomnia is detected in the elderly, it is incumbent upon the clinician to diagnose thoroughly and treat medical, psychiatric, and neurologic comorbidities that may be interfering with sleep.

DIAGNOSIS AND EVALUATION

As discussed in the previous sections, sleep disturbance is a common problem in the elderly. In this section, we will present a systematic approach to the diagnosis and evaluation of insomnia in the elderly, which takes into account the fact that the vast majority of insomnia symptoms in the elderly occur in the context of comorbid health conditions. Using the DSM-IV criteria for the diagnosis of primary insomnia as a guide, our proposed approach will systematically investigate and rule out the most common medical and psychiatric illnesses that contribute to insomnia, as well as consider other common causes of insomnia in the elderly.

Although numerous diagnostic tools are available to the clinician, the most important ones are a detailed clinical interview and physical examination, the goals of which are to identify medical and psychiatric comorbidities, and to generate a differential diagnosis. Often it will be important to interview not only the patient

---

Box 1 DSM-IV Diagnostic Criteria for Primary Insomnia

1. The predominant complaint is difficulty initiating or maintaining sleep, or nonrestorative sleep, for at least one month.
2. The sleep disturbance (or associated daytime fatigue) causes clinically significant distress or impairment in social, occupational, or other important areas of functioning.
3. The sleep disturbance does not occur exclusively during the course of narcolepsy, breathing-related sleep disorder, circadian rhythm sleep disorder, or a parasomnia.
4. The disturbance does not occur exclusively during the course of another mental disorder (e.g., major depressive disorder, generalized anxiety disorder, a delirium).
5. The disturbance is not due to the direct physiologic effects of a substance (e.g., a drug of abuse, a medication) or a general medical condition.

Source: from Ref. 87.

---

but his or her caregiver, who may be more aware of sleep disturbances during the night, as well as symptoms such as snoring, of which the patient may be unaware. In certain cases, additional testing has been shown to be helpful in ascertaining a definitive diagnosis. For example, multichannel sleep polysomnography studies can confirm diagnoses of primary sleep disorders such as sleep apneas, and sleep diaries can be helpful to detect circadian rhythm disorders. Wrist actigraphs, which measure nighttime movements, can be helpful to objectively document sleep/wake cycles, but clinicians should be aware that their use has not yet been fully validated for chronic insomnia (2).

In general, there is a strong need for validated diagnostic tools that are easy to administer, cross-culturally robust, and that can reliably measure the severity of sleep disturbance. Unfortunately, although various sleep questionnaires have been developed in response to this need, these instruments thus far suffer from lack of standardization, and most lack studies that demonstrate validity and reliability (2).

The diagnostic criteria for the DSM-IV diagnosis of primary insomnia are a useful guide for the clinician wishing to investigate sleep disturbances (see Box 1). "Primary insomnia" under the DSM-IV system is a diagnosis given to patients with insomnia symptoms, with clinically significant daytime functional impairment, and for which no medical comorbidity, psychiatric comorbidity, or primary sleep disorder can be found. Thus, diagnosing primary insomnia involves a systematic investigation to rule out various identifiable causes of sleep disturbance.

Following the criteria, firstly, the clinician must ascertain if the patient has a complaint of difficulty initiating or maintaining sleep, or has a complaint of nonrestorative sleep, lasting for at least one month. Secondly, the sleep disturbance must cause "clinically significant distress or impairment" during the day. The following are useful screening questions:

1. Do you have trouble falling asleep or staying asleep at night?
2. Does this cause problems for you during the day?
3. Do you feel extremely sleepy during the day or have trouble staying awake?

Once the presence of insomnia symptoms has been established with the first two criteria, the rest of the criteria guide us in ruling out various sleep-related conditions and comorbidities. The third criterion requires the clinician to rule out primary sleep disorders (which include narcolepsy, breathing-related sleep disorders, and circadian rhythm sleep disorders) and parasomnias.

Narcolepsy is a poorly understood disorder that is characterized by excessive sleepiness and is typically associated with cataplexy and REM sleep parasomnias, such as sleep paralysis and hypnagogic hallucinations. Polysomnographic studies can be useful in establishing a definitive diagnosis.

Breathing-related sleep disorders include OSA, central sleep apnea, and central alveolar hypoventilation syndrome. As a whole, breathing-related sleep disorders are much more common in the elderly. The prevalence in middle-aged adults (30–60 years old) is 4% to 9%, as compared with 45% to 62% in adults older than 60 (20). OSA, which is the most common breathing-related sleep disorder, is characterized by a distinctive snoring pattern caused by intermittent airway collapse, and consists of loud snores or brief gasps that alternate with episodes of silence lasting 20 to 30 seconds. During this time, respiration ceases and leads to sleep arousals, presumably due to arterial oxygen desaturation. Often the patient will not be aware of his or her snoring, and unaware of nighttime arousals, with the predominant complaint being excessive daytime sleepiness. In these cases, interviewing the patient's spouse or caregiver can be very useful. Sleep polysomnography studies can be helpful in establishing the diagnosis of breathing-related sleep disorders. Treatment of the breathing disorder can lead to resolution of sleep disturbances.

Circadian rhythm disorders are also quite common in the elderly. Of the various types, the most common in the elderly is called advanced sleep phase syndrome (ASPS) under the International Classification of Sleep Disorders, 2nd edition (ICSD-II) classification system (under the DSM-IV system, it is subsumed under the heading of "Circadian rhythm sleep disorder, unspecified type"). In this syndrome, patients have an advancement of their sleep/wake cycle such that they tend to fall asleep earlier and wake earlier than usual. Sleep diaries can be helpful in establishing this diagnosis. Interestingly, the increasing prevalence of this syndrome with age may be due in part to degeneration of neural circadian pacemakers such as the suprachiasmatic nucleus (20). Note that ASPS is not a medical disorder but rather a natural consequence of aging, and does not necessarily need to be treated unless it is causing discomfort in the patient's life. When indicated, treatment for this condition involves exposing patients to bright light (>10,000 lux) in late afternoon/early evening, which can shift circadian rhythms, so that patients feel sleepy later in the day.

RLS and PLMD are two primary sleep disorders that are not directly addressed in the DSM-IV criteria, but are important to the clinician, as prevalence increases with age to the point where it is quite common in the elderly. For example, the prevalence of PLMD in young adults is 5% to 6%, rising to 45% in older adults (20). Technically, both of these disorders are categorized in the DSM-IV system in the "dyssomnia not otherwise specified" category. PLMD is characterized by clusters of repeated limb jerks that lead to brief awakenings, of which the patient may not be aware. Additional information from the spouse or caregiver can be helpful in establishing this diagnosis. The primary complaint is usually unrefreshing sleep and daytime sleepiness. RLS is a disorder characterized by disagreeable leg sensations that occur at bedtime and interfere with sleep onset. The sensations are frequently described as "tingling," "crawling," and "aching," and are temporarily relieved by moving the legs. About 80% of patients with RLS have PLMS, and 30% with PLMS have RLS (20). There is controversy regarding whether PLMD and RLS represent two different disorders or are two different manifestations of the same underlying disorder. Although poorly understood, the dopaminergic system appears to be involved, as treatment with dopaminergic agonists such as pramipexole are effective (20).

Parasomnias are disorders that intrude into the sleep process but are not primarily disorders of sleep and wake states per se. Usually, they involve abnormal behavioral or physiologic events during sleep–wake transitions. Parasomnia diagnoses include sleep terror disorder, sleepwalking disorder, and REM-behavior sleep disorder (RBD). RBD is quite rare, but clinically relevant in the older population, as prevalence increases with age, affecting mostly men in their 60s or 70s. It is characterized by intermittent failure of sleep paralysis during REM sleep, often leading to violent motor activity related to dream mentation. Interestingly, RBD typically precedes the development of neurodegenerative conditions such as Parkinson's disease and Lewy body disease, suggesting that RBD represents the earliest clinical manifestation of an evolving neurodegenerative disorder (20).

The fourth criteria requires ruling out psychiatric comorbidities, especially major depression, which is the most common single diagnosis in individuals with insomnia (13). Clinicians should inquire whether their patients have been feeling sad or anxious, and whether they have risk factors for depression such as retirement, social isolation and bereavement. As mentioned earlier, because of the complex causal relationship between insomnia with mood disorders, treatment often involves treating both the mood disorder (e.g. with antidepressants) and insomnia symptoms (e.g. with hypnotics). Insomnia that persists after remission of depression substantially increases the risk of depressive relapse (9).

A further consideration about the relationship between insomnia and depression should also be noted. In patients who present with both symptoms of insomnia and major depression, under the DSM-IV system, two diagnostic pathways are possible. The first is simply a diagnosis of major depression, which features insomnia as one of its core symptoms. The other involves giving two separate diagnoses, one of major depression (to account for depressive symptoms), and the other of "insomnia related to another mental disorder" (in this case, major depression). How does the clinician choose which diagnosis is more appropriate for a given situation? The answer depends on the relative importance of insomnia symptoms compared with the rest of the depressive symptomatology. Patients that complain mostly about insomnia symptoms tend to see their depression as arising from the insomnia, and feel that if their insomnia resolved, their depression would resolve as well. Hence, clinicians would be inclined to diagnose insomnia, specifically "insomnia related to major depression," in addition to a separate "major depression" diagnosis. On the other hand, other patients may feel that their depressive symptoms are predominant and would tend to view their insomnia as arising from the depression. In this instance, clinicians would likely diagnose "major depression" without providing a separate diagnosis for insomnia.

The fifth criterion requires that the clinician rule out general medical conditions, medications, and drugs of abuse as contributing factors to insomnia. As discussed earlier, medical conditions are frequently associated with insomnia symptoms and in many cases are thought to play a role in causing or aggravating insomnia. Thus, it is imperative that the clinician first identify and treat medical comorbidities. Numerous medical conditions have been associated with insomnia (see the "Insomnia and Medical Illness" section of this chapter). Conceptually, they may be categorized as illnesses that give rise to respiratory distress (asthma, chronic obstructive pulmonary disease, pulmonary edema secondary to heart failure), pain (arthritis, rheumatic disease, musculoskeletal pain, chronic pain, heart disease, GERD, diabetes, malignancy), and neurodegenerative conditions (dementia, Parkinson's disease, stroke). Hypertension has also been linked to insomnia in the elderly, perhaps as a marker for autonomic hyperarousal, or as a consequence of activating anti-hypertensive medications. In older men especially, nocturia secondary to prostate conditions may be a prominent cause of difficulty maintaining sleep; reduced fluid intake before sleep may be helpful in these cases. Older women may be prone to postmenopausal hot flashes that may interfere with sleep. Despite optimal management of medical conditions, separate treatment for insomnia symptoms may also be necessary, a topic that is discussed in detail elsewhere in this book.

Numerous medications are thought to interfere with sleep. Activating medications include central nervous system stimulants, beta blockers, bronchodilators, calcium channel blockers, corticosteroids, decongestants, diuretics, stimulating antidepressants, and thyroid hormones (8). Changing the timing of administration of stimulating medications to earlier in the day will often improve sleep at night. The clinician should also assess for substance use. Caffeine and cigarette use both interfere with sleep (1), and their use should be minimized. As caffeine has a half-life from 3 to 10 hours (averaging 5 hours), caffeine intake should be restricted to earlier in the day. It may be important to remind patients that caffeine is found not only in coffee but in decaffeinated coffee, teas, and sodas.

The clinician should be aware that many people suffering from insomnia will use alcohol at night to help them sleep. Alcohol is a central nervous system depressant that does accelerate sleep onset. However, due to its short half-life, blood levels rapidly drop, causing awakening of sleep later in the night. In addition, there is rapid tolerance, such that prolonged use of alcohol at bedtime loses its effects on sleep onset, but sleep disruption remains (1). Patients should be counseled that the use of alcohol at night is counterproductive to good sleep and given other, more effective treatment options.

According to DSM-IV criteria, if a psychiatric, medical, neurologic, or medication- or substance-related cause for insomnia is not found, a diagnosis of "primary insomnia" is established. This is an atheoretical category that does not suggest a specific etiology for insomnia. It may be helpful at this point for the clinician to consider subcategories that are suggested by the more detailed ICSD-II classification system (22). Because diagnoses under the ICSD-II system have proposed pathophysiologies, specific treatments can then be considered. It should be noted, however, that the existence of many of the ICSD-II's more narrowly defined categories as distinct disease entities is controversial and for this reason have not yet been adopted in the DSM-IV system (26). The interested reader can learn more about these different classifications in the appendix at the end of this chapter.

When sleep experts were asked to diagnose insomniacs using both ICSD-II and DSM-IV classification systems, patients with primary insomnia (under the DSM-IV system) were most frequently categorized under the more detailed ICSD-II system as having psychophysiologic insomnia or inadequate sleep hygiene disorder (27). Psychophysiologic insomnia is thought to arise from learned associations that interfere with sleep. For example, patients that experience chronic insomnia due to a medical illness are likely to learn that poor sleep occurs in their bed, and the bed becomes a conditioned cue for poor sleep. Thus, even if the medical illness is fully resolved, patients may continue to suffer from insomnia due to this negative conditioning. Additional factors can perpetuate insomnia; for example, insomnia due to inadequate sleep hygiene is thought to arise from a variety of maladaptive voluntary behaviors that interfere with sleep at night, which include napping during the day, maintaining inconsistent sleep–wake times, and engaging in activities in bed other than sleeping or sex.

For patients suspected of having sleep hygiene and/or psychophysiologic insomnia, cognitive behavioral therapy (CBT) for insomnia may be especially helpful. CBT for insomnia, which combines stimulus control, sleep restriction, sleep hygiene, and cognitive restructuring, has been found to be at least as effective as prescription medications for the treatment of chronic insomnia (28), with an efficacy in older adults comparable to the benefits reported in middle-aged adults (29). For example, when temazepam was compared with CBT for the management of chronic, primary insomnia in the elderly, both treatments were found effective when measured at eight weeks. However, only the CBT groups (CBT alone, or CBT in combination with temazepam) maintained their clinical gains at 3, 12, and 24 month follow-ups (30). The NIH noted in its "state of the science" consensus statement (2) that while prescription hypnotics were found to be efficacious in the short-term management of insomnia, little data existed supporting long-term benefits. In addition, prescription hypnotics are associated with numerous side effects, including residual daytime sedation, cognitive impairment, and motor incoordination. As CBT does not appear to produce adverse effects, clinicians may wish to consider it as a more effective and potentially less harmful intervention for primary insomnia. The major drawback for CBT is the length of time needed, typically six to eight 50-minute sessions. However, abbreviated CBT, consisting of only two 25-minute sessions, has been shown to be highly effective and may be a more practical option for many patients (31).

HEALTH AND QUALITY OF LIFE CONSEQUENCES OF INSOMNIA IN THE OLDER ADULT

Thus far in this chapter we have emphasized the importance of medical and psychiatric comorbidities contributing to insomnia. Is the relationship bidirectional? That is, does insomnia negatively impact medical and psychiatric conditions? As discussed earlier, this clearly appears to be the case for psychiatric conditions. For example, insomniacs without depression are at much higher risk for the development of later depressive episodes (9). In the remainder of this chapter we will review evidence from a large variety of sources that supports the hypothesis that chronic insomnia has serious implications for quality of life and medical illness, especially in the elderly. First we will review economic studies that attempt to measure the public health burden of insomnia. These studies show that insomniacs utilize health care services more frequently than noninsomniacs, have poorer work performance, and are more often absent from work. These results will be put in the context of evidence that insomnia impairs daytime functioning, especially in the elderly, and of evidence that insomnia leads to increased risk of mortality and morbidity. Finally, the chapter will conclude with an investigation of several possible mechanisms by which sleep disturbances may lead to increased mortality and morbidity, which include the production of proinflammatory cytokines, increased activity of the sympathetic nervous system, and endocrine disturbances that lead to the development of glucose intolerance, obesity, and metabolic syndrome.

One of the challenges in determining the contribution of insomnia to health conditions is disentangling the role of insomnia per se from the comorbidities that usually accompany it. As reviewed earlier, chronic insomniacs as a population are sicker than noninsomniacs because insomnia usually occurs in the context of medical or psychiatric illness. How can we determine if differences between insomniacs and noninsomniacs are due to sleep disturbances or from comorbidities? The typical way this is handled in epidemiologic studies is by matching insomnia subjects with control subjects with the same level of medical and psychiatric illness, along with matching other variables such as age and gender. The reader should keep in mind that if insomnia does indeed worsen health conditions, this matching process will tend to underestimate the impact of insomnia on mortality and morbidity, as it masks differences in health status that may in fact be due to insomnia. Most of the studies that will be discussed here are cross-sectional epidemiologic studies that are subject to this potential underestimation bias. As a field, there is a strong need for more long-term prospective studies, which are less susceptible to this bias, as well as for interventional laboratory studies, which can more directly support causality.

Public Health Burden

Economists attempt to measure the economic impact of insomnia by considering direct and indirect costs. Direct costs reflect charges for medical care, which include the cost of doctor's visits, hospitalizations, emergency room visits, and treatments such as prescription medications. Indirect costs reflect charges that result from insomnia-related morbidity and mortality. In a sense, it attempts to measure the economic impact of functional impairments suffered by insomniacs. Examples of such costs would include costs related to decreased productivity at work, absenteeism, errors made at work, disability payments, and accidents on and off the job.

Numerous studies have established that insomniacs utilize the health care system at higher rates than noninsomniacs. In a survey of 1100 managed care enrollees in the United States, Hatoum et al. (32) found that individuals reporting insomnia had significantly more emergency room visits, more calls to the doctor, and more use of over-the-counter drugs than those without insomnia. This finding held constant even after controlling for demographic variables and medical and psychiatric comorbidities. Insomniacs also reported significantly worse health-related quality of life. Similarly, Simon and VonKorff (33) reported in a survey of primary care clinic patients that insomniacs had greater health care utilization, more days of disability due to health problems, and greater functional impairment as measured by self-reported physical and social disability; these associations persisted after controlling for medical and psychiatric comorbidities.

A recent study by Walsh and Engelhardt (34) estimated the annual direct costs for insomnia in 1995 to be $13.93 billion. This included costs for medications ($1.97 billion) and health care services related to insomnia ($11.96 billion). Somewhat surprisingly, the biggest expense in this analysis was nursing home costs, which totaled $10.9 billion, or 78% of total insomnia-related direct costs. Although this figure is seemingly high, Walsh argues that for a substantial percentage of caregivers, the main reason for institutionalization is an inability to accommodate the elderly family member's sleep disorder. A study by Pollak and Perlick (35), which interviewed caregivers in their decision to institutionalize elderly relatives, found that over 70% of caregivers cited sleep disturbances in their decision to institutionalize, often because their own sleep was affected, with 20% specifying sleep disturbance as their primary reason. Sleep problems of the elderly contribute heavily to the decision to institutionalize an elder.

Numerous studies have attempted to quantify the indirect costs of insomnia. Estimates of costs have ranged widely because of widely differing assumptions (e.g., using differing prevalence rates for insomnia), difficulty of measuring the variables (e.g., how does one measure "decreased productivity"?), and the difficulty of defining what the precise scope of indirect costs should be. Estimates of total (direct and indirect) insomnia-related costs in the United States alone range from $30 billion (36) to $107.5 billion annually (37). A recent study by Leger (38) in the French population found that, over a two-year period, insomniacs were nearly twice as likely to miss work compared with good sleepers and had over a twofold greater total duration of absenteeism in that time period (11.6 days vs. 4.8 days). A collaborative study by Godet-Cayré et al. (39) using data from the same population concluded that the cost of work absenteeism was 1.5 times greater for insomniacs than for controls. This study is noteworthy due to its rigorous definition of insomnia (using DSM-IV criteria) and the use of objective data, such as using employer-provided work attendance records to measure absenteeism, rather than relying on self-reports. However, it should be noted that medical comorbidities were not directly controlled for. Instead, subjects with chronic medical illnesses and any history of psychiatric illness were excluded, resulting in a fairly healthy, active subject population of employed workers.

Daytime Functional Impairment in Insomnia

One of the most robust findings in the literature is that people with insomnia feel that their insomnia impairs their ability to function in a variety of domains. Compared with noninsomniacs, they report feeling more fatigued during the day (40) and feel sleepier when driving a car (41). Interestingly, one of Leger's findings (38) was that in the two-year period studied, insomniacs were involved in twice as many serious car accidents as noninsomniacs, although this result did not quite reach statistical significance. A study by Chau et al. (42) found that the presence of a sleep disorder was one of most powerful independent factors in accidents in the construction industry. Among elderly insomniacs, sleeping difficulties contribute to slowed reaction times (43) and impaired balance (44), leading to a greater risk of falls in this population (45). This is a significant clinical issue, as the presence of falls in the community-dwelling, independently living older adult is a strong predictor of subsequent nursing home placement (46).

Insomniacs also complain that they have trouble remembering things (41), have trouble concentrating, and feel more often confused than noninsomniacs (47), which may be why they report significantly lower levels of self-esteem, job satisfaction, and efficiency at work (38). A study by Ohayon and Vecchierini (48) in the elderly population reported that the presence of excessive daytime sleepiness was a significant risk factor for cognitive impairment including attentional deficits, delayed recall, difficulties in orientation, and memory. These symptoms are of particular concern in older people, because they may be misinterpreted as symptoms of dementia or mild cognitive impairment.

Objective findings of memory deficits in insomniacs were confirmed in two rigorous studies, which used polysomnography to verify insomnia in its subjects. These studies found that compared with matched controls, insomniacs had deficits in short-term (47) and long-term memory (49). It should be noted, however, that there is a significant controversy in the field about the severity of daytime cognitive impairments among insomniacs, with many studies reporting the absence of objectively measurable differences on a variety of cognitive and psychomotor tasks. This may be due to subtleties of different methodologies used from study to study, as summarized in Riedel and Lichstein's excellent review article (50).

In addition to fatigue and cognitive deficits, insomniacs report a decreased ability to accomplish daily tasks and have decreased enjoyment of interpersonal relationships (51), resulting in a lowered quality of life (52). One study found that severe insomnia decreases quality of life comparable to severe medical conditions such as chronic heart failure (53). Not surprisingly, several studies have reported that insomniacs without psychiatric disorders nevertheless suffer from higher, albeit subclinical, levels of depression and anxiety compared with noninsomniacs (50).

Insomnia and Mortality

If insomnia worsens medical and psychiatric conditions and increases the chances of falls and accidents, one may expect that insomniacs would be at higher risk for premature death. What is the evidence for this? A prospective study by Kripke et al. (54) of over one million people in the general population concluded that sleep durations of less than six hours and more than eight hours were associated with a significantly increased risk of all-cause mortality over a six-year period. The best survival was found among those who slept seven hours a night, resulting in a U-shaped survival curve that has been replicated in other studies in the United States (55) and Japan (56,57). Kripke's study also reported that severity of insomnia was associated with shorter survival in a dose-dependent fashion, although this effect went away after controlling for comorbidities. This result suggests that insomnia per se does not affect mortality; rather, it affects mortality exclusively by worsening other health conditions. However, a significant limitation of this study was that insomnia was not well defined (participants were simply asked "How many times a month do you have insomnia?" without providing criteria for what constituted insomnia), limiting the conclusions one may draw about insomnia in this study.

A more recent prospective study by Dew et al. (58) among healthy community-dwelling elderly provides strong evidence that insomnia is associated with increased mortality, by providing an objective assessment of sleep disturbance using polysomnography. After controlling for age, gender, and medical burden, individuals with baseline sleep latencies of greater than 30 minutes were found to have 2.14 times greater risk of death over a mean follow-up of 12.8 years. Poor sleep efficiency and disturbed REM sleep were also found to be significantly correlated with greater risk of death. This study is remarkable in part due to the fact that sleep parameters were objectively measured with polysomnography for all 185 subjects, which differentiates it from earlier studies that used subjective self-reports to measure sleep disturbance, with similar results (59,60).

Unfortunately, although Kripke and Dew's studies could detect an association between sleep patterns and all-cause mortality, neither study had enough power and resolution to ascertain associations with specific causes of mortality. Deaths were ascertained in these studies with death certificates, which are limited in their accuracy and completeness. However, studies that have specifically looked at the relationship between sleep disturbance and cardiovascular disease (CVD) support the hypothesis that sleep disturbances increase mortality from CVD. The prospective study by Mallon et al. (61) in the Swedish population found that DIS was associated with a threefold greater risk of death from coronary artery disease in men over a 12-year period. Similarly,the prospective study by Newman et al. (62) in the U.S. population reported that daytime sleepiness was significantly associated with increased mortality and incident CVD.

Taken as a whole, the epidemiologic data support the hypothesis that insomniacs are at greater risk for premature death than noninsomniacs, even after controlling for medical and psychiatric morbidity, and that this is in part due to increased incidence of cardiovascular disease. Associational studies do not prove causality, however. Insomnia could either be a sensitive early marker of physical decline due to other causes, or it could play a more active role in contributing to a dysregulation of physiology, which ultimately leads to disease. To differentiate these two possibilities, interventional studies are needed to more directly prove causality, as noted in what follows.

Potential Mechanistic Pathways of Insomnia-Related Morbidity and Mortality

What are the possible biologic mechanisms by which insomnia may affect physical health? Three major pathophysiologic pathways are being studied as possible mechanisms through which insomnia may affect health: immunomodulation, sympathetic nervous system arousal, and endocrine changes leading to obesity and glucose intolerance. These mechanisms are not mutually exclusive and in fact may synergize in concert to diminish health.

Sleep has key consequences for expression of proinflammatory cytokines such as the pleiotropic cytokine interleukin-6 (IL-6). It has been well established that sleep loss and chronic insomnia lead to daytime increases in production and circulating levels of IL-6 (63–66) and C-reactive protein (CRP) (67), as well as increases in the expression cellular and genomic markers of inflammation (68). IL-6 is thought to influence the onset and course of a wide spectrum of age-associated diseases, including CVD, arthritis, type 2 diabetes, and certain cancers (69). Further data show that elevated levels of IL-6 prospectively predict future disability, declines of health status, and mortality risk in older adults (70,71). In humans, experimentally induced immune activation is associated with depressed mood, fatigue, and difficulty concentrating (72), and acute administration of IL-6 leads to fatigue and changes in EEG sleep (73), raising the possibility that this is one of the mechanisms by which insomnia may affect mood. The mechanisms by which disordered sleep induces changes in cytokines are not known, although nocturnal wakening produces increases of sympathetic activity (74), which is known to stimulate IL-6 secretion (75).

Substantial data in animals and humans reveal a dysregulation of sympathetic nervous system (SNS) activity in insomnia. Sleep plays a critical role in the homeostatic regulation of autonomic activity; sleep onset leads to nocturnal declines of sympathetic activity as measured by increases of pre-ejection period and decreases of circulating levels of catecholamines, heart rate, blood pressure, and single-fiber sympathetic output (74,76,77). In contrast, sleep deprivation and difficulties with sleep initiation or maintenance are associated with increases in sympathetic drive, as measured by higher circulating catecholamine levels (18,78,79), hypertension (80), decreased heart-rate variability (19), smaller pupils (81), and increased 24-hour oxygen consumption (which reflects metabolic rate) (47).

One of the most intriguing current lines of research is the emerging body of evidence that sleep deprivation induces endocrine changes that lead to obesity and glucose intolerance, which are well-known risk factors for the later development of diabetes (82). Sleep has long been known to play a role in glucose regulation. In normal, healthy individuals, insulin sensitivity varies throughout the day, peaking in the evening, and is at its lowest level in the middle of the night; this mechanism helps to maintain stable glucose levels during the extended overnight fast associated with sleep (83). Recent studies have confirmed that recurrent partial sleep deprivation impairs glucose tolerance. In the first laboratory study of its kind, Spiegel et al. (79) took healthy young men, subjected them to five nights of partial sleep deprivation (4 hours of sleep/night) followed by six nights of sleep recovery (12 hours sleep/night), and tested glucose tolerance on the last morning of each condition using an intravenous glucose tolerance test. In addition, levels of various hormones involved in glucose regulation, such as growth hormone and cortisol, were measured. They found that compared with the fully rested state, sleep-restricted subjects had substantially impaired glucose tolerance. Further analysis revealed that this impairment was multifactorial, with contributions due to decreased insulin release (possibly due to increased sympathetic activation), increases in circulating growth hormone and cortisol (which are counterregulatory to insulin), and increased insulin resistance due to increased levels of proinflammatory cytokines. The results of this study have recently been replicated (84).

One caveat about laboratory studies of sleep is that findings from acute sleep deprivation of healthy adults in the lab may not generalize to the kind of chronic insomnia found in the "real world." Indeed, in many ways acutely sleep-deprived individuals differ from individuals with chronic insomnia (16). However, a plethora of epidemiologic studies have shown a strong association between chronic sleep disturbance and diabetes risk, supporting the notion that findings of impaired glucose tolerance from acute sleep deprivation may indeed apply to chronic insomnia. The results of these studies, which encompass large populations in Japan, the United States, and Sweden, are summarized in an excellent review article by Knutson et al. (82).

In addition to promoting insulin resistance, which predisposes to increased adiposity and weight gain, sleep deprivation independently appears to alter the ability of the body to accurately signal caloric need by altering the production of the weight-regulating hormones leptin and ghrelin, thus promoting obesity. Appetite and energy expenditure are in part regulated by the production of leptin, which suppresses appetite and increases energy expenditure, and ghrelin, which stimulates appetite and decreases energy expenditure (82). These hormones are produced peripherally in the body and act on the arcuate nucleus of the hypothalamus, which integrates information regarding caloric need and effects behavior to promote weight homeostasis. Laboratory studies that involve sleep-depriving individuals and that measure their appetite and caloric intake have shown that sleep deprivation stimulates hunger and appetite, which appear due to decreased leptin and increased ghrelin production in these individuals (85,86). Interestingly, sleep loss has also been shown to increase the inflammatory marker C-reactive protein (CRP) (67), which is thought to promote leptin resistance and may be another pathway by which disturbed sleep promotes obesity. A large body of cross-sectional and prospective epidemiologic studies has confirmed a significant association between short sleep duration and obesity in the general population, as summarized by Knutson et al. in their review article (82).

In summary, insomnia is increasingly being recognized as a disorder of physiologic and emotional hyperarousal associated with characteristic immune and endocrine disturbances. Epidemiologic studies of poor sleepers in the general population and laboratory studies of sleep deprivation support the notion that persistent sleep disturbance induces a variety of physiologic changes in the body, which include immune modulation to proinflammatory states, increased autonomic arousal, and endocrine changes that promote glucose intolerance and obesity. In turn, these mechanisms may be responsible, at least in part, for the increased mortality and morbidity associated with insomnia.

SUMMARY

Insomnia is a complex phenomenon. It is a sensitive marker for medical and psychiatric illness and also appears to be an active participant in causing disease. Insomnia sits at the crossroads of multiple fundamental biologic mechanisms, through which it affects a dauntingly large array of illnesses, including some of the most urgent health epidemics of our time such as CVD, obesity, and diabetes. A note of hope for the clinician is that because insomnia is tied to so many fundamental disease processes, the application of effective treatments for insomnia may serve to have salutary effects on many of the conditions that are affected by it. The restoration of good sleep may prove to be a keystone in improving the health of our patients.

APPENDIX: MORE ON CLASSIFICATION SYSTEMS

There are currently three different disease classification systems in wide use today: the Diagnostic and Statistical Manual of Mental Disorders, currently in its fourth revision (DSM-IV) (87), the International Classification of Sleep Disorders, currently in its second edition (ICSD-II) (22), and the International Classification of Diseases, currently in its tenth edition (ICD-10) (88).

ICD-10, published by the World Health Organization (WHO), is mostly used for mortality and morbidity statistics, reimbursement systems, and automated decision support in medicine. It has limited utility for clinicians and insomnia researchers due to its limited number of sleep-related diagnoses compared with the other classification systems and is rarely used by clinicians.

ICSD-II is an etiology-based classification scheme developed primarily by the American Academy of Sleep Medicine. It contains over 40 narrowly defined insomnia diagnoses arranged by proposed pathophysiologies, such as "psychophysiologic insomnia," "altitude insomnia," and "insomnia due to inadequate sleep hygiene." Criteria for diagnoses are based on symptoms and polysomnographic data. ICSD-II is primarily used by sleep specialists.

The DSM-IV classification system was developed by the American Psychiatric Association, as a guide to diagnosing psychiatric disorders. As sleep disturbances are so often associated with psychiatric conditions, a classification scheme for sleep disorders was developed within this system. In both the DSM-IV and ICSD-II, sleep disorders are broadly divided into dyssomnias, parasomnias, and sleep disorders related to mental and physical illness. Dyssomnias are disorders that produce difficulty initiating or maintaining sleep (insomnia) or that lead to excessive sleepiness (hypersomnia), such as narcolepsy, circadian rhythm disorders, restless legs syndrome, obstructive sleep apnea, and insomnia with no evident cause ("primary insomnia" in the DSM-IV system, "idiopathic insomnia" in the ICSD-II system). Parasomnias are disorders that intrude into the sleep process but are not primarily disorders of sleep and wake states per se, such as sleep terrors, nightmares, and sleepwalking. The third category of "sleep disorders related to mental and physical illness" is a large category that reflects the finding that the vast majority of insomnia symptoms occur in the context of other medical and mental illness that affect sleep.

DSM-IV's complexity is somewhere between that of ICD-10 and ICSD-II. Unlike ICSD-II, DSM-IV is largely a non-etiology-based classification system; that is, many of DSM-IV's diagnostic categories are essentially atheoretical with regard to causation. For example, the diagnosis of "primary insomnia" in the DSM-IV system is applied to insomniacs without comorbid psychiatric or medical conditions. In the ICSD-II system, however, this condition could be categorized as "psychophysiologic insomnia," which invokes learned sleep-preventing associations; "inadequate sleep hygiene," which attributes causation to voluntary behaviors that interfere with sleep; or "idiopathic insomnia," which assumes an as-yet unidentified genetic or biologic component (27). Although the more narrowly defined, pathophysiology-based diagnoses in the ICSD-II system can be quite useful conceptually (e.g., in guiding specific treatments), it should be noted that most have not yet been adopted in the DSM system due to lack of sufficient evidence of each as disease entities that are distinct in terms of etiology, treatment, and pathophysiology (26). DSM-IV is primarily used by psychiatrists and, due to its relative simplicity compared with the ICSD-II, is the classification system most often used in epidemiologic studies and the majority of clinicians who are not sleep specialists.

ACKNOWLEDGMENTS
The authors have no financial gain related to the outcome of this research, and there are no potential conflicts of interest. This work was suported in part by grants T32-MH18399, HL 079955, AG 026364, CA 10014152, CA116778, RR00827, P30-AG028748, General Clinical Research Centers Program, the UCLA Cousins Center at the Semel Institute for Neurosciences, and the UCLA Older Americans Independence Center Inflammatory Biology Core.

REFERENCES

1. Ohayon MM. Epidemiology of insomnia: what we know and what we still need to learn. Sleep Med Rev 2002; 6(2):97–111.
2. National Institutes of Health. National Institutes of Health State of the Science Conference Statement on Manifestations and Management of Chronic Insomnia in Adults, June 13–15, 2005. Sleep 2005; 28(9):1049–1057.
3. Bixler EO, Kales A, Soldatos CR, et al. Prevalence of sleep disorders in the Los Angeles metropolitan area. Am J Psychiatry 1979; 136(10):1257–1262.

4. Ohayon MM, Roth T. What are the contributing factors for insomnia in the general population? J Psychosom Res 2001; 51(6):745–755.

5. Ohayon MM. Prevalence of DSM-IV diagnostic criteria of insomnia: distinguishing insomnia related to mental disorders from sleep disorders. J Psychiatr Res 1997; 31(3):333–346.

6. Bixler EO, Vgontzas AN, Lin HM, et al. Insomnia in central Pennsylvania. J Psychosom Res 2002; 53(1):589–592.

7. Ohayon MM, Roth T. Place of chronic insomnia in the course of depressive and anxiety disorders. J Psychiatr Res 2003; 37(1):9–15.

8. Ancoli-Israel S. Sleep and aging: prevalence of disturbed sleep and treatment considerations in older adults. J Clin Psychiatry 2005; 66(suppl 9):24–30.

9. Ford DE, Kamerow DB. Epidemiologic study of sleep disturbances and psychiatric disorders. An opportunity for prevention? JAMA 1989; 262(11):1479–1484.

10. Roberts RE, Shema SJ, Kaplan GA, et al. Sleep complaints and depression in an aging cohort: a prospective perspective. Am J Psychiatry 2000; 157(1):81–88.

11. Breslau N, Roth T, Rosenthal L, et al. Sleep disturbance and psychiatric disorders: a longitudinal epidemiological study of young adults. Biol Psychiatry 1996; 39(6):411–418.

12. Perlis ML, Smith LJ, Lyness JM, et al. Insomnia as a risk factor for onset of depression in the elderly. Behav Sleep Med 2006; 4(2):104–113.

13. Buysse DJ. Insomnia, depression and aging. Assessing sleep and mood interactions in older adults. Geriatrics 2004; 59(2):47–51.

14. Vgontzas AN. The diagnosis and treatment of chronic insomnia in adults. Sleep 2005; 28(9):1047–1048.

15. Vgontzas AN, Bixler EO, Lin HM, et al. Chronic insomnia is associated with nyctohemeral activation of the hypothalamic–pituitary–adrenal axis: clinical implications. J Clin Endocrinol Metab 2001; 86(8):3787–3794.

16. Vgontzas AN, Mastorakos G, Bixler EO, et al. Sleep deprivation effects on the activity of the hypothalamic–pituitary–adrenal and growth axes: potential clinical implications. Clin Endocrinol (Oxf) 1999; 51(2):205–215.

17. Vgontzas AN, Bixler EO, Wittman AM, et al. Middle-aged men show higher sensitivity of sleep to the arousing effects of corticotropin-releasing hormone than young men: clinical implications. J Clin Endocrinol Metab 2001; 86(4):1489–1495.

18. Irwin M, Clark C, Kennedy B, et al. Nocturnal catecholamines and immune function in insomniacs, depressed patients, and control subjects. Brain Behav Immun 2003; 17(5):365–372.

19. Bonnet MH, Arand DL. Heart rate variability in insomniacs and matched normal sleepers. Psychosom Med 1998; 60(5):610–615.

20. Ancoli-Israel S, Cooke JR. Prevalence and comorbidity of insomnia and effect on functioning in elderly populations. J Am Geriatr Soc 2005; 53(suppl 7):S264–S271.

21. Savard J, Simard S, Blanchet J, et al. Prevalence, clinical characteristics, and risk factors for insomnia in the context of breast cancer. Sleep 2001; 24(5):583–590.

22. American Academy of Sleep Medicine. The International Classification of Sleep Disorders, 2nd edn. Westchester, IL: American Academy of Sleep Medicine, 2005.

23. Ohayon MM, Carskadon MA, Guilleminault C, et al. Meta-analysis of quantitative sleep parameters from childhood to old age in healthy individuals: developing normative sleep values across the human lifespan. Sleep 2004; 27(7):1255–1273.

24. Foley DJ, Monjan AA, Brown SL, et al. Sleep complaints among elderly persons: an epidemiologic study of three communities. Sleep 1995; 18(6):425–432.

25. Foley D, Ancoli-Israel S, Britz P, et al. Sleep disturbances and chronic disease in older adults: results of the 2003 National Sleep Foundation Sleep in America Survey. J Psychosom Res 2004; 56(5):497–502.

26. Reynolds CF 3rd, Kupfer DJ, Buysse DJ, et al. Subtyping DSM-III-R primary insomnia: a literature review by the DSM-IV Work Group on Sleep Disorders. Am J Psychiatry 1991; 148(4):432–438.

27. Buysse DJ, Reynolds CF 3rd, Kupfer DJ, et al. Clinical diagnoses in 216 insomnia patients using the International Classification of Sleep Disorders (ICSD), DSM-IV and

ICD-10 categories: a report from the APA/NIMH DSM-IV Field Trial. Sleep 1994; 17(7):630–637.

28. Cooke JR, Ancoli-Israel S. Sleep and its disorders in older adults. Psychiatr Clin North Am 2006; 29(4):1077–1093.

29. Irwin MR, Cole JC, Nicassio PM. Comparative meta-analysis of behavioral interventions for insomnia and their efficacy in middle-aged adults and in older adults 55 +years of age. Health Psychol 2006; 25(1):3–14.

30. Morin CM, Colecchi C, Stone J, et al. Behavioral and pharmacological therapies for late-life insomnia: a randomized controlled trial. JAMA 1999; 281(11):991–999.

31. Edinger JD, Sampson WS. A primary care "friendly" cognitive behavioral insomnia therapy. Sleep 2003; 26(2):177–182.

32. Hatoum HT, Kong SX, Kania CM, et al. Insomnia, health-related quality of life and healthcare resource consumption. A study of managed-care organisation enrollees. Pharmacoeconomics 1998; 14(6):629–637.

33. Simon GE, VonKorff M. Prevalence, burden, and treatment of insomnia in primary care. Am J Psychiatry 1997; 154(10):1417–1423.

34. Walsh JK, Engelhardt CL. The direct economic costs of insomnia in the United States for 1995. Sleep 1999; 22(suppl 2):S386–S393.

35. Pollak CP, Perlick D. Sleep problems and institutionalization of the elderly. J Geriatr Psychiatry Neurol 1991; 4(4):204–210.

36. Chilcott LA, Shapiro CM. The socioeconomic impact of insomnia. An overview. Pharmacoeconomics 1996; 10(suppl 1):1–14.

37. Stoller MK. Economic effects of insomnia. Clin Ther 1994; 16(5):873–897.

38. Léger D, Massuel MA, Metlaine A, et al. Professional correlates of insomnia. Sleep 2006; 29(2):171–178.

39. Godet-Cayré V, Pelletier-Fleury N, Le Vaillant M, et al. Insomnia and absenteeism at work. Who pays the cost? Sleep 2006; 29(2):179–184.

40. Lichstein KL, Means MK, Noe SL, et al. Fatigue and sleep disorders. Behav Res Ther 1997; 35(8):733–740.

41. Balter MB, Uhlenhuth EH. The beneficial and adverse effects of hypnotics. J Clin Psychiatry 1991; 52(suppl):16–23.

42. Chau N, Mur JM, Benamghar L, et al. Relationships between certain individual characteristics and occupational injuries for various jobs in the construction industry: a case–control study. Am J Ind Med 2004; 45(1):84–92.

43. Crenshaw MC, Edinger JD. Slow-wave sleep and waking cognitive performance among older adults with and without insomnia complaints. Physiol Behav 1999; 66(3):485–492.

44. Hauri PJ. Cognitive deficits in insomnia patients. Acta Neurol Belg 1997; 97(2):113–17.

45. Brassington GS, King AC, Bliwise DL. Sleep problems as a risk factor for falls in a sample of community-dwelling adults aged 64–99 years. J Am Geriatr Soc 2000; 48(10):1234–1240.

46. Tinetti ME, Williams CS. Falls, injuries due to falls, and the risk of admission to a nursing home. N Engl J Med 1997; 337(18):1279–1284.

47. Bonnet MH, Arand DL. 24-Hour metabolic rate in insomniacs and matched normal sleepers. Sleep 1995; 18(7):581–588.

48. Ohayon MM, Vecchierini MF. Daytime sleepiness and cognitive impairment in the elderly population. Arch Intern Med 2002; 162(2):201–208.

49. Mendelson WB, Garnett D, Gillin JC, et al. The experience of insomnia and daytime and nighttime functioning. Psychiatry Res 1984; 12(3):235–250.

50. Riedel BW, Lichstein KL. Insomnia and daytime functioning. Sleep Med Rev 2000; 4(3):277–298.

51. Roth T, Ancoli-Israel S. Daytime consequences and correlates of insomnia in the United States: results of the 1991 National Sleep Foundation Survey. II. Sleep 1999; 22(suppl 2):S354–S358.

52. Zammit GK, Weiner J, Damato N, et al. Quality of life in people with insomnia. Sleep 1999; 22(suppl 2):S379–S385.

53. Katz DA, McHorney CA. The relationship between insomnia and health-related quality of life in patients with chronic illness. J Fam Pract 2002; 51(3):229–235.
54. Kripke DF, Garfinkel L, Wingard DL, et al. Mortality associated with sleep duration and insomnia. Arch Gen Psychiatry 2002; 59(2):131–136.
55. Wingard DL, Berkman LF. Mortality risk associated with sleeping patterns among adults. Sleep 1983; 6(2):102–107.
56. Kojima M, Wakai K, Kawamura T, et al. Sleep patterns and total mortality: a 12-year follow-up study in Japan. J Epidemiol 2000; 10(2):87–93.
57. Tamakoshi A, Ohno Y, JACC Study Group. Self-reported sleep duration as a predictor of all-cause mortality: results from the JACC study, Japan. Sleep 2004; 27(1):51–54.
58. Dew MA, Hoch CC, Buysse DJ, et al. Healthy older adults' sleep predicts all-cause mortality at 4 to 19 years of follow-up. Psychosom Med 2003; 65(1):63–73. Erratum in: Psychosom Med 2003; 65(2):210.
59. Pollak CP, Perlick D, Linsner JP, et al. Sleep problems in the community elderly as predictors of death and nursing home placement. J Community Health 1990; 15(2):123–135.
60. Manabe K, Matsui T, Yamaya M, et al. Sleep patterns and mortality among elderly patients in a geriatric hospital. Gerontology 2000; 46(6):318–322.
61. Mallon L, Broman JE, Hetta J. Sleep complaints predict coronary artery disease mortality in males: a 12-year follow-up study of a middle-aged Swedish population. J Intern Med 2002; 251(3):207–216.
62. Newman AB, Spiekerman CF, Enright P, et al. Daytime sleepiness predicts mortality and cardiovascular disease in older adults. The Cardiovascular Health Study Research Group. J Am Geriatr Soc 2000; 48(2):115–123.
63. Redwine L, Dang J, Hall M, et al. Disordered sleep, nocturnal cytokines, and immunity in alcoholics. Psychosom Med 2003; 65(1):75–85.
64. Redwine L, Hauger RL, Gillin JC, et al. Effects of sleep and sleep deprivation on interleukin-6, growth hormone, cortisol, and melatonin levels in humans. J Clin Endocrinol Metab 2000; 85(10):3597–3603.
65. Vgontzas AN, Papanicolaou DA, Bixler EO, et al. Circadian interleukin-6 secretion and quantity and depth of sleep. J Clin Endocrinol Metab 1999; 84(8):2603–2607.
66. Shearer WT, Reuben JM, Mullington JM, et al. Soluble TNF-alpha receptor 1 and IL-6 plasma levels in humans subjected to the sleep deprivation model of spaceflight. J Allergy Clin Immunol 2001; 107(1):165–170.
67. Meier-Ewert HK, Ridker PM, Rifai N, et al. Effect of sleep loss on C-reactive protein, an inflammatory marker of cardiovascular risk. J Am Coll Cardiol 2004; 43(4):678–683.
68. Irwin MR, Wang M, Campomayor CO, et al. Sleep deprivation and activation of morning levels of cellular and genomic markers of inflammation. Arch Intern Med 2006; 166(16):1756–1762.
69. Ferrucci L, Harris TB, Guralnik JM, et al. Serum IL-6 level and the development of disability in older persons. J Am Geriatr Soc 1999; 47(6):639–646.
70. Volpato S, Guralnik JM, Ferrucci L, et al. Cardiovascular disease, interleukin-6, and risk of mortality in older women: the women's health and aging study. Circulation 2001; 103(7):947–953.
71. Reuben DB, Cheh AI, Harris TB, et al. Peripheral blood markers of inflammation predict mortality and functional decline in high-functioning community-dwelling older persons. J Am Geriatr Soc 2002; 50(4):638–644.
72. Reichenberg A, Yirmiya R, Schuld A, et al. Cytokine-associated emotional and cognitive disturbances in humans. Arch Gen Psychiatry 2001; 58(5):445–452.
73. Späth-Schwalbe E, Hansen K, Schmidt F, et al. Acute effects of recombinant human interleukin-6 on endocrine and central nervous sleep functions in healthy men. J Clin Endocrinol Metab 1998; 83(5):1573–1579.
74. Irwin M, Thompson J, Miller C, et al. Effects of sleep and sleep deprivation on catecholamine and interleukin-2 levels in humans: clinical implications. J Clin Endocrinol Metab 1999; 84(6):1979–1985.

75. Sanders VM, Straub RH. Norepinephrine, the beta-adrenergic receptor, and immunity. Brain Behav Immun 2002; 16(4):290–332.
76. Dodt C, Breckling U, Derad I, et al. Plasma epinephrine and norepinephrine concentrations of healthy humans associated with nighttime sleep and morning arousal. Hypertension 1997; 30(1 Pt 1):71–76.
77. Somers VK, Dyken ME, Mark AL, et al. Sympathetic-nerve activity during sleep in normal subjects. N Engl J Med 1993; 328(5):303–307.
78. Dimsdale JE, Coy T, Ziegler MG, et al. The effect of sleep apnea on plasma and urinary catecholamines. Sleep 1995; 18(5):377–381.
79. Spiegel K, Leproult R, Van Cauter E. Impact of sleep debt on metabolic and endocrine function. Lancet 1999; 354(9188):1435–1439.
80. Tochikubo O, Ikeda A, Miyajima E, et al. Effects of insufficient sleep on blood pressure monitored by a new multibiomedical recorder. Hypertension 1996; 27(6):1318–1324.
81. Lichstein KL, Johnson RS, Sen Gupta S, et al. Are insomniacs sleepy during the day? A pupillometric assessment. Behav Res Ther 1992; 30(3):283–292.
82. Knutson KL, Spiegel K, Penev P, et al. The metabolic consequences of sleep deprivation. Sleep Med Rev 2007; 11(3):163–178.
83. Van Cauter E, Polonsky KS, Scheen AJ. Roles of circadian rhythmicity and sleep in human glucose regulation. Endocr Rev 1997; 18(5):716–738.
84. Spiegel K, Knutson K, Leproult R, et al. Sleep loss: a novel risk factor for insulin resistance and Type 2 diabetes. J Appl Physiol 2005; 99(5):2008–2019.
85. Spiegel K, Leproult R, L'hermite-Balériaux M, et al. Leptin levels are dependent on sleep duration: relationships with sympathovagal balance, carbohydrate regulation, cortisol, and thyrotropin. J Clin Endocrinol Metab 2004; 89(11):5762–5771.
86. Spiegel K, Tasali E, Penev P, et al. Brief communication: sleep curtailment in healthy young men is associated with decreased leptin levels, elevated ghrelin levels, and increased hunger and appetite. Ann Intern Med 2004; 141(11):846–850.
87. American Psychiatric Association. Diagnostic and Statistical Manual of Mental Disorders: DSM-IV-TR, 4th edn., text revision. Washington, DC: American Psychiatric Association, 2000.
88. World Health Organization. International Statistical Classification of Diseases and Related Health Problems, 10th revision. Geneva: World Health Organization, 1992.

6 Pharmacologic Therapy of Chronic Insomnia in Older Adults

Teofilo Lee-Chiong and John Harrington

National Jewish Medical and Research Center, Denver, Colorado, U.S.A.

INTRODUCTION

Insomnia is commonly defined as repeated difficulty with either initially falling asleep (sleep onset insomnia) or remaining asleep (sleep maintenance insomnia). This occurs despite adequate opportunity, condition, and time for sleep to occur and is associated with impairment of daytime function. Patients with insomnia may describe frequent extended periods of wakefulness during the sleep period or persistent morning awakenings that are earlier than desired (terminal insomnia). Insomnia can be divided on the basis of its duration into transient or short-term (lasting only a few days to three to four weeks) or chronic (persisting for more than one to three months). This chapter on pharmacologic therapy of sleep disturbance will be limited to the treatment of chronic insomnia.

Polysomnographically, insomnia is defined by most investigators as a sleep latency of ≥ 30 minutes, wake time after sleep onset of ≥ 30 minutes, sleep efficiency of less than 85%, or total sleep time of less than 6 to 6.5 hours, occurring on at least three nights a week. It must be noted, however, that patients with insomnia often report greater subjective sleep disturbance than changes in objective polysomnographic measures of sleep and have a greater likelihood of reporting, when awakened from polysomnographically defined sleep, of being awake all along, compared with those without insomnia.

Consequences of untreated insomnia include an increased risk of developing new-onset psychiatric illness, daytime sleepiness, fatigue, cognitive impairment, alterations in mood, increased likelihood of accidents, diminished quality of life, and greater healthcare utilization. Recent investigations have increasingly demonstrated that the daytime consequences of insomnia are due to several factors, including disturbed nighttime sleep, associated sleep deprivation, and a constant state of somatic and cognitive hyperarousal that is present throughout the 24-hour day. Without effective therapy, chronic insomnia tends to persist with no significant remission of symptoms over time.

INSOMNIA IN OLDER ADULTS

Significant changes may occur during sleep with aging. The ability to fall asleep and achieve consolidated sleep may decline. There is a reduction in melatonin levels, dampening of circadian sleep–wake rhythms, tendency for phase advancement of circadian rhythms, decreased strength of homeostatic sleep drive, greater sleep fragmentation, and increased likelihood of sleep disorders, including obstructive sleep apnea, restless legs syndrome, and rapid eye movement (REM) behavior disorder.

Older adults often have longer sleep latencies, lower sleep efficiencies, more nighttime awakenings, greater time spent awake while in bed, higher percentage of light stage 1 nonrapid eye movement (NREM) sleep, and less stages 3 and 4 NREM sleep. Greater nighttime sleep disturbance may lead to daytime sleepiness and more frequent daytime napping.

Insomnia is the most common sleep complaint among older adults. Prevalence of insomnia in older adults is estimated to be between 20% and 40% compared with 9% to 15% in the general adult population. In all age groups, women are more likely to have insomnia than men. Insomnia is rarely exclusively due to aging per se but is more often the result of other underlying medical, neurological (e.g., dementia, Parkinson's disease, and cerebral degenerative disorders), or psychiatric disorders. In addition, sleep disturbances in older adults can result from a variety of chronic pain syndromes, menopause, nocturia, and stress (e.g., loss of spouse or retirement). It is also commonly noted in residents of long-term care facilities, who are more likely to remain inactive during the day, nap more frequently, and receive minimal light exposure compared with their community-dwelling peers. A reason for poor sleep in nursing homes is probably due to environmental factors that are less conducive to sleep, such as excessive noise and nursing care practices at night.

Aging is associated with a greater likelihood that insomnia becomes chronic. In addition, older insomniacs may be at a higher risk for early institutionalization. Treatment for these symptoms among older adults is also not without consequences. The use of hypnotic agents in this population is associated with increased frequency of accidents and falls and, possibly, greater mortality risk.

THERAPY OF INSOMNIA

The primary goals of insomnia therapy include the alleviation of nighttime sleep disturbance and the relief of its daytime consequences. Pharmacotherapy and non-pharmacologic interventions, such as sleep hygiene education, are the principal treatment modalities employed for this condition. In cases where the sleep disturbance is clearly associated with an underlying medical, neurological, or psychiatric disorder or medication use or withdrawal, appropriate corrective measures can lead to improvements in sleep. Further, any comorbid sleep disorders, such as obstructive sleep apnea or restless legs syndrome, along with chronic pain syndromes or mood disorders that can produce insomnia, should be identified and managed accordingly. All patients with chronic insomnia should be provided with behavioral therapy as well as instructions on proper sleep hygiene.

HYPNOTIC USE AMONG OLDER ADULTS

Hypnotic agents are primarily indicated for the treatment of transient sleep disruption such as adjustment sleep disorder or that caused by acute stressors. They are also commonly used for primary chronic insomnia, which has failed to respond to behavioral therapy, or for secondary insomnia, which persists despite resolution of the underlying causes of sleep disturbance.

The *ideal* hypnotic agent for older adults with chronic insomnia should (1) be able to induce sleep rapidly, (2) have no adverse effects on normal sleep architecture, (3) demonstrate no significant residual effects, (4) be safe in patients with respiratory and cardiac conditions, (5) have minimal effects on memory,

(6) not impair functioning, (7) have no risk of tolerance or rebound insomnia, (8) be safe during overdose, and (9) possess no potential for abuse or dependence. Unfortunately, such a drug is not currently available. Selection among the numerous available compounds should be based on the nature of the sleep disturbance (sleep onset, sleep maintenance, or terminal insomnia), characteristics of the patient (presence of underlying medical or psychiatric disorders, and medication use) and specific drug profile (absorption and elimination kinetics, abuse potential, and possible drug interactions). Among older adults, presence of any underlying neurocognitive impairment, greater sensitivity to the hypnotic effects of medications, and altered hepatic and renal clearance mechanisms require alterations in drug dosing.

The potential benefits and possible risks of hypnotic use should be determined for each patient. Ideally, hypnotics should be limited to short-term use or used intermittently if required long term. It is advisable to use the lowest effective dose. The need for continuing hypnotic therapy must be reassessed frequently. Adverse effects to the medication, as well as changes in medical or psychiatric status, should be closely monitored.

Available medications for the treatment of insomnia include barbiturates, chloral hydrate, benzodiazepines, non-benzodiazepine benzodiazepine receptor agonists, sedating antidepressants, and the nonprescription hypnotic agents (e.g., antihistamine agents, melatonin, and botanical compounds) (Table 1). In a retrospective analysis conducted in 1996, 4.8% (1.5 million) of community-dwelling elderly persons aged 65 and older used sedative-hypnotic medications during the year. The use of sedative-hypnotic agents was related to both health status and the availability of insurance (1). Another prospective study involving 1627 individuals aged 65 and over in a rural community showed that the use of prescription sedative-hypnotic agents, primarily benzodiazepines, remained relatively stable (from 1.8% to 3.1%), whereas over-the-counter sedative use, principally diphenhydramine, increased substantially (from 0.4% to 7.6%) as the subjects aged over a 10-year period (2).

There is no role for chloral hydrate and barbiturates in the therapy of older adults with chronic insomnia. Chloral hydrate is associated with rapid development of tolerance and can cause rashes, gastric discomfort, and hepatic toxicity. Barbiturates can induce psychological and physical dependency, and overdosage is an ever-present danger given its relatively narrow therapeutic-toxic window.

Benzodiazepines

Benzodiazepines act by binding to the supramolecular gamma-aminobutyric acid–benzodiazepine (GABA-BZ) receptor complex. The GABA-BZ receptor subunits differ in their action, with BZ1 responsible for its hypnotic and amnesic actions and BZ2 and BZ3 receptors accounting for its muscle relaxation, and antiseizure and antianxiety properties. Benzodiazepines bind nonselectively to the different GABA-BZ receptor subunits. Thus, in addition to their soporific properties, these agents also possess anxiolytic, myorelaxant, and anticonvulsant actions.

Benzodiazepines can be classified based on duration of action into short-acting (triazolam), intermediate-acting (estazolam and temazepam), and long-acting (flurazepam and quazepam) agents. The half-lives are less than 3 to 4 hours, 8 to 24 hours, and greater than 24 hours for short-, intermediate-, and long-acting medications, respectively. Duration of action can be used to select the appropriate agent for specific types of sleep disturbance. Short-acting agents are helpful

TABLE 1 Hypnotic Medications

Agent	Dose in older adults	Primary metabolism/excretion	Important adverse effects	Comments
Estazolam	0.5 mg at bedtime	Hepatic/renal	Dizziness, drowsiness, headache	Intermediate-acting benzodiazepine
Eszopiclone	1–2 mg immediately prior to bedtime	Hepatic/renal	Headache, unpleasant taste, xerostomia	Non-benzodiazepine benzodiazepine receptor agonist; tablet should not be crushed or broken; avoid taking after a heavy meal
Flurazepam	15 mg at bedtime	Hepatic/renal	Dizziness, drowsiness, headache, residual sedation in the morning after nighttime administration	Long-acting benzodiazepine
Ramelteon	8 mg at bedtime	Hepatic/renal	Dizziness, fatigue, headaches, sleepiness	Melatonin MT1 and MT2 receptor agonist
Quazepam	7.5 mg at bedtime	Hepatic/renal	Dizziness, drowsiness, fatigue	Long-acting benzodiazepine
Temazepam	7.5 mg at bedtime	Hepatic/renal	Dizziness, drowsiness, fatigue, headache	Intermediate-acting benzodiazepine
Triazolam	0.125 mg at bedtime	Hepatic/renal	Confusion, drowsiness, fatigue, headache	Short-acting benzodiazepine
Zaleplon	5 mg at bedtime	Hepatic/renal/gastrointestinal	Dizziness, headache, somnolence	Non-benzodiazepine benzodiazepine receptor agonist; short-acting
Zolpidem	5 mg at bedtime	Hepatic/renal	Dizziness, drowsiness, headache, nausea	Non-benzodiazepine benzodiazepine receptor agonist

for patients with sleep-onset insomnia, whereas recurrent awakenings during the evening can be managed with drugs with intermediate action. Long-acting medications are indicated for patients with terminal insomnia and daytime anxiety. Short-acting agents generally have minimal residual sedation on the morning after nighttime administration. Onset of action also differs among the various benzodiazepines. Both flurazepam and quazepam have a rapid onset of action and are given immediately at bedtime. The onset of action of temazepam, in contrast, is delayed following ingestion.

As a class, benzodiazepines are associated with several adverse effects, including memory impairment, confusion, rebound insomnia, development of tolerance and withdrawal symptoms, and the risk for dependence and abuse. Tolerance refers to the need for increasingly higher dosages to attain comparable therapeutic benefits with chronic use. Discontinuation can result in withdrawal symptoms such as anxiety, irritability and restlessness; relapse with recurrence of sleep disturbance; or worsening of sleep compared with pretreatment baseline levels (rebound insomnia). The severity of withdrawal syndrome is related to the dosage used, duration of treatment, and the rapidity of drug tapering (3). There may be significant night-to-night variation in the deterioration of sleep after hypnotic drug withdrawal — symptoms may not become apparent for a few days in some patients and may last longer in others (4). High-dose benzodiazepines users and those with poor general health perception predict the risk of relapse (5). Rebound insomnia is more common with short-acting and intermediate acting agents and can be minimized by gradual dose reduction (4). Risk of dependency can be significant in patients with a prior history of dependency to related compounds. Short-acting agents may cause rebound daytime anxiety following cessation of their use. The effect of agents with long elimination half-lives may persist into the following day, producing daytime sleepiness, poor motor coordination, delayed reaction times, and cognitive impairment. Patients should be advised against operating motor vehicles when using these medications.

Dose adjustment should be made for older adults and those with significant renal or hepatic impairment. Older adults may be more susceptible to the hypnotic and sedative effects of benzodiazepines, which may give rise to greater risk of confusion and falls. Accordingly, both therapeutic benefit and adverse effects should be monitored closely in this population. Age-related changes in medication clearance may require that initial doses of benzodiazepines be reduced in older adults. Benzodiazepines can suppress respiration and should be avoided in patients with untreated obstructive sleep apnea and severe respiratory compromise.

Polysomnographic changes that accompany benzodiazepine use in patients with insomnia consist of a decrease in sleep latency, increase in total sleep time, decrease in frequency of awakenings, increase in stage 2 NREM sleep, greater sleep spindles, and decreased stages 3 and 4 NREM sleep and REM sleep. Spectral analysis of polysomnographic data demonstrated significant changes in sleep microstructure (e.g., less delta and theta activity) among older adults with insomnia who were taking benzodiazepines chronically compared with drug-free insomnia sufferers and good sleepers (6).

Estazolam

Estazolam is an intermediate-acting benzodiazepine. It undergoes hepatic metabolism and is excreted renally. Its serum half-life ranges from 10 to 24 hours.

Important drug interactions include azole antifungals, barbiturates, muscle relaxants, opioid analgesics, and sodium oxybate. It should be used cautiously in older adults and in debilitated patients and is not recommended for those with a history of severe depression, drug abuse, chronic pulmonary insufficiency, or sleep apnea. Adverse effects include dizziness, sleepiness, and impairment of neurocognition and coordination. Recommended dose for older adults is 0.5 mg at bedtime.

Flurazepam

A long-acting benzodiazepine agent with a duration of sedative action of 10 to 30 hours, flurazepam is indicated primarily for the treatment of sleep maintenance insomnia. The agent undergoes extensive hepatic metabolism before it is excreted renally. Use should be avoided when using alcohol, azole antifungals, barbiturates, muscle relaxants, opioid analgesics, ritonavir, and sodium oxybate. It is also not recommended in patients with severe depression, untreated sleep apnea, and chronic respiratory insufficiency. Chronic use is associated with the development of tolerance, a potential for dependency, and rebound insomnia and withdrawal symptoms following abrupt discontinuation. Patients taking flurazepam have reported dizziness, sleepiness, lightheadedness, headaches, depression, and confusion. Residual sleepiness can lead to daytime impairment following nighttime use due to its prolonged elimination half-life. Finally, it can worsen obstructive sleep apnea and chronic pulmonary insufficiency. Flurazepam is given at a dose of 15 mg at bedtime for older adults.

Quazepam

Quazepam is a rapid-onset, long-acting benzodiazepine with an elimination half-life up to 41 hours. Drugs that can interact with quazepam include alcohol, azole antifungals, barbiturates, muscle relaxants, and opioid analgesics. Adverse effects, including sleepiness, dizziness, headaches, fatigue, and incoordination, are common with concurrent use of alcohol and central nervous system depressants. It is less likely to cause rebound insomnia with abrupt drug discontinuation but more prone to produce sedative effects the following morning compared with shorter-acting benzodiazepines. Tolerance and withdrawal symptoms can develop. The liver metabolizes quazepam and doses should be reduced in patients with severe hepatic disease. As with other agents in its class, quazepam should be avoided in patients with severe respiratory disorders and sleep apnea. For older adults, quazepam is administered at a dose of 7.5 mg at bedtime.

Temazepam

Temazepam is an intermediate-acting benzodiazepine. Its use should be monitored closely when given in combination with central nervous system depressants (alcohol, muscle relaxants, opioid analgesics, and sodium oxybate) and azole antifungals, especially to patients with obstructive sleep apnea, chronic pulmonary insufficiency or severe depression. Temazepam administration is associated with a detrimental effect on psychomotor performance in healthy elderly subjects (7). However, because it has no active metabolites, there is minimal accumulation of temazepam compared with other benzodiazepines. In a study involving 75 convalescent-home older adults, temazepam had significantly less drug hangover both on awakening and during the entire day after nighttime treatment than did patients receiving flurazepam (8). Withdrawal symptoms can develop after abrupt discontinuation. Initial recommended dose for older adults is 15 mg at bedtime.

Triazolam

Triazolam is a short-acting benzodiazepine agent with a half-life of approximately 1.5 to 5 hours. Onset of action is rapid and is usually within 30 minutes. It is metabolized in the liver and excreted in the urine. Its use should be avoided in patients with prior benzodiazepine abuse, chronic pulmonary insufficiency, severe depression, and severe liver dysfunction. Important drug interactions include azole antifungals, barbiturates, and several anti-retroviral agents, including efavirenz, macrolide antibiotics, muscle relaxants, nefazodone, opioid analgesics, protease inhibitors, and sodium oxybate. Adverse effects include fatigue, drowsiness, amnesia, rebound insomnia with abrupt drug discontinuation, cognitive dysfunction, respiratory depression, and worsening of obstructive sleep apnea. It is associated with a potential for addiction and dependency as well as drug tolerance. The recommended dose of triazolam for older adults is 0.125 mg at bedtime. Maximum recommended dose is 0.25 mg daily.

Non-Benzodiazepine Benzodiazepine Receptor Agonists

These agents, like benzodiazepines, bind to the GABA-BZ receptor complex. The hypnosedative action of the non-benzodiazepine benzodiazepine receptor agonists (NBBRA) is comparable with that of benzodiazepines. They have relative selectivity for the GABA$_A$ receptor subtype BZ1, which accounts for its sedative and amnesic properties. Therefore, the NBBRAs have no significant anxiolytic, myorelaxant, or anticonvulsant activity. NBBRAs appear to be safer in older adults compared with benzodiazepine hypnotic agents. The risks of tolerance and dependency are low, and abuse potential is generally minimal but remains a concern in patients with a history of abuse or dependence and those with psychiatric disorders (9–11). These agents are less likely than benzodiazepines to impair daytime performance and memory due to their relatively shorter duration of action and their low potential for residual effect. Drug interactions have been reported with several medications, including rifampin, ketoconazole, erythromycin, cimetidine, and ethanol (12).

Both regular preparation zolpidem and zaleplon are indicated for sleep-onset insomnia, whereas eszopiclone and extended-release zolpidem are preferred for difficulties related to sleep maintenance. When taking NBBRAs, patients should be cautioned against driving or participating in activities that require full alertness.

Eszopiclone

Eszopiclone, an s-isomer of the cyclopyrrolone hypnosedative zopiclone, possesses the longest duration of any currently available unmodified preparations of NBBRAs. It has a half-life of about four to six hours. Eszopiclone is generally considered to be as effective as the benzodiazepines in the therapy of insomnia. Long-term administration over a six-month period in subjects with chronic primary insomnia has demonstrated significant and sustained improvements in sleep latency, wake time after sleep onset, number of awakenings, total sleep time, quality of sleep, next-day function, alertness, and sense of physical well-being compared with placebo (13). In a randomized, placebo-controlled study, eszopiclone (1 and 2 mg) was well tolerated and significantly reduced subjective sleep onset compared with placebo in healthy older adults [aged 65 to 85 years [mean age

72.3 years)] with primary insomnia. Eszopiclone 2 mg also increased total sleep time, decreased subjective wake time after sleep onset, resulted in higher ratings of sleep quality and sleep depth, and improved daytime alertness compared with placebo (14). Eszopiclone possesses minimal tolerance potential and is associated with a low risk of residual clinical effects, daytime sedation, or withdrawal reactions. Although rebound of insomnia has been described after drug withdrawal, this does not appear to be common (15). Treatment-related adverse events include unpleasant taste. It should be avoided in patients with severe hepatic impairment. Eszopiclone can interact with several agents, including azole antifungals, clarithromycin, ciprofloxacin, diclofenac, doxycycline, erythromycin, ethanol, isoniazid, ketoconazole, nefazodone, olanzapine, quinidine, and verapamil. Tablets should not be crushed or broken or taken with other hypnotic drugs or alcohol. Initial dose of eszopiclone for older adults is 1 mg immediately prior to bedtime. Maximum recommended dose is 2 mg for elderly patients.

Zaleplon

Zaleplon has the shortest elimination half-life (about 1 hour) of all the currently available NBBRAs. It had been shown to reduce subjective sleep latency and improve subjective sleep quality in older adults with insomnia (16). Aside from a reduction of sleep latency and an increase in sleep duration, zaleplon has minimal effect on sleep architecture. No evidence of significant undesired effects or clinically significant rebound insomnia has occurred after discontinuation of treatment in older subjects with insomnia (17). There is also no evidence of tolerance to its sleep promoting effects and no rebound insomnia upon its discontinuation (18). Drug interactions include cimetidine, ethanol, and rifampin. Initial recommended dose is 5 mg at bedtime for older adults. It may also be given during prolonged middle-of-the-night awakenings as long as there is at least four hours remaining prior to rising time.

Zolpidem

Zolpidem binds preferentially to the BZ1 receptor and, thus, possesses no anticonvulsant or muscle relaxant activity. It has a quick onset of action and has a short half-life of approximately 2.4 hours. Its metabolites are inactive and readily excreted. Zolpidem lacks any appreciable potential for addiction, tolerance, withdrawal symptoms, rebound insomnia, or residual daytime cognitive impairment. In a study of elderly psychiatric patients with severe insomnia, treatment with 20 mg zolpidem resulted in significant improvements in total sleep time, sleep efficiency, and REM sleep percentage. Stage 1 NREM decreases were accompanied by increases in stages 2, 3, and 4 NREM sleep during active treatment (19). Administration has also been shown to reduce sleep latency, decrease the frequency of awakenings, and delay REM sleep onset. It is less likely to disrupt normal sleep architecture compared with the benzodiazepines. Side effects are generally mild and include headaches, dizziness, drowsiness, and nausea. Zolpidem interacts with antidepressants, ethanol, ketoconazole, rifampin, and ritonavir, and their concurrent use should be avoided. The dose of zolpidem for older adults is commonly 5 mg (or 6.25 mg of the sustained release preparation) at bedtime.

Melatonin Receptor Agonists

Ramelteon is a selective MT1/MT2 receptor agonist that is indicated for the treatment of insomnia. MT1 and MT2 receptors are believed to mediate the effects of melatonin on circadian rhythms and are located primarily in the cells of the suprachiasmatic nucleus. It reduces sleep latency to persistent sleep, improves sleep efficiency, and increases total sleep time (20,21). In a randomized control study of older adults with chronic insomnia, nightly ramelteon administration resulted in reductions in sleep latency and increases in total sleep time. Reductions in sleep latency were more pronounced in patients with greater sleep disturbances. There was no evidence of significant rebound insomnia or withdrawal effects following discontinuation of treatment (22).

Sedating Antidepressants

Off-label prescriptions of sedating antidepressants are commonly given to treat primary insomnia despite limited published data on their use among patients without comorbid mood disorders. Tricyclic antidepressants, such as amitriptyline, doxepin, nortriptyline, and trimipramine, can give rise to cardiac arrhythmias, orthostatic hypotension, and other anticholinergic effects (e.g., constipation or dry outh) and cannot be recommended as first-line therapy of insomnia in older adults. Tricyclic antidepressants can also exacerbate symptoms of restless legs and periodic limb movements during sleep. Finally, these agents should be used with caution in patients with glaucoma, seizures, or cardiac conduction disorders.

Trazodone

A sedating antidepressant, trazodone is widely used in the treatment of chronic insomnia. It antagonizes 5-HT(2) and alpha(1) receptors. Trazodone has been shown to increase sleep efficiency, total sleep time, and stages 3 and 4 NREM sleep and to decrease wakefulness, early morning awakening, and stages 1 and 2 NREM sleep in patients with insomnia related to depression or other antidepressant therapy (e.g., selective serotonin reuptake inhibitors) compared with placebo (23,24). REM latency is lengthened with a decrease in REM sleep duration. There are limited data on its use among patients with insomnia unrelated to affective disorders, and there are no randomized controlled studies assessing its efficacy and safety among older adults. Although it appears to have fewer adverse effects than the older tricyclic antidepressants, arrhythmias, blurring of vision, delirium, dizziness, hypotension, priapism, and sleepiness can occur. Therefore, it is not recommended for use in patients with significant cardiac disease or arrhythmias. Coadministration with nefazodone can result in the serotonin syndrome. There is no significant tolerance potential or risk of dependency. Important drug interactions include antihypertensive agents, chlorpromazine, droperidol, trifluoperazine, and warfarin. It is excreted in the urine after it undergoes hepatic metabolism. Trazodone may be given at an initial dose of 25 to 50 mg at bedtime. However, patients should be informed that trazodone is not approved by the Food and Drug Administration (FDA) for the treatment of insomnia.

Other Agents

Mirtazapine is a noradrenergic and specific serotonergic antidepressant that can cause sedation. In patients with major depression and insomnia, it has been shown to improve sleep latency, sleep efficiency, and sleep continuity (25). Side effects include weight gain and nausea. Nefazodone is a serotonin receptor blocker and mild serotonin reuptake inhibitor. Administration is associated with either no change in REM sleep parameters or a decrease in REM sleep latency and increase in REM sleep. Adverse effects include rare liver toxicity.

Nonprescription Hypnotic Agents
Older adults with insomnia commonly self-administer nonprescription sleep agents, including antihistamines, melatonin, or botanical compounds, to aid with their sleep. A survey conducted on ambulatory elderly adults (aged 60 years or more) revealed that 48% of respondents had reported using one or more therapies for sleep within the past year. Nonprescription products accounted for 50% of therapies. Prescription products were used in 17% and nonpharmacologic activities such as walking or drinking milk were reported in the remaining 34%. The most frequently used nonprescription products were dimenhydrinate (21%), acetaminophen (19%), diphenhydramine (15%), alcohol (13%), and herbal products (11%). Thirty-two percent took them daily and 79% took them at least one day per week (26).

Histamine Antagonists
Many over-the-counter hypnotic agents contain first generation histamine H1 antagonists. These agents, which may also act on serotonergic, cholinergic, and central alpha-adrenergic receptors, include diphenhydramine and chlorpheniramine. Saitou et al. observed that the order of potency, from greatest to least, of first-generation histamine H1 antagonists for the reduction in sleep latency was promethazine > chlorpheniramine > diphenhydramine and pyrilamine. Chlorpheniramine was the most potent in inducing an increase in sleep duration, followed by promethazine, then diphenhydramine and pyrilamine (27). Second-generation agents, such as loratadine and fexofenadine, are less able to cross the blood–brain barrier and, thus, less likely to cause sedation. As a class, antihistamines are relatively weak soporific agents and are ineffective for anything more than mild insomnia. In one randomized controlled study, 17 nursing home residents with sleeping problems were given either temazepam (15 mg), diphenhydramine (50 mg), or placebo. Diphenhydramine use was associated with a shorter sleep latency compared with placebo, and longer duration of sleep than temazepam (28). Tolerance to the hypnotic effects of diphenhydramine may develop rapidly. Polysomnographic changes related to first-generation histamine H1 antagonists include an increase in stages 3 and 4 NREM sleep (27,29). Diphenhydramine administration can have a detrimental effect on psychomotor performance and daytime alertness (7). Other adverse effects of histamine antagonists include confusion, cognitive decline, delirium, abnormal psychomotor activity, dizziness, blurring of vision, dry mouth, urinary retention, and constipation.

Melatonin
Melatonin is a hormone produced under the control of the suprachiasmatic nucleus during darkness in the pineal gland. A reduction in sleep latency has been described with nighttime administration of melatonin. It has been used primarily for the management of sleep disturbances secondary to circadian rhythm sleep disorders (e.g., delayed sleep phase syndrome). The FDA has not approved it for this purpose.

Older adults appear to have lower endogenous melatonin levels. Several studies have shown that melatonin is able to restore sleep efficiency and reduce wake time after sleep onset in older adults with insomnia (30,31).

Botanical Compounds

Except for valerian, none of the herbal preparations, such as kava (*Piper methysticum*), passion flower (*Passiflora incarnata*), and skullcap (*Scutellaria laterifolia*), which have been described for the alleviation of sleep disturbance, have been studied in older adults with chronic insomnia. Kava is a psychoactive agent belonging to the pepper family. Adverse effects include dizziness, mild gastrointestinal disturbances, and skin reactions (i.e., a scaly dermatitis referred to as kava dermopathy) (32). Kava has been removed from the market in a number of countries because of concerns about hepatotoxicity.

Valerian (*Valeriana officinalis*) is included as one of the ingredients in herbal compounds marketed for the therapy of insomnia. Polysomnography demonstrates variable effects on sleep efficiency, sleep onset, wake time after sleep onset, and REM sleep. Valerian has been reported to increase stages 3 and 4 NREM sleep and decrease stage 1 NREM sleep (33). A subjective decrease in sleep latency and reduction in wake time after sleep onset has been described. However, a systematic review of nine randomized clinical trials demonstrated no conclusive evidence for the efficacy of valerian in the treatment of insomnia (34). Overdoses with valerian can cause abdominal pain, chest tightness, tremor, lightheadedness, mydriasis, and fine hand tremors (32).

SUMMARY

Because insomnia may be due to many causes, one should attempt to identify any factor that may precipitate or perpetuate these complaints, and initiate appropriate corrective measures. Most patients benefit from a combination of sleep hygiene counseling, behavior modification, and the judicious administration of hypnotic agents. Pharmacotherapeutic management is generally effective for transient insomnia due to jet lag or acute stressors. It may also be used intermittently in patients with more chronic complaints. The selection of a particular hypnotic medication should be based on the characteristics of the patient, his or her particular sleep disturbance, and the hypnotic agent. In the elderly, it is advisable to use the lowest effective dose and to monitor carefully both therapeutic response and side effects.

REFERENCES

1. Aparasu RR, Mort JR, Brandt H. Psychotropic prescription use by community-dwelling elderly in the United States. J Am Geriatr Soc 2003; 51:671–677.
2. Basu R, Dodge H, Stoehr GP, et al. Sedative-hypnotic use of diphenhydramine in a rural, older adult, community-based cohort: effects on cognition. Am J Geriatr Psychiatry 2003; 11:205–213.
3. Schweizer E, Rickels K. Benzodiazepine dependence and withdrawal: a review of the syndrome and its clinical management. Acta Psychiatr Scand Suppl 1998; 393:95–101.

4. Hajak G, Clarenbach P, Fischer W, et al. Rebound insomnia after hypnotic withdrawal in insomniac outpatients. Eur Arch Psychiatry Clin Neurosci 1998; 248:148–156.

5. Voshaar RO, Gorgels W, Mol A, et al. Predictors of relapse after discontinuation of long-term benzodiazepine use by minimal intervention: a 2-year follow-up study. Fam Pract 2003; 20(4):370–372.

6. Bastien CH, LeBlanc M, Carrier J, et al. Sleep EEG power spectra, insomnia, and chronic use of benzodiazepines. Sleep 2003; 26:313–317.

7. Glass JR, Sproule BA, Herrmann N, et al. Acute pharmacological effects of temazepam, diphenhydramine, and valerian in healthy elderly subjects. J Clin Psychopharmacol 2003; 23(3):260–268.

8. Fillingim JM. Double-blind evaluation of temazepam, flurazepam, and placebo in geriatric insomniacs. Clin Ther 1982; 4:369–380.

9. Voderholzer U, Riemann D, Hornyak M, et al. A double-blind, randomized and placebo-controlled study on the polysomnographic withdrawal effects of zopiclone, zolpidem and triazolam in healthy subjects. Eur Arch Psychiatry Clin Neurosci 2001; 251(3):117–123.

10. Hajak G. A comparative assessment of the risks and benefits of zopiclone: a review of 15 years' clinical experience. Drug Saf 1999; 21(6):457–469.

11. Hajak G, Muller WE, Wittchen HU, et al. Abuse and dependence potential for the non-benzodiazepine hypnotics zolpidem and zopiclone: a review of case reports and epidemiological data. Addiction 2003; 98(10):1371–1378.

12. Hesse LM, von Moltke LL, Greenblatt DJ. Clinically important drug interactions with zopiclone, zolpidem and zaleplon. CNS Drugs 2003; 17(7):513–532.

13. Krystal AD, Walsh JK, Laska E, et al. Sustained efficacy of eszopiclone over 6 months of nightly treatment: results of a randomized, double-blind, placebo-controlled study in adults with chronic insomnia. Sleep 2003; 26(7):793–799.

14. Scharf M, Erman M, Rosenberg R, et al. A 2-week efficacy and safety study of eszopiclone in elderly patients with primary insomnia. Sleep 2005; 28(6):720–727.

15. Noble S, Langtry HD, Lamb HM. Zopiclone. An update of its pharmacology, clinical efficacy and tolerability in the treatment of insomnia. Drugs 1998; 55(2):277–302.

16. Hedner J, Yaeche R, Emilien G, et al. Zaleplon shortens subjective sleep latency and improves subjective sleep quality in elderly patients with insomnia. The Zaleplon Clinical Investigator Study Group. Int J Geriatr Psychiatry 2000; 15:704–712.

17. Ancoli-Israel S, Walsh JK, Mangano RM, et al. Zaleplon, a novel nonbenzodiazepine hypnotic, effectively treats insomnia in elderly patients without causing rebound effects. Prim Care Companion J Clin Psychiatry 1999;1(4):114–120.

18. Walsh JK, Vogel GW, Scharf M, et al. A five week, polysomnographic assessment of zaleplon 10 mg for the treatment of primary insomnia. Sleep Med 2000; 1:41–49.

19. Kummer J, Guendel L, Linden J, et al. Long-term polysomnographic study of the efficacy and safety of zolpidem in elderly psychiatric in-patients with insomnia. J Int Med Res 1993; 21:171–184.

20. Roth T, Walsh J. Phase II study of the selective ML-1 receptor agonist TAK-375 in a first night effect model of transient insomnia [abstract]. Sleep 2003; 26(suppl):A294.

21. Erman M, Seiden D, Zammit G. Phase II study of the selective ML-1 receptor agonist TAK-375 in subjects with primary chronic insomnia [abstract]. Sleep. 2003; 26(suppl):A298.

22. Roth T, Seiden D, Sainati S, et al. Effects of ramelteon on patient-reported sleep latency in older adults with chronic insomnia. Sleep Med 2006; 7:312–318.

23. Saletu-Zyhlarz GM, Abu-Bakr MH, Anderer P, et al. Insomnia in depression: differences in objective and subjective sleep and awakening quality to normal controls and acute effects of trazodone. Prog Neuropsychopharmacol Biol Psychiatry 2002; 26(2):249–260.

24. Kaynak H, Kaynak D, Gozukirmizi E, et al. The effects of trazodone on sleep in patients treated with stimulant antidepressants. Sleep Med 2004; 5(1):15–20.

25. Winokur A, DeMartinis NA 3rd, McNally DP, et al. Comparative effects of mirtazapine and fluoxetine on sleep physiology measures in patients with major depression and insomnia. J Clin Psychiatry 2003; 64(10):1224–1229.

26. Sproule BA, Busto UE, Buckle C, et al. The use of non-prescription sleep products in the elderly. Int J Geriatr Psychiatry 1999; 14(10):851–857.
27. Saitou K, Kaneko Y, Sugimoto Y, et al. Slow wave sleep-inducing effects of first generation H1-antagonists. Biol Pharm Bull 1999; 22(10):1079–1082.
28. Meuleman JR, Nelson RC, Clark RL Jr. Evaluation of temazepam and diphenhydramine as hypnotics in a nursing-home population. Drug Intell Clin Pharm 1987; 21(9):716–720.
29. Rickels K, Morris RJ, Newman H, et al. Diphenhydramine in insomniac family practice patients: a double-blind study. J Clin Pharmacol 1983; 23(5–6):234–242.
30. Zhdanova IV, Wurtman RJ, Regan MM, et al. Melatonin treatment for age-related insomnia. J Clin Endocrinol Metab 2001; 86:4727–4730.
31. Garfinkel D, Laudon M, Nof D, et al. Improvement of sleep quality in elderly people by controlled-release melatonin. Lancet 1995; 346:541–544.
32. Fugh-Berman A, Jerry M. Cott J. Dietary Supplements and Natural Products as Psychotherapeutic Agents. Psychosomatic Medicine 1999; 61:712–728.
33. Donath F, Quispe S, Diefenbach K, et al. Critical evaluation of the effect of valerian extract on sleep structure and sleep quality. Pharmacopsychiatry 2000; 33:47–53.
34. Stevinson C, Ernst E. Valerian for insomnia: a systematic review of randomized clinical trials. Sleep Medicine 2000; 1:91–99.

7 Cognitive-Behavioral Treatment of Insomnia in Older Adults

Charles M. Morin and Lynda Bélanger

École de Psychologie, Université Laval Québec, Québec, Canada

INTRODUCTION

Insomnia is a prevalent condition in the elderly population, and it is often associated with significant medical and psychological morbidity (1,2). Insomnia complaints in older adults do not always receive adequate clinical attention, perhaps due to a tendency to normalize such symptoms in the aging individual. When treatment is initiated, it is predominantly pharmacological in nature. Despite its clinical benefits in the short-term management of insomnia, medication is not always an acceptable treatment option among older individuals, and it may be contraindicated for some patients due to the increased risks of adverse effects and interactions with other medications. Thus, it is important to consider alternative nonpharmacological interventions that may prove safer than and as effective as pharmacotherapy.

Cognitive-behavioral therapy (CBT) of insomnia is receiving increasing attention from the research community. Whereas older adults were systematically excluded from clinical trials of insomnia therapies in the 1970s and 1980s, there has been a recent shift of interest, with more investigations examining treatment response specifically in older adults (3–5). Significant advances have been made in documenting the efficacy and effectiveness of behavioral and psychological interventions for insomnia in older adults. Despite such progress, insomnia remains for the most part untreated and behavioral interventions underutilized by health care providers (6).

This chapter presents the main therapeutic components of multimodal CBT for insomnia in older adults. First, a conceptual model of chronic insomnia is presented, followed by a description of the main components of CBT adapted to the aging individual. A summary of the evidence supporting the efficacy of CBT for insomnia in older adults follows, with a concluding section discussing the main advantages and limitations of this treatment approach.

A CONCEPTUAL MODEL OF CHRONIC INSOMNIA

Several predisposing, precipitating, and perpetuating factors are involved at different times during the course of insomnia (7). Increasing age, female gender, hyperarousal, prior history of insomnia, and an anxiety-prone personality represent some of those factors that may predispose to insomnia. Sleep disturbances are often precipitated by stressful life events such as the death of a loved one, medical illness, retirement, separation, or hospitalization. Sleep usually normalizes after the stressor has faded away or the person has adapted to its more enduring presence. For some individuals, however, perhaps those who are more vulnerable to insomnia, sleep disturbances will develop a chronic course. A cardinal assumption of this model is

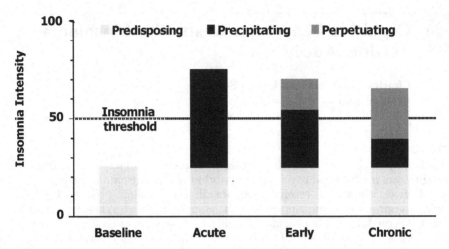

FIGURE 1 A model showing how different factors contribute to the course of chronic insomnia. *Source*: Adapted from Ref. 7.

that insomnia may become functionally independent from the original precipitating event (see Fig. 1). For example, although pain is a common precipitating factor of sleep disturbances in older adults, spending excessive amounts of time in bed or napping during the day may perpetuate the sleep problem over time. Treatment should then focus on these maintaining factors, even if the precipitating factors may still be instrumental in maintaining the sleep difficulties.

According to this model, behavioral and psychological factors are almost always involved in perpetuating insomnia over time, regardless of the nature of the precipitating event. In older adults, as in any age group, such features may include poor sleep habits, irregular sleep–wake schedules, and misconceptions and unrealistic expectations about normal sleep. Figure 2 schematizes the interplay of different behavioral and cognitive factors hypothesized to maintain insomnia and how they interact to form a vicious cycle.

COGNITIVE-BEHAVIORAL THERAPY FOR INSOMNIA

Several behavioral, cognitive, and psychological interventions have been validated for the treatment of insomnia in later life: sleep restriction, stimulus control therapy, relaxation-based interventions, cognitive therapy, and combined CBT. These interventions are not incompatible with each other and multicomponent therapy such as CBT, which typically combines a behavioral intervention (i.e., stimulus control, sleep restriction, and, sometimes, relaxation), a cognitive (cognitive restructuring therapy), and an educational component (sleep hygiene), is becoming the standard approach to treating insomnia (3–5,8,9). CBT thus aims at curtailing sleep-incompatible behaviors, attenuating arousal, and altering sleep-related dysfunctional cognitions and thoughts, all of which are hypothesized to play a major role in maintaining and exacerbating insomnia over time.

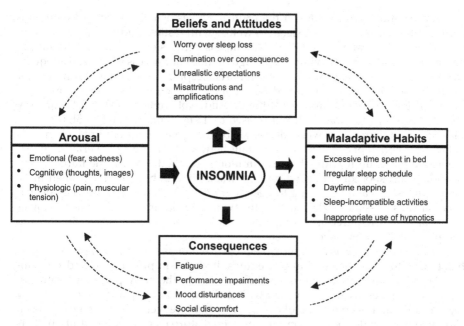

FIGURE 2 A microanalytic model of chronic insomnia showing how maladaptive sleep habits and dysfunctional beliefs and attitudes can contribute to perpetuate insomnia. *Source*: Adapted from Ref. 27.

Sleep Restriction

In response to poor sleep, a common reaction is to increase time in bed. However, this misguided effort to provide more opportunity for sleep is a strategy that is more likely to result in fragmented and poor-quality sleep. Sleep restriction therapy consists of curtailing the amount of time spent in bed to the actual amount of time asleep (10). After sleep efficiency (SE) improves, time in bed is gradually increased until optimal sleep duration is achieved. The presumed underlying mechanisms involve a mild sleep deprivation which strengthens the homeostatic drive and consolidates the total amount of sleep over a shorter period of time. In addition, sleep restriction often produces a paradoxical shift of attention from apprehension and worrying about not being able to fall asleep at the desired time to one of concern about staying awake until the prescribed bedtime.

The following example illustrates how to implement this procedure. John is a 67-year-old man who presents with a 12-year history of mixed sleep-onset and maintenance insomnia. According to his daily sleep diaries kept for a two-week baseline period, his usual bedtime is 9:30 p.m. and he typically arises around 6:00 a.m., for a nightly mean of 8.5 hours spent in bed. He takes an average of 60 minutes to fall asleep and is awake for 45 minutes in the middle of the night and for an additional 45 minutes at the end of the sleep period before getting out of bed. The summation of these three variables (i.e., sleep-onset latency, wake after sleep onset, and early-morning awakening) yields a total wake time of 2.5 hours, leaving only six hours of sleep out of 8.5 spent in bed, for a global SE of 71% (SE = total sleep time/total time in bed × 100).

An SE index which is lower than 80% to 85% is usually associated with diffi-culties initiating/maintaining sleep, as well as with restless and unsatisfying sleep. Conversely, SE greater than 85% to 90% means better sleep initiation/ continuity and more sound and satisfying sleep. High SE does not necessarily mean adequate sleep duration. In this example, John reports sleeping an average of 6 hours per night out of 8.5 hours spent in bed, so the initial prescribed "sleep window" (i.e., from bedtime to arising time) is six hours. Allowable time in bed is subsequently adjusted contingent upon SE. It is increased by 15 to 20 minutes when SE is greater than 85% for the previous week, decreased by the same amount of time when SE is below 80%, and kept constant when SE falls between 80% and 85%. Periodic adjust-ments are made until optimal sleep duration is reached. Ideally, the initial "sleep window" and subsequent changes in allowable time in bed are determined in an empirical fashion and according to sleep diary data. In clinical practice, however, it is not always possible or desirable to follow these rules in a rigid fashion. Adjust-ments are often required as a function of patients' acceptance and willingness to comply with the prescribed regimen.

This procedure has been shown effective, either as a mono therapy or in com-bination with other behavioral procedures, both for improving SE and continu-ity. Despite a small reduction in total sleep time in the early phase of treatment, patients are generally more satisfied with their initial sleep quality and eventually regain additional sleep time at follow-up (11–14). Moreover, this treatment has been shown to meet evidence-based criteria of sleep disturbances in older adults, both as a stand-alone intervention and when combined with other interventions (4,5).

Stimulus Control Therapy
Stimulus control treatment is based on the assumption that insomnia is the result of maladaptive conditioning between environmental (bed/bedroom) and tempo-ral (bedtime) stimuli and sleep-incompatible behaviors (e.g., worrying, reading, or watching TV in bed). According to this paradigm, these stimuli (bed, bedtime, and bedroom) have lost their discriminative properties previously associated with sleep. The main therapeutic goal is to reestablish or strengthen the associations between sleep and the stimulus conditions under which it typically occurs. This is accomplished by minimizing the amount of time awake in bed, by eliminating sleep-interfering activities, and by regulating the sleep–wake schedule. The basic principles operating are analogous to those implicated with other clinical dysfunc-tions (e.g., obesity, substance abuse) in that the objective is to alter the relation-ship between a particular behavior (sleep) and the stimulus conditions (bed, bed-time, bedroom) controlling it. Stimulus control instructions for insomnia include (i) postponing bedtime until sleep is imminent, i.e. when the person feels sleepy (as opposed to feeling tired); (ii) getting out of bed when unable to fall back to sleep quickly during the night; (iii) eliminating all nonsleeping activities (e.g., reading, watching TV, working) from the bedroom; (iv) keeping a regular arising time in the morning; and (v) avoiding daytime naps (15). These recommendations are par-ticularly relevant to some older adults who may engage more frequently in sleep-incompatible activities in the bedroom due to physical discomfort and restricted range of movement. Daytime napping is also a common practice and may decrease the homeostatic drive when scheduled too close to bedtime.

Controlled studies indicate that stimulus control, singly or in combination, is effective for both sleep-onset and sleep-maintenance insomnia in older adults

(16–21). However, results from a recent review examining evidence-based psychological treatments for older adults suggest that this approach, although well validated with younger adults, only partially meets criteria for an evidence-based intervention in older adults (4). This may be due to the fact that recent clinical studies conducted with older adults have typically combined these procedures with other behavioral and cognitive procedures.

Relaxation-Based Interventions

There are several types of relaxation-based interventions (22), with some methods aimed at reducing muscle tension (e.g., progressive-muscle relaxation), whereas attention-focusing procedures target mental arousal in the forms of worries or intrusive thoughts (e.g., imagery training). A more passive form of relaxation may be preferable with older adults experiencing physical discomfort or pain (13,20,23). Relaxation requires training and daily practice for at least two to four weeks and professional guidance is often necessary at the initial stage of treatment. Relaxation has been shown to be effective for insomnia in younger adults with few differences across methods, but less so with older individuals (12,13,18).

Cognitive Therapy

Insomnia can be exacerbated by excessive preoccupation with sleep and by apprehensions of the next day consequences, all of which can heighten arousal and interfere with sleep (see Fig. 2). Some older adults may struggle to maintain sleep patterns that are unrealistic for their age groups, whereas others believe that insomnia is an inevitable fact of aging. Cognitive therapy seeks to alter such beliefs, expectations, or attributions either through the use of formal cognitive restructuring (24) or through education about changing some of these sleep/insomnia misconceptions. The basic premise of this approach is that appraisal of a given situation (sleeplessness) can trigger negative emotions (anxiety, frustration) which are incompatible with sleep. For example, when a person is unable to sleep at night and begins thinking about the possible consequences of sleep loss on the next day's performance, this can set off a spiral reaction and feed into the cycle of insomnia, emotional distress, and more sleep disturbances. Cognitive therapy for insomnia is designed to short-circuit the self-fulfilling nature of this cycle (25). A more didactic approach can be used to provide basic facts about individual differences in sleep needs and developmental changes in sleep physiology over the course of the life span. This information is useful to distinguish age-related changes in sleep patterns from clinical insomnia. Cognitive therapy has become a standard component of most insomnia interventions (26–30), although its specific contribution to outcomes remains to be evaluated in older adults (4).

Sleep Hygiene Education

Sleep hygiene education is concerned with health practices (e.g., diet, exercise, substance use) and environmental factors (e.g., light, noise, temperature) that may interfere with sleep. Although these factors are seldom of sufficient severity to be the primary cause of insomnia, they may exacerbate sleep difficulties caused by other factors. Several recommendations can be made to minimize interference from poor sleep hygiene practices: avoidance of stimulants (e.g., caffeine, nicotine) and alcohol, exercising regularly, and minimizing noise, light, and excessive temperature. Although sleep hygiene education alone is often not sufficient for treating insomnia successfully (17), a regular exercise regimen has been found useful for insomnia in older adults (31).

EVIDENCE FOR TREATMENT EFFICACY AND EFFECTIVENESS IN OLDER ADULTS

Evidence regarding the efficacy of psychological and behavioral treatments has been summarized in several meta-analyses and systematic reviews (3–5,9,29,32–34). Estimates of effect sizes, across all age groups, indicate that treatment produces reliable changes in several sleep parameters including sleep latency (average effect size of 0.88), number of awakenings (0.53–0.63), duration of awakenings (0.65), total sleep time (0.42–0.49), and sleep-quality ratings (0.94). These effect sizes are similar to those obtained for hypnotic medications (34) with a slight advantage for behavioral treatment on measures of sleep latency and quality, and for medication on total sleep time. These estimates are based on all behavioral therapies and across all age groups and insomnia diagnoses.

As sleep becomes more fragmented with advancing age and given the higher rate of medical comorbidity associated with insomnia in late life, it cannot be assumed that older adults would respond to treatment in the same way as younger adults do. Recognizing this gap in knowledge and the importance of better understanding the treatment needs in older adults, two systematic reviews have recently focused on this population. In a comparison of studies conducted with middle-aged adults versus older adults (55+ years of age), Irwin et al. (3) found moderate to large effect sizes (0.5–0.79) on subjective measures of sleep latency, wake after sleep onset, and sleep quality in both groups. However, smaller effects were obtained on measures of SE and total sleep time for the older relative to younger age group. A systematic review applying American Psychological Association evidence-based criteria (35) was recently conducted to evaluate the benefits of psychological treatments for insomnia in older adults specifically (4). Only two treatments met criteria for evidence-based psychological treatments for insomnia in older adults – sleep restriction and multicomponent CBT, which contrasts with another systematic review of studies conducted with all age groups that found several therapies (stimulus control, sleep restriction, relaxation, CBT, paradoxical intention) to meet these same criteria (5).

While older adults were often excluded from earlier clinical trials, increasing attention to the aging individual has been emerging in recent clinical trials of behavioral interventions for insomnia. For example, in a systematic review of the evidence for the period of 1998–2004 (5), 9 out of 37 reviewed studies were conducted with older adults (average age > 60 years old), which contrast with only eight studies reported for the previous two decades (1978–1997) (29). Another important shift in focus is that earlier studies mostly included otherwise healthy and medication-free older adults, whereas recent investigations have been evaluating insomnia treatment in comorbid conditions and associated with chronic use of hypnotics.

Among the most recent investigations with older adults, four focused on primary insomnia (11,13,29,36), four on insomnia associated with medical or psychiatric illnesses (30,37–39), one included a mix of patients with primary and secondary insomnia (20), two evaluated the impact of behavioral interventions in older adults who were chronic users of hypnotic medications (26,28), and one study (40) examined the moderating role of upper airway resistance syndrome in the treatment of postmenopausal insomnia. With one exception (20), all these investigations were randomized clinical trials.

Primary Insomnia

In a study of 89 older adults with primary insomnia (13), sleep restriction and relaxation were both more effective than a psychological placebo for reducing time awake after sleep onset; changes were identical (67–43 minutes) for the two treatment groups at the end of the six-week treatment phase, but sleep restriction produced the best outcome at the one-year follow-up. No significant changes were obtained on polysomnography (PSG) measures. All three conditions, including placebo control, showed improvements on secondary measures of fatigue and a measure of insomnia impact. In a comparison of sleep restriction, with and without an optional daytime nap, with sleep education alone (11), both sleep restriction conditions produced greater SE increase, with reduced time spent in bed, relative to the control condition. There was no significant group difference on actigraphy or PSG measures; total sleep time was reduced for the sleep restriction conditions at posttreatment and returned toward baseline values at the three-month follow-up. There was a mild increase in physiological sleepiness (as measured by the multiple sleep latency test [MSLT]) but no change in subjective sleepiness. Results of a study comparing a multimodal CBT intervention to pharmacotherapy and placebo interventions in 46 adults with chronic primary insomnia (36) suggested that CBT improved short-term and long-term outcomes compared with pharmacotherapy in three out of four measures. Results also showed that participants in the CBT group spent more time in slow-wave sleep compared with those in other groups and spent less time awake during the night.

Comorbid Insomnia

At least five studies have now produced evidence that older adults with insomnia and comorbid medical disorders can benefit from sleep-specific behavioral interventions (20,30,37–39). In a study of 51 older adults with insomnia associated with medical illness (30), CBT and relaxation conditions were more effective than control on diary measures of wake after sleep onset and SE, as well as on a measure of overall sleep quality (PSQI); the relaxation group had a greater increase in total sleep time than CBT and controls. A higher proportion of treated patients relative to controls achieved clinically significant improvements. There were no differential group effects on actigraphy, medication use, or other secondary measures of anxiety, depression, and quality of life. In a study of 49 older adults with insomnia associated with medical and psychiatric conditions (38), a combined intervention of stimulus control, relaxation, and education reduced wake after sleep onset by 25 minutes and increased SE by 11% at posttreatment. Fifty-seven percent of treated patients achieved clinically significant improvements relative to 19% of control patients; there was no significant change in secondary measures of anxiety, depression, and impact of insomnia. Outcomes were similar for individuals with insomnia associated with a medical condition and those with insomnia related to a psychiatric disorder. In a study of older adults presenting osteoarthritis, coronary artery disease, or pulmonary disease (39), 92 individuals were randomly allocated to either classroom CBT or stress management placebo. Compared with participants of the placebo conditions, CBT participants showed larger improvements in 8 out of 10 self-report measures of sleep; the type of chronic disease had no impact on the sleep outcomes. These latter results provide indirect evidence that psychological factors are likely involved in insomnia. Furthermore, this is especially important for the older adults, because they are at increased risk of having chronic physical conditions. Targeting insomnia-maintaining factors can provide relief for a condition which was thought as more refractory or contingent only of the physical condition's remission.

In a study of older adults with mixed primary and secondary insomnia (20), a combination of sleep education plus stimulus control was as effective as sleep education plus relaxation, and more effective than a wait-list control; there were modest improvements of daytime measures for both active conditions. Finally, a brief behavioral intervention implemented in the context of two consultation visits in primary care was found of benefits to older adults (mean age = 70.2 years) with medical and psychiatric comorbidities (37). Treatment was associated with significant improvements in sleep and daytime symptoms of anxiety and depression. Of the 17 individuals who received the intervention, 12 met criteria for a treatment response and 9 for remission.

Combined Behavioral and Pharmacological Approaches

Combined behavioral and drug interventions should theoretically optimize treatment outcome by capitalizing on the more rapid relief produced by medication and the more sustained effects of behavioral therapy. Several studies have contrasted the separate and combined effects of behavioral and pharmacological therapies for insomnia, but only two of these were conducted with older adults (29,36). In the first study (29), 76 older adults treated with CBT, medication (temazepam), or combined CBT plus medication improved more on the main outcome measures of SE and wake after sleep onset than those receiving placebo. PSG comparisons yielded improvements in the same direction, albeit of smaller magnitude, than those reported on sleep diaries. A greater proportion of patients treated with CBT, alone or combined with medication, achieved clinically significant improvements (i.e., SE > 85%) compared with those receiving medication alone or placebo. In the second study (36), described in the "Primary Insomnia" section earlier, 46 adults (mean age = 60.8 years) with chronic primary insomnia received CBT, sleep medication (zopiclone, 7.5 mg HS), or a pill-placebo. The results showed that CBT produced better outcomes than medication on three of the four main endpoints (SE, total wake time, slow-wave sleep), both at the six-week postassessment and six-month follow-up. There was no difference in total sleep time.

Evidence from these investigations and other studies conducted with younger and middle-aged adults (34) indicate that both treatment modalities are effective in the short term, with drug therapy producing quicker and slightly better results in the acute phase (first week) of treatment, whereas behavioral and drug therapies are equally effective in the short-term interval (4–8 weeks). Combined interventions appear to have a slight advantage over single treatment modality during the initial course of treatment, but it is unclear whether a combined approach produces a better long-term outcome than behavioral therapy alone. For instance, the Morin et al. (29) study (1999) showed that sleep improvements were well sustained after behavioral treatment, while those obtained with a benzodiazepine hypnotic were gradually lost after discontinuation of the medication. Long-term effects of combined behavioral and pharmacological approaches were more variable. Thus, despite the intuitive appeal in combining drug and nondrug interventions, it is not entirely clear when, how, and for whom this is indicated. In light of the mediating role of psychological factors in chronic insomnia, behavioral and psychological/attitudinal changes appear essential to sustain improvements in sleep patterns. Additional research is needed to evaluate the effects of combined treatments for insomnia and to examine mechanisms of changes mediating short- and long-term outcomes.

Treatment of Insomnia in Chronic Hypnotic Users

Hypnotic discontinuation can be a challenging task for some people, particularly after prolonged use, which is frequent in older adult populations. Two investigations have investigated the efficacy of behavioral interventions for insomnia in the context of chronic hypnotic usage in older adults (26,28). In a study of 209 chronic hypnotic users (26), CBT was associated with improved subjective sleep quality and reductions of hypnotic use at three-month and six-month follow-ups. A greater percentage of patients treated with CBT for insomnia (39%) relative to no treatment controls (11%) achieved at least a 50% reduction in hypnotic use relative to baseline at the six-month follow-up. A cost-offset analysis revealed that when CBT was added to the initial treatment cost, there was a significant cost offset at follow-up resulting from a reduction of sleep medication use. In another study comparing a supervised medication withdrawal program, alone and combined with CBT for insomnia, with CBT alone (28), all three interventions produced significant reductions in both the quantity (90%) and frequency (80%) of benzodiazepine use, and more patients in the combined approach (85%) were medication free at post-treatment than those receiving the taper schedule alone (48%) or CBT alone (54%). There were modest changes in sleep patterns during the initial 10-week withdrawal phase, but CBT-treated patients reported greater sleep improvements relative to those receiving the medication withdrawal alone. Several improvements were also reported in secondary measures of insomnia severity, anxiety, and depressive symptoms.

Insomnia in Special Populations

Treatment outcome evidence has been derived predominantly from clinical studies conducted with ambulatory outpatient populations in relatively good health. Sleep disturbances are probably more prevalent and more incapacitating among elderly patients with dementia and those living in nursing homes. A multicomponent intervention restricting the amount of time spent in bed during the daytime, combined with daily sunlight exposure, increased physical activity, and structured bedtime routine has yielded some promising results in improving sleep/wake rhythms and social life among nursing home residents (41,42). A similar behavioral program was also found beneficial for patients with dementia living at home with their family caregivers (43). An earlier study by McCurry et al. (44) had also found that a behavioral intervention involving sleep and stress management could also benefit elderly caregivers of dementia patients.

ADVANTAGES AND LIMITATIONS OF CBT WITH OLDER ADULTS

When the clinician has to select a treatment option for managing insomnia in the elderly patient, several advantages and limitations must be considered to weigh the different options. The main advantages of CBT include its safety, acceptance by patients, and durability of clinical improvements. Indeed, CBT is a safer treatment option than most hypnotics, which are all associated with some risks of adverse

TABLE 1   Psychological and Behavioral Treatments for Insomnia

Therapy	Description
Stimulus control therapy	A set of instructions designed to reassociate the bed/bedroom with sleep and to re-establish a consistent sleep–wake schedule: go to bed only when sleepy; get out of bed when unable to sleep; use the bed/bedroom for sleep only (no reading, watching TV, etc.); arise at the same time every morning; no napping
Sleep restriction therapy	A method to curtail time in bed to the actual sleep time, thereby creating mild sleep deprivation, which results in more consolidated and more efficient sleep
Relaxation training	Clinical procedures aimed at reducing somatic tension (e.g., progressive muscle relaxation, autogenic training) or intrusive thoughts (e.g., imagery training, meditation) interfering with sleep
Cognitive therapy	Psychotherapeutic method aimed at changing faulty beliefs, attitudes, misconceptions, or unrealistic expectations about sleep, insomnia, and the next day consequences
Sleep hygiene education	General guidelines about health practices (e.g., diet, exercise, substance use) and environmental factors (e.g., light, noise, temperature) that may promote or interfere with sleep

effects, tolerance, dependence, and interactions with other drugs. This safety issue becomes particularly important when insomnia is comorbid with other medical conditions. The most significant advantage of CBT is that it produces treatment gains that are well sustained over time; although it requires more time and efforts, CBT produces sleep improvements that are more durable than medication. Finally, unlike most hypnotic medications, which can alter the sleep architecture, CBT improves sleep continuity without altering sleep stages and one study (36) actually showed some increase in slow-wave sleep. Despite these advantages, CBT is not a panacea for all older adults with insomnia. It does require motivation and time, from both patients and clinicians and, although it is generally well accepted, compliance with behavioral recommendations is not always optimal. Some old habits and beliefs about sleep are strongly engrained and may represent a real barrier to compliance. There are also some educational, psychological, and physical (cognitive and physical limitations), as well as contextual factors (residential care facilities) that might limit the use of behavioral interventions. Accessibility to therapists with expertise in providing behavioral intervention for insomnia is another important limiting factor. Innovative training programs for nurses or mental-health therapists to implement brief behavioral interventions in primary care and mental health clinics have recently been pilot-tested in small clinical studies and the results are promising (37,45). Additional translational research is warranted.

CONCLUSIONS
Insomnia is a prevalent and costly health problem which is often left untreated, especially in older adults. Significant advances have been made in the management of insomnia and recent investigations have documented the benefits of CBT for older adults with primary insomnia, comorbid insomnia, and among chronic users of hypnotics. Thus, the presence of comorbid medical or psychiatric conditions is not a contraindication to using CBT and, in many cases, CBT should be the first-line

approach to treating persistent insomnia. The magnitude of treatment response is generally comparable with that obtained with younger adults, particularly when patients are screened for other sleep disorders (e.g., sleep apnea). Although few older adults resume "normal sleep" with treatment, CBT-treated patients are usually more satisfied with their sleep, use less medication, and report lower psychological distress and concerns with sleep. Most importantly, CBT produces sleep improvements that are well sustained over time. An important challenge for the future will be to promote wider dissemination and utilization of this approach among health care providers and make it more readily accessible to seniors.

REFERENCES

1. Foley DJ, Monjan AA, Brown SL, et al. Sleep complaints among elderly persons: an epidemiologic study of three communities. Sleep 1995; 18:425–432.
2. Hohagen F, Kappler C, Schramm E, et al. Prevalence of insomnia in elderly general practice attenders and the current treatment modalities. Acta Psychiatr Scand 1994; 90:102–108.
3. Irwin MR, Cole JC, Nicassio PM. Comparative meta-analysis of behavioral interventions for insomnia and their efficacy in middle-aged adults and in older adults 55+ years of age. Health Psychol 2006; 25:3–14.
4. McCurry SM, Logsdon RG, Teri L, et al. Evidence-based psychological treatments for insomnia in older adults. Psychol Aging 2007; 22:18–27.
5. Morin CM, Bootzin RR, Buysse DJ, et al. Psychological and behavioral treatment of insomnia: update of the recent evidence (1998–2004). Sleep 2006; 29:1398–1414.
6. National Institutes of Health. Manifestations and management of chronic insomnia in adults. Sleep 2005; 28:1049–1057.
7. Spielman AJ, Conroy D, Glovinsky PB. Evaluation of insomnia. In: Perlis ML, Lichstein KL, eds. Treating Sleep Disorders: Principles and Practice of Behavioral Sleep Medicine. New York: Wiley, 2003:190–213.
8. Lichstein KL, Morin CM. Treatment of Late-Life Insomnia. Thousand Oaks, CA: Sage Publications, 2000.
9. Nau SD, McCrae CS, Cook KG, et al. Treatment of insomnia in older adults. Clin Psychol Rev 2005; 25:645–672.
10. Spielman AJ, Saskin P, Thorpy MJ. Treatment of chronic insomnia by restriction of time in bed. Sleep 1987; 10:45–56.
11. Friedman L, Benson K, Noda A, et al. An actigraphic comparison of sleep restriction and sleep hygiene treatments for insomnia in older adults. J Geriatr Psychiatry Neurol 2000; 13:17–27.
12. Friedman L, Bliwise DL, Yesavage JA, et al. A preliminary study comparing sleep restriction and relaxation treatments for insomnia in older adults. J Gerontol 1991; 46:1–8.
13. Lichstein KL, Riedel BW, Wilson NM, et al. Relaxation and sleep compression for late-life insomnia: a placebo-controlled trial. J Consult Clin Psychol 2001; 69:227–239.
14. Riedel BW, Lichstein KL, Dwyer WO. Sleep compression and sleep education for older insomniacs: self-help versus therapist guidance. Psychol Aging 1995; 10:54–63.
15. Bootzin RR, Epstein D. Stimulus control. In: Lichstein KL, Morin CM, eds. Treatment of Late-Life Insomnia. Thousand Oaks, CA: Sage Publications, 1991:167–184.
16. Davies R, Lacks P, Storandt M, et al. Counter-control treatment of sleep-maintenance insomnia in relation to age. Psychol Aging 1986; 1:233–238.
17. Engle-Friedman M, Bootzin RR, Hazlewood L, et al. An evaluation of behavioral treatments for insomnia in the older adult. J Clin Psychol 1992; 48:77–90.
18. Morin CM, Azrin NH. Behavioral and cognitive treatments of geriatric insomnia. J Consult Clin Psychol 1988; 56:748–753.

19. Morin CM, Kowatch RA, Barry T, et al. Cognitive behavior therapy for late-life insomnia. J Consult Clin Psychol 1993; 1:137–146.
20. Pallesen S, Nordhus IH, Kvale G, et al. Behavioral treatment of insomnia in older adults: an open clinical trial comparing two interventions. Behav Res Ther 2003; 41:31–48.
21. Puder R, Lacks P, Bertelson AD, et al. Short-term stimulus control treatment of insomnia in older adults. Behav Ther 1983; 14:424–429.
22. Manber R, Kuo TF. Cognitive-behavioral therapies for insomnia. In: Lee-Chiong TL, Sateia ML, Carskadon MA, eds. Sleep Medicine. Philadelphia: Hanley & Belfus, 2002:177–185.
23. Lichstein KL, Johnson RS. Relaxation for insomnia and hypnotic medication use in older women. Psychol Aging 1993; 8:103–111.
24. Beck JS. Cognitive therapy: basics and beyond. New York: The Guilford Press, 1995.
25. Bélanger L, Savard J, Morin CM. Clinical management of insomnia using cognitive therapy. Behav Sleep Med 2006; 4:179–202.
26. Morgan K, Dixon S, Mathers N, et al. Psychological treatment for insomnia in the management of long-term hypnotic drug use: a pragmatic randomised controlled trial. Br J Gen Pract 2003; 53:923–928.
27. Morin CM. Insomnia: psychological assessment and management. New York, NY: The Guilford Press, 1993.
28. Morin CM, Bastien CH, Guay B, et al. Randomized clinical trial of supervised tapering and cognitive-behavior therapy to facilitate benzodiazepine discontinuation in older adults with chronic insomnia. Am J Psychiatry 2004; 161:332–342.
29. Morin CM, Colecchi C, Stone J, et al. Behavioral and pharmacological therapies for late-life insomnia: a randomized clinical trial. JAMA 1999; 281:991–999.
30. Rybarczyk B, Lopez M, Benson R, et al. Efficacy of two behavioral treatment programs for comorbid geriatric insomnia. Psychol Aging 2002; 17:288–298.
31. King AC, Oman RF, Brassington GS, et al. Moderate-intensity exercise and self-rated quality of sleep in older adults. A randomized controlled trial. JAMA 1997; 277:32–37.
32. Montgomery P, Dennis J. A systematic review of non-pharmacological therapies for sleep problems in later life. Sleep Med Rev 2004; 8:47–62.
33. Pallesen S, Nordhus IH, Kvale G. Nonpharmacological interventions for insomnia in older adults: a meta-analysis of treatment efficacy. Psychotherapy 1998; 35:472–482.
34. Smith MT, Perlis ML, Park A, et al. Comparative meta-analysis of pharmacotherapy and behavior therapy for persistent insomnia. Am J Psychiatry 2002; 159:5–11.
35. American Psychological Association Presidential Task Force on Evidence-Based Practice. Evidence-based practice in psychology. Am Psychol 2006; 61:271–285.
36. Sivertsen B, Omvik S, Pallesen S, et al. Cognitive behavioral therapy vs zopiclone for treatment of chronic primary insomnia in older adults: a randomized controlled trial. JAMA 2006; 295:2851–2858.
37. Germain A, Moul DE, Franzen PL, et al. Effects of a brief behavioral treatment for late-life insomnia: preliminary findings. J Clin Sleep Med 2006; 15:403–406.
38. Lichstein KL, Wilson NM, Johnson CT. Psychological treatment of secondary insomnia. Psychol Aging 2000; 15:232–240.
39. Rybarczyk B, Stepanski E, Fogg L, et al. A placebo-controlled test of cognitive-behavioral therapy for co-morbid insomnia in older adults. J Consult Clin Psychol 2005; 73:1164–1174.
40. Guilleminault C, Palombini L, Poyares D, et al. Chronic insomnia, premenopausal women and sleep disordered breathing. Part 2. Comparison of nondrug treatment trials in normal breathing and UARS post menopausal women complaining of chronic insomnia. J Psychosom Res 2002; 53:617–623.
41. Alessi CA, Martin JL, Webber AP, et al. Randomized, controlled trial of a nonpharmacological intervention to improve abnormal sleep wake patterns in nursing home residents. J Am Geriatr Soc 2005; 53:803–810.
42. Martin JL, Marler MR, Harker JO, et al. A multicomponent nonpharmacological intervention improves activity rhythms among nursing home residents with disrupted sleep/wake patterns. J Gerontol A Biol Sci Med Sci 2007; 62:67–72.

43. McCurry SM, Gibbons LE, Logsdon RG, et al. Nighttime insomnia treatment and education for Alzheimer's disease: a randomized, controlled trial. J Am Geriatr Soc 2005; 53:793–802.
44. McCurry SM, Logsdon RG, Vitiello MV, et al. Successful behavioral treatment for reported sleep problems in elderly caregivers of dementia patients: a controlled study. J Gerontol B Psychol Sci Soc Sci 1998; 53:122–129.
45. McCrae CS, McGovern R, Lukefahr R, et al. Research evaluating brief behavioral sleep treatments for rural elderly (RESTORE): a preliminary examination of effectiveness. Am J Geriatr Psychiatry 2007; 15:979–982.

Sleep-Related Breathing Disorders in Aging

Nalaka S. Gooneratne

Division of Geriatric Medicine and the Center for Sleep and Respiratory Neurobiology, University of Pennsylvania School of Medicine, Philadelphia, Pennsylvania, U.S.A.

INTRODUCTION

Obstructive sleep apnea is a common entity in older adults that can lead to significant impairments in sleep quality and daytime functioning. It is often under-diagnosed, however, because of both an underappreciation of its prevalence and consequences in older adults as well as an inconstant presentation of signs and symptoms. In addition, relatively few studies have focused on obstructive sleep apnea in the older population. As a result, much of our knowledge base on obstructive sleep apnea in older adults is based on extrapolation of findings from younger populations. Whenever possible, this review will attempt to cite literature that focuses on older adults and will specifically identify these studies as such; however, in most cases, data from younger cohorts will be discussed, as these remain the only data available.

MANIFESTATIONS AND CONSEQUENCES

Definition

Obstructive sleep apnea is characterized by recurrent upper airway obstruction that occurs during the sleep period (1). These episodes can lead to intermittent nocturnal oxyhemoglobin desaturation, episodes of central nervous system arousal, or fragmented sleep (1,2).

Obstructive sleep apnea is often quantified by the apnea–hypopnea index (AHI), which refers to the number of apneas or hypopneas that occur each hour of sleep. An apnea is formally defined as a cessation (a 90% or more reduction in breathing) for at least 10 seconds (93). A hypopnea is defined as a greater than 4% drop in oxyhemoglobin saturation, which is due to either a 30% reduction in thoracic or abdominal effort, or a 30% reduction in airflow (1).

The clinical diagnosis of obstructive sleep apnea is established when a patient meets either of the following criteria: (1) an AHI>5 events/hr with associated symptoms, such as daytime sleepiness, insomnia, nocturnal awakening due to abnormal breathing, or witnessed apneas/loud snoring, or (2) an AHI>15 events/hr (1). While the current International Classification of Sleep Disorders does not propose severity criteria, one approach is to classify patients who have 5 to 15 events/hr as having mild obstructive sleep apnea; 15 to 30 events/hr, as having moderate obstructive sleep apnea; and more than 30 events/hr, as having severe obstructive sleep apnea.

Subtypes of Obstructive Sleep Apnea

Rapid eye movement (REM)-related sleep apnea refers to cases where the abnormal breathing episodes occur primarily during the REM phase of sleep. These patients may have relatively normal breathing during non-REM sleep or may have only a slightly elevated AHI during non-REM sleep. Positional sleep apnea, in contrast, occurs primarily when the patient is in the supine position. Other diagnostic groups that have some similarities to obstructive sleep apnea include central sleep apnea (discussed in a later chapter), obesity-hypoventilation syndrome, and upper airway resistance syndrome. Obesity-hypoventilation syndrome is characterized by the presence of obstructive sleep apnea in the setting of impaired ventilatory drive and is usually associated with hypercapnia. Since neurologic abnormalities play a key role, this disorder is generally classified under central hypoventilation disorder (1). Patients with upper airway resistance syndrome often do not have frank recurrent upper airway obstruction as noted on flow monitors, but have recurrent arousals due to increased airway resistance. These events are referred to as respiratory effort-related arousals (RERAs) (1). It is a diagnosis that is not universally accepted and can be difficult to establish without the use of esophageal manometry in addition to the standard polysomnography montage. Upper airway resistance syndrome is generally included under the diagnosis code for obstructive sleep apnea (1). Primary snoring could also be viewed as an abnormal breathing pattern; however, it is not associated with apneas, or hypopneas, and does not lead to oxyhemoglobin desaturation or arousals; thus it is a relatively benign condition.

While a distinct entity referred to as "geriatric sleep apnea" has been proposed (3), this is not yet a widely accepted term. The term geriatric sleep apnea may be relevant because obstructive sleep apnea in older adults can have different manifestations and sequelae than in younger populations. However, it is not clear if it represents a distinct diagnostic entity or rather a continuum of disease (4). The same criteria for obstructive sleep apnea are generally applied to young, middle-aged and aged populations, although some have argued that the threshold for obstructive sleep apnea should be higher in older populations (5).

The term "sleep-related breathing disorder" (SRBD) is a related term that is often used in research studies that rely on polysomnography criteria alone (independent of a physician evaluation). This term often includes obstructive apneas, hypopneas, and central apneas, and the definition for hypopneas, in particular, may vary from study to study. We will use the term sleep-related breathing disorders when referring to research studies that specifically mention SRBDs, but will otherwise use the term obstructive sleep apnea consistent with the International Classification of Sleep Disorders, 2nd edition, criteria (1). The term sleep apnea will be used if a manuscript does not distinguish between central or obstructive sleep apnea. It is also worth noting that the severity of SRBDs can be described by the respiratory disturbance index (RDI), which may include "respiratory event related arousals" in addition to apneas and hypopneas; this differs from the AHI, which only includes apneas and hypopneas. The term RDI or AHI will be used in this review in a manner similar to that used by the original study authors when presenting research findings.

Manifestations

History

Obstructive sleep apnea in younger populations is often associated with a characteristic history that can aid in diagnosis. Typical symptoms include loud snoring, witnessed apneas, nocturnal choking or gasping, or dry mouth (1,6). In older populations, however, these symptoms have a weaker association to sleep apnea. For example, witnessed breathing pauses in subjects aged <40 years had an odds ratio of >10 for SRBDs, while in subjects >60 years, the odds ratio had decreased to <5 (6). There are several possible explanations for this. First, older adults are more likely to be single; in these cases, the history of sleep symptoms is less accurate and patients are more likely to respond that they "don't know" (7). Additional useful history can be obtained from family members or friends who may notice snoring or apneas during nap episodes or visits. Central sleep apnea may also be more frequent in older adults, especially if they have comorbid conditions such as heart failure. The absence of respiratory effort during a central apnea (which would otherwise lead to snoring or gasping) may make it more difficult to detect by an observer.

The identification of obstructive sleep apnea is further complicated by the fact that daytime symptoms, such as daytime sleepiness, may also be difficult to discern. For example, daytime sleepiness may be a frequent complaint in older adults due to reasons other than sleep disorders (8); these include comorbid medical illnesses such as heart failure or hypothyroidism, and the effects of medications, such as clonidine (8).

While some of the signs and symptoms used to identify obstructive sleep apnea in younger patients may be less reliable in older adults, it is also possible that older adults may present with different types of complaints. Nocturia or nocturnal falls may be important manifestations of obstructive sleep apnea in older adults, for example (4).

Physical Exam

There are several findings that are suggestive of obstructive sleep apnea on physical exam. These include the following: (1) neck circumference >40 cm (approximately 15.5 inches), (2) body mass index (BMI) >25 kg/mm^2, (3) low-lying soft palate, (4) elongated or large uvula, (5) large tongue (often noted by the presence of tongue edge crenations), or (6) large tonsils or narrow distance between the tonsillar pillars (9–11). Nasal abnormalities, such as nasal septal deviation, may also contribute (11). The association between these exam findings and obstructive sleep apnea may weaken with age: the odds ratio for having sleep-related breathing disorder in the presence of an increased BMI was 2.0 for at age 40, but decreased to 1.3 by age 80 (6). In older adults, an additional risk factor is the edentulous state. When patients remove their dentures at night, this leads to a reduction in the vertical dimension that increases the occurrence of upper airway obstructive events (12).

Underdiagnosis in Older Adults

Sleep disorders, in general, are often not evaluated in older adults: sleep histories are rarely obtained during routine clinical encounters, and when evaluating symptomatic older adults, polysomnographies were rarely or never ordered 80% of the

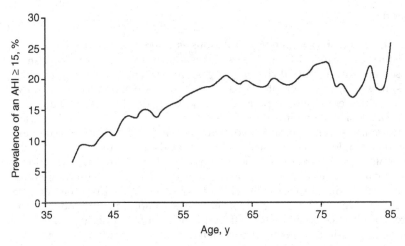

FIGURE 1 Prevalence of sleep-related breathing disorder (AHI = 15 events/hr) as a function of age (smoothed plot). *Source*: From Ref. 6.

time (13). The challenges noted above in discerning symptoms and signs suggestive of obstructive sleep apnea may contribute to this tendency toward underdiagnosis. Women, across all ages, tend to be less frequently referred for evaluation of obstructive sleep apnea symptoms than men (14) and are less likely to be diagnosed with obstructive sleep apnea despite having symptoms (15).

Epidemiology
Several studies have examined the prevalence of obstructive sleep apnea in older adult populations. The Sleep Heart Health Study of 5615 subjects drawn from six existing cardiovascular/pulmonary studies noted that sleep-disordered breathing was common in older adults, with approximately 20% of subjects aged 60 or above having an AHI = 15 events/hr (6). Furthermore, this prevalence rate was higher than in younger subjects, where only 10% of subjects aged 39 to 49 had SRBD (6). These prevalence rates are based on cross-sectional data, and thus may be influenced by the survivorship effect: subjects with more severe disease may pass away and no longer be represented in the cross-sectional analysis. This is suggested by the observation that the prevalence rate appears to "plateau" after the age of 60 (Fig. 1).

There are also ethnic differences in the prevalence of obstructive sleep apnea. Asians, due to craniofacial differences, are more likely to have obstructive sleep apnea in the absence of obesity (16). African-Americans may also have elevated rates of severe sleep-related breathing disorder (RDI > 30) relative to Caucasians (17). Obstructive sleep apnea clusters in families, most likely due to genetic factors such as obesity and craniofacial structure (18).

Institutionalized Patients
While prevalence rates of obstructive sleep apnea are more common in older adults, the prevalence rate is potentially even higher in institutionalized patients. This is discussed in more detail in the chapter "Sleep in Nursing Homes." One factor that

may contribute to the high prevalence rate of obstructive sleep apnea in institutionalized patients is the high rate of dementia in these populations: Dementia is strongly associated with sleep apnea (19). The mean RDI for patients with no dementia, mild dementia, or moderate dementia was 15.8 ± 14.5 events/hr, while in patients with severe dementia, it was 25.8 ± 24.0 events/hr (20). These data are from cross-sectional studies; thus it is unclear if dementia is a risk factor for obstructive sleep apnea or vice versa (see the "Consequences" section). One mechanism by which dementia may contribute to the development of obstructive sleep apnea is by loss of upper motor neurons as part of the degenerative disease process, thus resulting in reduced upper airway muscle tone.

Other Etiologic Considerations

Age-related changes may occur in the upper airway that could increase the proclivity toward obstructive sleep apnea (21,22). Upper airway muscle changes may contribute to this process. Aged Wistar rats, for example, have altered genioglossus (tongue) fiber-type distribution that leads to an increased risk of obstructive sleep apnea due to decreased muscle endurance (23). Repetitive barotrauma due to many years of apnea events could also be a risk factor with advancing age.

CONSEQUENCES

Obstructive sleep apnea is associated with a myriad range of adverse consequences. Of note, obstructive sleep apnea has a weaker association with some of these conditions in older adults than in younger subjects. This may be related to the effect of "competing morbidities" where other age-related processes may attenuate the risk of any one specific condition on specific domains.

Cardiovascular

Hypertension

Hypertension has often been associated with obstructive sleep apnea because of increased sympathetic tone and the loss of the nocturnal "dip" in blood pressure. With advancing age, there may be an attenuation of the risk of hypertension in patients with sleep apnea. In subjects under the age of 65, the Sleep Heart Health Study investigators noted that the odds ratio for having hypertension in the setting of sleep-related breathing disorder (as defined by an AHI = 30 events/hr) was 1.64 in an adjusted model, while in subjects over the age of 65, the odds ratio decreased to 1.23 and was no longer statistically significant (24).

One of the most robust ways to demonstrate a causal link between a risk factor and an outcome is by demonstrating a treatment response. Treatment of obstructive sleep apnea with positive airway pressure (PAP, described in more detail later) has been found to improve hypertension in adults with moderate or severe sleep apnea to a greater extent than sham PAP or supplemental oxygen alone (25). A recent meta-analysis confirmed the presence of small but statistically significant improvement of 2.22 mmHg in mean arterial pressure with PAP (26). It is possible that the benefits for PAP therapy are most prominent in patients who have daytime sleepiness in addition to hypertension (27). However, many of these studies have not been repeated in older adults, and it is unclear if the benefit from PAP will be present in an older adult population.

Other Cardiovascular Diseases

Patients with obstructive sleep apnea may be at higher risk of atrial fibrillation. Gami et al. examined the risk of atrial fibrillation in a retrospective study, where they noted that for subjects under the age of 65 years, nocturnal desaturation (presumably in part from obstructive sleep apnea) and obesity were risk factors for new-onset atrial fibrillation, while in subjects over 65 years of age, obstructive sleep apnea was not a risk factor (28).

Other cardiovascular diseases may also be associated with sleep-related breathing disorders as noted in cross-sectional studies, including congestive heart failure (29) and coronary artery disease (30). Longitudinal research has demonstrated an increased risk of cardiovascular events in patients with untreated obstructive sleep apnea (31). Mortality may also be increased due to elevated rates of sudden cardiac death, with one study showing that in patients with a mean age of 70.1 years, the relative risk of sudden cardiac death from midnight to 6:00 AM was 2.61 in those with an AHI = 40 events/hr compared with those without obstructive sleep apnea (32).

Cerebrovascular Events

The recurrent nocturnal oxyhemoglobin desaturation and other physiologic changes that can occur with obstructive sleep apnea may also increase the risk of cerebrovascular events. Sleep-related breathing disorder, for example, is a risk factor for increased mortality after an acute cerebrovascular event (33). Yaggi et al., in a longitudinal study with a mean follow-up of 3.4 years, also noted an increased risk of stroke or death in patients with obstructive sleep apnea (34). Clinical trial data in this context have had mixed findings. One study comparing patients post cerebrovascular event who were compliant with PAP to those who were not compliant found a significant reduction in recurrent stroke (35). In general, the major limiting factor is patient compliance, with only 29.4% of patients able to tolerate PAP. Indeed, another study found no benefit of PAP therapy in part due to a 22% compliance rate with continuous positive airway pressure (CPAP) therapy (36).

Cognitive Effects

A growing body of literature suggests that obstructive sleep apnea has adverse effects on cognitive function in older adults. While the mechanism for this may be nocturnal hypoxia, it has also been suggested that other factors, such as recurrent nocturnal respiratory arousals or daytime fatigue, may play a role (37). Imaging studies have demonstrated areas of gray matter loss in patients with obstructive sleep apnea relative to controls, especially in areas related to cognitive function (38). Patients who are carriers of APOE epsilon4 may be at particular risk of these cognitive impairments (39).

Recent work has extended these findings by attempting to treat obstructive sleep apnea using PAP therapy. Digital vigilance time improved with PAP therapy in one placebo-controlled trial; however, global metrics of cognitive function were unchanged (40). One frequently cited concern regarding the use of PAP in patients with cognitive impairment is that of compliance. A recent clinical trial of PAP therapy in patients with mild-moderate Alzheimer's disease observed that compliance rates could remain high (41). Caregiver involvement was a key factor in promoting compliance, while depression in the Alzheimer's disease patients reduced compliance (41).

Daytime Sleepiness

Daytime sleepiness and fatigue are frequently cited as key elements in the morbidity of obstructive sleep apnea (1). Older adults, in particular, are susceptible to functional impairment across many domains from daytime sleepiness (42). Treatment of sleep apnea with PAP can improve these functional impairments, as noted in one study of sleep apnea patients ranging from age 28 to 74 (43). Elderly patients with cognitive impairment from mild-moderate Alzheimer's disease can have improvements in daytime sleepiness as well with PAP treatment relative to sham PAP (44). The risk of driving accidents, one particularly important manifestation of daytime sleepiness, can be reduced by obstructive sleep apnea treatment (45).

Gastroesophageal Reflux Disease

Obstructive sleep apnea has also been implicated as a risk factor for gastroesophageal reflux disease (GERD). The significant intrathoracic pressure shifts that occur during an apnea episode may increase the likelihood of gastric acid moving up into the esophagus. Treatment with PAP therapy has been found to significantly reduce the 24-hour acid contact time in patients with GERD and severe obstructive sleep apnea (46).

Urogenital

Nocturia/Incontinence

The prevalence of nocturia increases with advancing age, affecting 72% of men and 91% of women over the age of 80 years (47). Risk factors for nocturia and incontinence include bed rest, congestive heart failure, bladder outlet obstruction and bladder atony, urinary tract infection, and poorly controlled type 2 diabetes, among others. In addition, obstructive sleep apnea may increase the risk of nocturia and incontinence. Abdominal pressure fluctuations during an apneic episode may increase pressure on the bladder and lead to involuntary voiding (48). In addition, apnea episodes may lead to cardiac atria distention or increased right atrium transmural pressure (49). This results in increased production of atrial natriuretic factor, which in turn promotes sodium and water excretion from the kidneys (50); patients with obstructive sleep apnea produce nearly 300 cc more of urine per night than do nonapneic patients (50). Treatment of sleep apnea with PAP therapy can reduce atrial natriuritic peptide levels and improve nocturia (51,52).

Impotence

Patients with severe obstructive sleep apnea, as defined by a respiratory disturbance index >40 events/hr, are more likely to have erectile dysfunction (53). Nocturnal oxyhemoglobin desaturation may be a key element of this process (54). Treatment with PAP therapy was noted to lead to remission of erectile dysfunction in 75% of patients in one uncontrolled trial (54).

Depression

Depression can affect up to 21.8% of patients with obstructive sleep apnea across all age groups (19). Other mood disorders are more common as well (19). The pattern of depression symptoms can vary, with obstructive sleep apnea patients tending to manifest depression symptomatology in the somatic domain as opposed to the cognitive domain of the Beck Depression Index (55). Treatment studies with PAP have had no effect on depression scores according to one meta-analysis (56); however,

PAP did improve global psychological symptom distress as measured by the Brief Symptom Inventory (57).

Comorbid Insomnia and Sleep Apnea

The frequent nocturnal arousals associated with obstructive sleep apnea can increase the risk of insomnia: Up to 51% of patients with sleep-related breathing disorders in one clinic-based cohort had insomnia symptoms (58). The pattern of insomnia complaints tends to be difficulty maintaining sleep, as opposed to difficulty initiating sleep (59). In this context, it is interesting to note that advanced age is associated more so with difficulty maintaining sleep than sleep initiation (60).

It is also possible that the excessive sleepiness that may occur as a consequence of sleep-related breathing disorder may reduce the likelihood of insomnia (9). However, this is a consequence of an adverse effect of obstructive sleep apnea, namely, increased sleepiness. Furthermore, patients with both insomnia and sleep-related breathing disorder are at higher risk of functional impairments than those with either condition alone (9).

DIAGNOSIS AND EVIDENCE-BASED REVIEW OF THERAPY

Diagnosis

The gold-standard method for the diagnosis of obstructive sleep apnea is nocturnal polysomnography (61). A standard polysomnography montage will measure electrooculograms (to assess eye movements), electroencephalograms (to determine arousal events), electromyelograms (to screen for leg or arm movements and muscle tone), electrocardiograms, airflow (to detect obstruction or reduction in airflow), oximetry, chest and abdominal effort, and snoring levels. For assessing sleep apnea, most patients undergo a single night of polysomnography (61). However, there can be significant night-to-night variability in sleep apnea severity (62,63), with approximately 15.5% to 23% of older adults crossing the clinical threshold of an AHI of 5 events/hr from one night to the next (63). Factors associated with increased variability include male gender (64) and nasal obstruction/septal deviation (63). For these reasons, it has been suggested that patients whose clinical complaints do not match their polysomnography findings should undergo a repeat sleep study (62).

Older adults with the signs or symptoms of obstructive sleep apnea clearly warrant evaluation. As noted earlier, though, in many cases the presentation is less apparent. In certain cases, such as patients with significant comorbidites that may be related to sleep apnea, such as coronary artery disease, congestive heart failure, stroke, or poorly controlled hypertension, an evaluation to screen for obstructive sleep apnea may be justified even in the absence of a typical presentation.

Alternate methods of diagnosis have also been proposed. These include oximetry, peripheral arterial tonometry, and limited polysomnography montages. These approaches may be especially useful in cases where limitations in functional status (impairments in activities of daily living) may prevent a patient from coming for an in-lab overnight sleep study. In these cases, it may be possible to request a caregiver to assist overnight with the sleep study if the sleep lab can accommodate a guest. In other situations, though, an alternate study method, such as oximetry or limited montage at-home polysomnographies, may be used. However, there is in adequate evidence at present to recommend these diagnostic modalities for clinical

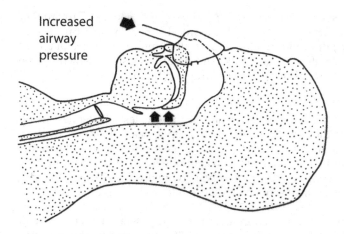

Increased
airway
pressure

FIGURE 2 Diagram demonstrating the effect of PAP therapy on upper airway anatomy. *Source*: Image courtesy of Dr. Sam Kuna.

purposes (65), and they are usually not covered by Medicare or supplemental insurance policies.

Treatment of Sleep Apnea
Obstructive sleep apnea can be treated using a variety of modalities that ultimately act to improve upper airway patency. Most of these methods have been studied in young and middle-aged subjects. There is a marked paucity of data available regarding the efficacy of these techniques in older adults, however.

Positive Airway Pressure
PAP therapy relies on the noninvasive application of increased air pressure from a flow generator to maintain upper airway patency throughout the sleep cycle (Fig. 2). Several studies have examined the effects of PAP relative to the adverse consequences of obstructive sleep apnea (62). These were reviewed earlier as part of the discussion of specific obstructive sleep apnea consequences. A recent Cochrane Database review of PAP therapy for obstructive sleep apnea concluded that PAP therapy was effective in reducing daytime sleepiness and improving quality of life in patients with moderate to severe obstructive sleep apnea (56).

Alternative forms of PAP delivery have also been developed, including autotitrating PAP machines, which adjust the pressure during the course of the night on the basis of a continuous analysis of airflow. In some cases, patients may prefer the autotitrating PAP devices because these devices provide a more tailored pressure profile that may reflect varying pressure needs during the night (especially in cases where the sleep apnea is worse in REM sleep or in the supine position) (66). Close monitoring of the compliance and device-derived apnea-hypopnea data from these devices is warranted in case patients have suboptimal treatment. Another form of PAP is bilevel PAP, in which the airway pressure is reduced during the exhalation phase in order to increase patient tolerance.

Most side effects from PAP therapy result from the physical aspects of therapy (56). These include the following: discomfort from the pressure of the mask on the face, with skin pressure sores or excoriations developing in severe cases (treatment involves changing mask type or patient education); dry nose, which can in rare cases lead to nosebleeds; dry mouth, often as a result of mouth leak (use of a chin strap can reduce this side effect); mask leak; and nasal congestion, which can be treated in some cases with nasal steroids or ipratropium bromide.

PAP Compliance
Ensuring compliance with PAP therapy is one of the greatest challenges facing health care providers as they treat patients with sleep apnea. The initial week of therapy is a crucial period in this regard (67). Overall, nearly 30% to 40% of patients stop using PAP, and many of the patients who continue to use PAP use it for only limited numbers of hours each night or for only a few nights a week (68). In older patients, such as older adult males, noncompliance rates as high as 39% have been reported (69).

Several factors have been studied in regard to their possible association with PAP compliance. A history of "recent life-events" or "living alone" has been associated with reduced PAP compliance (70). Additional history of active cigarette smoking (69) and nocturia (69) have also been noted to reduce PAP compliance. In regard to the patient's obstructive sleep apnea, the presence of mild or moderate sleep apnea (71) and minimal daytime sleepiness symptoms at presentation (71) may lead to reduced compliance. Treatment-related factors include whether the patient had resolution of sleep apnea symptoms with treatment (69) or the need for higher PAP pressures (71). Increasing age has been associated with greater degrees of noncompliance in univariate analysis but, when controlling for other factors, was no longer found to be significant (71). This is possibly due to the limited sample size of the studies that have focused on older subjects.

Patients with insomnia may also have particular difficulty adapting to positive pressure ventilation (72). These patients spend considerable portions of the night awake and thus have a heightened awareness of the discomfort of the equipment (58). For these reasons, treatment of insomnia may help to improve compliance with CPAP (58); however, standardized paradigms have not yet been established.

Patient comfort with PAP can be improved by careful selection of a PAP mask, with particular focus on any disabilities the older adult patient may have that could limit use, such as rotator cuff tears that may limit upper arm mobility. The use of a humidification unit can be helpful on the basis of anecdotal experience, but is not routinely required (73). Increasing a patient's understanding of sleep apnea may also improve compliance; two 45-minute education sessions were found to improve compliance in one study in older adults with obstructive sleep apnea (74). With proper support, older adults can have PAP compliance rates of up to 70% that are similar to patients less than 65 years of age (75).

Medical Therapy
Medical therapy for obstructive sleep apnea consists primarily of treatment for the consequences of obstructive sleep apnea, such as daytime sleepiness. Modafenil was effective in improving both objective and subjective measures of sleepiness in patients with persistent daytime sleepiness despite compliance with PAP (76). Armodafenil has also been tested as an adjunct for patients with obstructive sleep apnea and residual daytime sleepiness (77). While the use of modafenil or

armodafenil for the treatment of residual daytime sleepiness in patients who are being effectively treated for their sleep apnea is well established, its role in patients who are noncompliant with PAP treatment is less clear.

Pharmacotherapy has also been attempted to treat obstructive sleep apnea directly (78). Commonly used agents include protriptyline, mirtazapine, and acetazolamide; while these agents have been associated with improvements in certain areas, side effects limit their use (79). For these reasons, pharmacotherapy is currently not recommended to treat obstructive sleep apnea.

Oral Appliances
Oral appliances improve upper airway patency by advancing the mandible. Commonly used oral appliances include the Herbst and Klearway, but several other models exist as well. Most studies suggest that the AHI is reduced by half with the use of oral appliances (80) and that oral appliances can improve daytime sleepiness (81). While beneficial, oral appliances are generally not recommended over PAP as first-line therapy for obstructive sleep apnea (82).

Most patients prefer oral appliances to PAP therapy; however, adherence rates may be lower for oral appliances (56). Long-term compliance is estimated at 56% to 68% (83). Risk factors for noncompliance with an oral appliance devices include insomnia or the presence of significant comorbidities, such as gastric or neurologic disease (84). Side effects include teeth discomfort, temperomandibular joint disorder, and excessive salivation (83). Patients with dentures or bridges may not be able to use an oral appliance. In some cases, cost may be a limiting factor as oral appliances are not covered by all health insurance policies.

Atrial Overdrive Pacing
In patients with a cardiac pacemaker for cardiac dysrhythmias, such as sinus bradycardia, and sleep apnea, increasing the atrial rate by 15 beats/min has been proposed as a means of reducing the AHI (85). However, subsequent studies have found a small effect (86) or no effect (87,88). Further research is needed to clarify what subtypes of sleep apnea may respond most favorably to this modality.

Behavioral Modification
Two commonly used behavioral modification modalities for the treatment of obstructive sleep apnea include positional therapy and weight loss. Positional therapy consists of techniques intended to increase the time spent in the lateral sleeping position as opposed to the supine position. These include propping a pillow against the back or sewing a ball into the back of the pajama shirt in order to make the supine position more uncomfortable. While frequently recommended for the treatment of positional sleep apnea (i.e., obstructive sleep apnea that is worse in the supine position), little research has been done to evaluate its efficacy, and no studies have been done in older adults. Jokic et al. compared positional therapy to PAP: they noted that positional therapy was as effective as PAP for improving daytime sleepiness and perceived quality of sleep, but that positional therapy was less effective in decreasing the AHI (89).

Weight loss is also frequently suggested as a therapeutic option. However, data from the Sleep Heart Health Study longitudinal analysis suggest that sleep-related breathing disorder severity tends to increase more with weight gain than it decreases with weight loss (90). In addition, these effects vary by gender, with men two to five times more likely to reduce their AHI than women (90). Chakravorty et al. compared PAP to a lifestyle intervention consisting of weight loss counseling, exercise and sleep hygiene techniques (91). Participants had an average weight loss of 1.85 kg, which led to a significant hange in REM AHI from 42 ± 17.7 to 26 ± 19.6 events/hr; however, there was no change in the overall AHI (91). Sleepiness scores also improved, but less than with PAP (91).

Surgery

A variety of surgical procedures have been proposed to treat obstructive sleep apnea, utilizing interventions ranging from mandibular advancement to removal of excess tissue in the posterior oropharynx. In approximately 5% to 10% of cases, these procedures are associated with side effects such as dysphagia or nasal regurgitation; these symptoms tend to resolve over time (92). A 2005 Cochrane Database review concluded that there is currently inadequate evidence to support the routine use of surgical therapy for sleep apnea (92). Older adults are generally excluded from these studies; thus little data exist regarding efficacy for elders.

CONCLUSION

Obstructive sleep apnea is a highly prevalent condition affecting up to 20% of older adults. The signs and symptoms in elders may be more difficult to ascertain, especially because of the reduced associations with snoring and obesity. However, the detection of obstructive sleep apnea is crucial to the effective care of older adults because of the numerous potential sequelae of untreated disease, including daytime sleepiness, cognitive impairment, hypertension, and mortality. Several treatment options exist for obstructive sleep apnea, with the preponderence of data demonstrating that PAP is an effective modality; however, compliance remains a major challenge. PAP can also be successfully utilized in patients with mild to moderate cognitive impairment and may benefit these patients across several domains.

REFERENCES

1. American Academy of Sleep Medicine. International Classification of Sleep Disorders: Diagnostic and Coding Manual. 2nd ed. Westchester, IL: American Academy of Sleep Medicine; 2005.
2. Redline S, Budhiraja R, Kapur V, et al. The scoring of respiratory events in sleep: reliability and validity. J Clin Sleep Med 2007; 3(2):169–200.
3. Berry DT, Phillips BA, Cook YR, et al. Geriatric sleep apnea syndrome: a preliminary description. J Gerontol 1990; 45(5):M169–M174.
4. Launois SH, Pepin JL, Levy P. Sleep apnea in the elderly: a specific entity? Sleep Med Rev 2007; 11(2):87–97.
5. Bixler E, Vgontzas A, Ten H, et al. Effects of age on sleep apnea in men: I. Prevalence and severity. AJRCCM 1998; 157(1):144–148.
6. Young T, Shahar E, Nieto FJ, et al. Predictors of sleep-disordered breathing in community-dwelling adults: the Sleep Heart Health Study. Arch Intern Med 2002; 162(8):893–900.
7. Enright PL, Newman AB, Wahl PW, et al. Prevalence and correlates of snoring and observed apneas in 5,201 older adults. Sleep 1996; 19(7):531–538.

8. Bixler EO, Vgontzas AN, Lin HM, et al. Excessive daytime sleepiness in a general population sample: the role of sleep apnea, age, obesity, diabetes, and depression. J Clin Endocrinol Metab 2005; 90(8):4510–4515.

9. Gooneratne NS, Gehrman PR, Nkwuo JE, et al. Consequences of comorbid insomnia symptoms and sleep-related breathing disorder in elderly subjects. Arch Intern Med 2006; 166(16):1732–1738.

10. Kushida CA, Efron B, Guilleminault C. A predictive morphometric model for the obstructive sleep apnea syndrome. Ann Intern Med 1997; 127(8 Pt 1):581–587.

11. Zonato AI, Martinho FL, Bittencourt LR, et al. Head and neck physical examination: comparison between nonapneic and obstructive sleep apnea patients. Laryngoscope 2005; 115(6):1030–1034.

12. Bucca C, Cicolin A, Brussino L, et al. Tooth loss and obstructive sleep apnoea. Respir Res 2006; 7:8.

13. Haponik EF. Sleep disturbances of older persons: physicians' attitudes. Sleep 1992; 15(2):168–172.

14. Larsson LG, Lindberg A, Franklin KA, et al. Gender differences in symptoms related to sleep apnea in a general population and in relation to referral to sleep clinic. Chest 2003; 124(1):204–211.

15. Kapur V, Strohl KP, Redline S, et al. Underdiagnosis of sleep apnea syndrome in U.S. communities. Sleep Breath 2002; 6(2):49–54.

16. Li KK, Kushida C, Powell NB, et al. Obstructive sleep apnea syndrome: a comparison between Far-East Asian and white men. Laryngoscope 2000; 110(10 pt 1):1689–1693.

17. Ancoli-Israel S, Klauber MR, Stepnowsky C, et al. Sleep-disordered breathing in African-American elderly. Am J Respir Crit Care Med 1995; 152(6 pt 1):1946–1949.

18. Buxbaum SG, Elston RC, Tishler PV, et al. Genetics of the apnea hypopnea index in Caucasians and African Americans: I. Segregation analysis. Genet Epidemiol 2002; 22(3):243–253.

19. Sharafkhaneh A, Giray N, Richardson P, et al. Association of psychiatric disorders and sleep apnea in a large cohort. Sleep 2005; 28(11):1405–1411.

20. Ancoli-Israel S, Klauber MR, Butters N, et al. Dementia in institutionalized elderly: relation to sleep apnea. J Am Geriatr Soc 1991; 39(3):258–263.

21. Martin SE, Mathur R, Marshall I, et al. The effect of age, sex, obesity and posture on upper airway size. Eur Respir J 1997; 10(9):2087–2090.

22. Huang J, Shen H, Takahashi M, et al. Pharyngeal cross-sectional area and pharyngeal compliance in normal males and females. Respiration 1998; 65(6):458–468.

23. Oliven A, Carmi N, Coleman R, et al. Age-related changes in upper airway muscles morphological and oxidative properties. Exp Gerontol 2001; 36(10):1673–1686.

24. Nieto FJ, Young TB, Lind BK, et al. Association of sleep-disordered breathing, sleep apnea, and hypertension in a large community-based study. Sleep Heart Health Study. JAMA 2000; 283(14):1829–1836.

25. Norman D, Loredo JS, Nelesen RA, et al. Effects of continuous positive airway pressure versus supplemental oxygen on 24-hour ambulatory blood pressure. Hypertension 2006; 47(5):840–845.

26. Bazzano LA, Khan Z, Reynolds K, et al. Effect of nocturnal nasal continuous positive airway pressure on blood pressure in obstructive sleep apnea. Hypertension 2007; 50(2):417–423.

27. Robinson GV, Smith DM, Langford BA, et al. Continuous positive airway pressure does not reduce blood pressure in nonsleepy hypertensive OSA patients. Eur Respir J 2006; 27(6):1229–1235.

28. Gami AS, Hodge DO, Herges RM, et al. Obstructive sleep apnea, obesity, and the risk of incident atrial fibrillation. J Am Coll Cardiol 2007; 49(5):565–571.

29. Shahar E, Whitney CW, Redline S, et al. Sleep-disordered breathing and cardiovascular disease: cross-sectional results of the Sleep Heart Health Study. Am J Respir Crit Care Med 2001; 163(1):19–25.

30. Baldwin CM, Bell IR, Guerra S, et al. Obstructive sleep apnea and ischemic heart disease in southwestern US veterans: implications for clinical practice. Sleep Breath 2005; 9(3):111–118.
31. Peker Y, Hedner J, Kraiczi H, et al. Respiratory disturbance index: an independent predictor of mortality in coronary artery disease. Am J Respir Crit Care Med 2000; 162(1):81–86.
32. Gami AS, Howard DE, Olson EJ, et al. Day-night pattern of sudden death in obstructive sleep apnea. N Engl J Med 2005; 352(12):1206–1214.
33. Parra O, Arboix A, Montserrat JM, et al. Sleep-related breathing disorders: impact on mortality of cerebrovascular disease. Eur Respir J 2004; 24(2):267–272.
34. Yaggi HK, Concato J, Kernan WN, et al. Obstructive sleep apnea as a risk factor for stroke and death. N Engl J Med 2005; 353(19):2034–2041.
35. Martinez-Garcia MA, Galiano-Blancart R, Roman-Sanchez P, et al. Continuous positive airway pressure treatment in sleep apnea prevents new vascular events after ischemic stroke. Chest 2005; 128(4):2123–2129.
36. Palombini L, Guilleminault C. Stroke and treatment with nasal CPAP. Eur J Neurol 2006; 13(2):198–200.
37. Cohen-Zion M, Stepnowsky C, Johnson S, et al. Cognitive changes and sleep disordered breathing in elderly: differences in race. J Psychosom Res 2004; 56(5):549–553.
38. Macey PM, Henderson LA, Macey KE, et al. Brain morphology associated with obstructive sleep apnea. Am J Respir Crit Care Med 2002; 166(10):1382–1387.
39. O'Hara R, Schroder CM, Kraemer HC, et al. Nocturnal sleep apnea/hypopnea is associated with lower memory performance in APOE epsilon4 carriers. Neurology 2005; 65(4):642–644.
40. Lim W, Bardwell WA, Loredo JS, et al. Neuropsychological effects of 2-week continuous positive airway pressure treatment and supplemental oxygen in patients with obstructive sleep apnea: a randomized placebo-controlled study. J Clin Sleep Med 2007; 3(4):380–386.
41. Ayalon L, Ancoli-Israel S, Stepnowsky C, et al. Adherence to continuous positive airway pressure treatment in patients with Alzheimer's disease and obstructive sleep apnea. Am J Geriatr Psychiatry 2006; 14(2):176–180.
42. Gooneratne NS, Weaver TE, Cater JR, et al. Functional outcomes of excessive daytime sleepiness in older adults. J Am Geriatr Soc 2003; 51(5):642–649.
43. Montserrat JM, Ferrer M, Hernandez L, et al. Effectiveness of CPAP treatment in daytime function in sleep apnea syndrome: a randomized controlled study with an optimized placebo. Am J Respir Crit Care Med 2001; 164(4):608–613.
44. Chong MS, Ayalon L, Marler M, et al. Continuous positive airway pressure reduces subjective daytime sleepiness in patients with mild to moderate Alzheimer's disease with sleep disordered breathing. J Am Geriatr Soc 2006; 54(5):777–781.
45. Hack M, Davies RJ, Mullins R, et al. Randomised prospective parallel trial of therapeutic versus subtherapeutic nasal continuous positive airway pressure on simulated steering performance in patients with obstructive sleep apnoea. Thorax 2000; 55(3):224–231.
46. Tawk M, Goodrich S, Kinasewitz G, et al. The effect of 1 week of continuous positive airway pressure treatment in obstructive sleep apnea patients with concomitant gastroesophageal reflux. Chest 2006; 130(4):1003–1008.
47. Middelkoop HA, Smilde-van den Doel DA, Neven AK, et al. Subjective sleep characteristics of 1,485 males and females aged 50–93: effects of sex and age, and factors related to self-evaluated quality of sleep. J Gerontol A Biol Sci Med Sci 1996; 51(3):M108–M115.
48. Bliwise DL, Adelman CL, Ouslander JG. Polysomnographic correlates of spontaneous nocturnal wetness episodes in incontinent geriatric patients. Sleep 2004; 27(1):153–157.
49. Yalkut D, Lee LY, Grider J, et al. Mechanism of atrial natriuretic peptide release with increased inspiratory resistance. J Lab Clin Med 1996; 128(3):322–328.
50. Umlauf MG, Chasens ER. Sleep disordered breathing and nocturnal polyuria: nocturia and enuresis. Sleep Med Rev 2003; 7(5):403–411.
51. Baruzzi A, Riva R, Cirignotta F, et al. Atrial natriuretic peptide and catecholamines in obstructive sleep apnea syndrome. Sleep 1991; 14(1):83–86.

52. Liu S, Liu L. Effect of treatment with continuous positive airway pressure on nocturnal polyuria in patients with obstructive sleep apnea syndrome. Zhonghua Jie He He Hu Xi Za Zhi 2001; 24(3):158–160.
53. Margel D, Cohen M, Livne PM, et al. Severe, but not mild, obstructive sleep apnea syndrome is associated with erectile dysfunction. Urology 2004; 63(3):545–549.
54. Goncalves MA, Guilleminault C, Ramos E, et al. Erectile dysfunction, obstructive sleep apnea syndrome and nasal CPAP treatment. Sleep Med 2005; 6(4):333–339.
55. Aloia MS, Arnedt JT, Smith L, et al. Examining the construct of depression in obstructive sleep apnea syndrome. Sleep Med 2005; 6(2):115–121.
56. Giles TL, Lasserson TJ, Smith BH, et al. Continuous positive airways pressure for obstructive sleep apnoea in adults. Cochrane Database Syst Rev 2006; 3:CD001106.
57. Bardwell WA, Norman D, Ancoli-Israel S, et al. Effects of 2-week nocturnal oxygen supplementation and continuous positive airway pressure treatment on psychological symptoms in patients with obstructive sleep apnea: a randomized placebo-controlled study. Behav Sleep Med 2007; 5(1):21–38.
58. Krakow B, Melendrez D, Ferreira E, et al. Prevalence of insomnia symptoms in patients with sleep-disordered breathing. Chest 2001; 120(6):1923–1929.
59. Chung KF. Insomnia subtypes and their relationships to daytime sleepiness in patients with obstructive sleep apnea. Respiration 2005; 72(5):460–465.
60. Ohayon MM, Carskadon MA, Guilleminault C, et al. Meta-analysis of quantitative sleep parameters from childhood to old age in healthy individuals: developing normative sleep values across the human lifespan. Sleep 2004; 27(7):1255–1273.
61. Kushida CA, Littner MR, Morgenthaler T, et al. Practice parameters for the indications for polysomnography and related procedures: an update for 2005. Sleep 2005; 28(4):499–521.
62. Weaver TE, Chasens ER. Continuous positive airway pressure treatment for sleep apnea in older adults. Sleep Med Rev 2007; 11(2):99–111.
63. Bliwise DL, Benkert RE, Ingham RH. Factors associated with nightly variability in sleep-disordered breathing in the elderly. Chest 1991; 100(4):973–976.
64. Pittsley M, Gehrman P, Cohen-Zion M, et al. Comparing night-to-night variability of sleep measures in elderly African Americans and Whites. Behav Sleep Med 2005; 3(2):63–72.
65. ATS/ACCP/AASM Taskforce Steering Committee. Executive summary on the systematic review and practice parameters for portable monitoring in the investigation of suspected sleep apnea in adults. Am J Respir Crit Care Med 2004; 169(10):1160–1163.
66. Nussbaumer Y, Bloch KE, Genser T, et al. Equivalence of autoadjusted and constant continuous positive airway pressure in home treatment of sleep apnea. Chest 2006; 129(3):638–643.
67. Weaver TE, Kribbs NB, Pack AI, et al. Night-to-night variability in CPAP use over the first three months of treatment. Sleep 1997; 20(4):278–283.
68. DeMolles DA, Sparrow D, Gottlieb DJ, et al. A pilot trial of a telecommunications system in sleep apnea management. Med Care 2004; 42(8):764–769.
69. Russo-Magno P, O'Brien A, Panciera T, et al. Compliance with CPAP therapy in older men with obstructive sleep apnea. J Am Geriatr Soc 2001; 49(9):1205–1211.
70. Lewis KE, Seale L, Bartle IE, et al. Early predictors of CPAP use for the treatment of obstructive sleep apnea. Sleep 2004; 27(1):134–138.
71. Pelletier-Fleury N, Rakotonanahary D, Fleury B. The age and other factors in the evaluation of compliance with nasal continuous positive airway pressure for obstructive sleep apnea syndrome. A Cox's proportional hazard analysis. Sleep Med 2001; 2(3):225–232.
72. Haynes PL. The role of behavioral sleep medicine in the assessment and treatment of sleep disordered breathing. Clin Psychol Rev 2005; 25(5):673–705.
73. Duong M, Jayaram L, Camfferman D, et al. Use of heated humidification during nasal CPAP titration in obstructive sleep apnoea syndrome. Eur Respir J 2005; 26(4):679–685.
74. Aloia MS, Di Dio L, Ilniczky N, et al. Improving compliance with nasal CPAP and vigilance in older adults with OAHS. Sleep Breath 2001; 5(1):13–21.

75. Parish JM, Lyng PJ, Wisbey J. Compliance with CPAP in elderly patients with OSA. 2000; 1(3):209–214.

76. Dinges DF, Weaver TE. Effects of modafinil on sustained attention performance and quality of life in OSA patients with residual sleepiness while being treated with nCPAP. Sleep Med 2003; 4(5):393–402.

77. Hirshkowitz M, Black JE, Wesnes K, et al. Adjunct armodafinil improves wakefulness and memory in obstructive sleep apnea/hypopnea syndrome. Respir Med 2007; 101(3):616–627.

78. Smith IE, Quinnell TG. Pharmacotherapies for obstructive sleep apnoea: where are we now? Drugs 2004; 64(13):1385–1399.

79. Carley DW, Olopade C, Ruigt GS, et al. Efficacy of mirtazapine in obstructive sleep apnea syndrome. Sleep 2007; 30(1):35–41.

80. Chan AS, Lee RW, Cistulli PA. Dental appliance treatment for obstructive sleep apnea. Chest 2007; 132(2):693–699.

81. Naismith SL, Winter VR, Hickie IB, et al. Effect of oral appliance therapy on neurobehavioral functioning in obstructive sleep apnea: a randomized controlled trial. J Clin Sleep Med 2005; 1(4):374–380.

82. Engleman HM, McDonald JP, Graham D, et al. Randomized crossover trial of two treatments for sleep apnea/hypopnea syndrome: continuous positive airway pressure and mandibular repositioning splint. Am J Respir Crit Care Med 2002; 166(6):855–859.

83. Hoffstein V. Review of oral appliances for treatment of sleep-disordered breathing. Sleep Breath 2007; 11(1):1–22.

84. Machado MA, de Carvalho LB, Juliano ML, et al. Clinical co-morbidities in obstructive sleep apnea syndrome treated with mandibular repositioning appliance. Respir Med 2006; 100(6):988–995.

85. Garrigue S, Bordier P, Jais P, et al. Benefit of atrial pacing in sleep apnea syndrome. N Engl J Med 2002; 346(6):404–412.

86. Sharafkhaneh A, Sharafkhaneh H, Bredikus A, et al. Effect of atrial overdrive pacing on obstructive sleep apnea in patients with systolic heart failure. Sleep Med 2007; 8(1):31–36.

87. Krahn AD, Yee R, Erickson MK, et al. Physiologic pacing in patients with obstructive sleep apnea: a prospective, randomized crossover trial. J Am Coll Cardiol 2006; 47(2):379–383.

88. Shalaby AA, Atwood CW, Hansen C, et al. Analysis of interaction of acute atrial overdrive pacing with sleep-related breathing disorder. Am J Cardiol 2007; 99(4):573–578.

89. Jokic R, Klimaszewski A, Crossley M, et al. Positional treatment vs continuous positive airway pressure in patients with positional obstructive sleep apnea syndrome. Chest 1999; 115(3):771–781.

90. Newman AB, Foster G, Givelber R, et al. Progression and regression of sleep-disordered breathing with changes in weight: the sleep heart health study. Arch Intern Med 2005; 165(20):2408–2413.

91. Chakravorty I, Cayton RM, Szczepura A. Health utilities in evaluating intervention in the sleep apnoea/hypopnoea syndrome. Eur Respir J 2002; 20(5):1233–1238.

92. Sundaram S, Bridgman SA, Lim J, et al. Surgery for obstructive sleep apnoea. Cochrane Database Syst Rev 2005(4):CD001004.

93. Iber C., Ancoli-Israel S., Chesson A., Quan S., eds., AASM Manual for the Scoring of Sleep and Associated Events: Rules, Terminology and Technical Specifications. 2007, American Academy of Sleep Medicine: Westchester, Ill.

9   Central Sleep Apnea

Susmita Chowdhuri and M. Safwan Badr

John D. Dingell Veterans Affairs Medical Center and Wayne State University, Detroit, Michigan, U.S.A.

INTRODUCTION

Central sleep apnea (CSA) is characterized by cessation of breathing during sleep due to absent ventilatory drive. On the basis of etiology, CSA in the older population can be broadly classified as primary CSA, Cheyne–Stokes breathing pattern in heart failure, and CSA in neurodegenerative disease and stroke. In older individuals, literature about the prevalence of CSA in the different subcategories is scarce, although some data on the prevalence of Cheyne–Stokes breathing pattern in heart failure are available. While a few epidemiologic studies have attempted to study the prevalence of the disorder in the general population, information on the pathogenesis and treatment of CSA in the older population is insufficient. This chapter describes the accumulating evidence on the pathogenesis, prevalence, and treatment modalities for CSA, specifically as it pertains to older people. The different types of presentations of CSA in the geriatric population are discussed below.

PATHOPHYSIOLOGY OF CENTRAL SLEEP APNEA

On polysomnographic recording, CSA is characterized by the cessation of airflow and ventilatory effort lasting 10 seconds or longer, with central apneas occurring at a rate of five or more per hour (1). The patient may report symptoms of excessive daytime sleepiness, insomnia, or frequent arousals. A discussion regarding the pathophysiology is important as it underpins the rationale behind current and evolving therapy. Central apneas can occur through two broad pathophysiologic patterns, either post-hyperventilation or post-hypoventilation.

Central Apnea Secondary to Hyperventilation

The removal of the wakefulness drive to breathe renders ventilation dependent on the prevailing chemical stimuli and unmasks a highly sensitive hypocapnic apneic threshold. Central apnea occurs if $PaCO_2$ (arterial CO_2) falls below a highly reproducible hypocapnic apneic threshold. Patients with post-hyperventilation central apnea are typically free of neuromuscular or pulmonary disorders and have a normal or exaggerated response to hypercapnia (2). Thus, there is no evidence of daytime alveolar hypoventilation, implicating a transient instability of the ventilatory control system.

How does the first apnea begin? Oscillation in sleep state (3), transient hypoxia possibly due to retention of secretions, or reduced lung volumes in obese supine patients may be primary precipitating events of CSA episodes. For example, hypoxia stimulates ventilation, subsequently leading to hypocapnia and, subsequently, apnea. The occurrence of apnea initiates the *repetitive process of apnea-hyperpnea* and leads to sustained breathing instability, manifested as periodic breathing. Post-hyperventilation central apnea is a heterogeneous entity that may be an idiopathic phenomenon or a secondary condition, as described below. The pathogenesis may vary depending on the clinical condition.

How is central sleep apnea related to obstructive sleep apnea? CSA may also induce obstructive sleep apnea (OSA). There is evidence that patients with sleep apnea and snorers with evidence of inspiratory flow limitation are dependent on ventilatory motor output to preserve upper airway patency (4–5). In these individuals, pharyngeal obstruction occurs when ventilatory drive reaches a nadir during induced periodic breathing (4–6). Likewise, using fiberoptic nasopharyngoscopy, Badr et al. (7) have shown that central apnea is associated with pharyngeal narrowing or occlusion early (<10 sec) during the central apneic period and even in the absence of inspiratory efforts. In addition, many OSA patients display an enhanced controller gain during sleep, which would predispose to periodic breathing (8). Furthermore, the ability of the patient with severe OSA to effectively compensate (via effective neural control of the respiratory muscles of both the upper airway and the pump, without EEG arousal) for airway narrowing and increased mechanical load was shown, by correlational analysis, to be a more important determinant of the degree of cycling behavior of airway patency and ventilation than was the inherent passive collapsibility of the airway (9). An implication of these clinical data is that although an inherently collapsible airway may allow for significant airway narrowing and even obstruction during sleep, any repetitive cycling behavior in airway patency and ventilation is critically dependent on neurochemical control mechanisms.

In summary, differences in ventilatory control stability during sleep may contribute to CSA in older people; however, the few available investigations that have described age-related changes in ventilatory control during sleep have reported conflicting findings (described below). In addition, increased prevalence of comorbid conditions such as thyroid disease, congestive heart failure, atrial fibrillation, and cerebrovascular disease may also contribute to increased susceptibility to develop central apnea in older adults. Increased sleep state oscillations may also precipitate central apneas in older adults. Therapy is aimed at treating the underlying condition, and often, addition of nasal continuous positive airway pressure (CPAP) and/or supplemental oxygen and carbon dioxide (Figure 1).

Central Sleep Apnea Secondary to Hypoventilation

The transition from wakefulness to sleep is associated with decreased ventilatory motor output, a fall in ventilation, and increased PCO_2, likely due to the combination of decreased ventilatory motor output and increased upper airway resistance. Therefore, increased PCO_2 by 3 to 6 mmHg during sleep is a physiologic event. Similarly, REM sleep (especially phasic REM) is associated with hypoventilation and hence increased PCO_2. Hypoventilation during sleep may be inconsequential in a healthy individual but leads to significant reduction in alveolar ventilation. However, in patients with chronic ventilatory failure, neuromuscular disease, or chest wall disease, these changes may manifest as central apnea or hypopnea. This is particularly noted in patients who suffer from central nervous system (CNS) disease (e.g., encephalitis), neuromuscular disease, or severe abnormalities in pulmonary mechanics [e.g., kyphoscoliosis (10)]. Thus, central apnea due to hypoventilation is due to the removal of the wakefulness stimulus to breathe or to phasic REM-related hypoventilation. This type of central apnea does not necessarily meet the strict

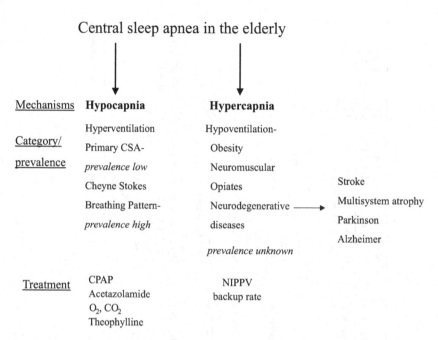

FIGURE 1   Summary of the classification of central sleep apnea in the elderly based on pathogenesis, prevalence, and potential treatment modalities.

definition of "apnea," as ventilatory motor output is severely reduced and therefore insufficient to preserve alveolar ventilation. Likewise, it may not meet the definition of "central" in patients with respiratory muscle disease or skeletal deformities.

Older patients may be at a high risk for developing episodic hypoventilation and related apnea-hypopnea given the high prevalence of neurologic disease in this group (see the section "Etiologic Classification of CSA in the Older Adult"). The clinical presentation may be of nocturnal ventilatory failure, particularly in patients with marginal ventilatory status or worsening of existing chronic ventilatory failure. Arousal from sleep restores alveolar ventilation to a variable degree, while resumption of sleep reduces ventilation in a cyclical fashion. Consequently, the presenting clinical picture includes both features of the underlying ventilatory insufficiency (e.g., morning headache, cor pulmonale, peripheral edema, polycythemia, and abnormal pulmonary function tests) and features of the sleep apnea-hypopnea syndrome (e.g., poor nocturnal sleep, snoring, and daytime sleepiness). The mechanism(s) responsible for CSA in a given patient influence(s) the management strategy aimed at restoration of effective alveolar ventilation during sleep. Treatment of choice in such patients is assisted ventilation (Figure 1). Nasal CPAP and supplemental oxygen are *unlikely* to alleviate the condition.

EPIDEMIOLOGY OF CSA IN THE OLDER ADULT

Epidemiologic studies suggest a high prevalence of both obstructive and central sleep apneas in older adults (11–19,52,53) (Table 1), with a significant association

TABLE 1 Prevalence of Sleep Apnea in the Elderly

Author (reference)	Population, n	Age range (yr)	SDB measurements	Prevalence (definition of sleep apnea based on AHI)	Prevalence of CSA reported: Yes/No
Ancoli-Israel (11,14,16)	Community dwellers, 427 Hospital, 350 Nursing home residents, 200	65–95	4-channel portable sleep recording	AI ≥ 5/hr: 24%, AHI ≥ 10/h: 62%, community dwellers AI ≥ 5/hr: 33% acute-care patients, 42% nursing home patients	Yes
Hoch (17)	Population based, 555	30–70	Polysomnography	AI ≥ 5: 3%, 33%, and 39%, at ages 60, 70, and 80 yr, respectively	No
Phillips (18)	Normal volunteers, 256	50–80	Polysomnography	AHI ≥ 5/hr 15% in elderly	No
Bixler (12)	Population based, 1731, 20–100 years	65–100 vs 45–64	Polysomnography	AHI ≥ 10/hr: 24% vs. 3%, central apneas: 1.1% vs. 0.4%	Yes
Bliwise (15)	Community dwellers, 198	75–91	Polysomnography	Significant association with age and AHI > 10/hr	Unspecified RDI reported
Duran (19)	Spanish cohort, 555	71–100	Portable sleep recording	AHI ≥ 5/hr: 80%, increased with age with an odds ratio of 2.2 for each 10-year increase	No

Abbreviations: AHI, apnea-hypopnea index; AI, apnea index; CSA, central sleep apnea; n, sample size; RDI, respiratory disturbance index; SDB, sleep-disordered breathing.

between age and the apnea-hypopnea index (AHI, number of apneas and hypopneas per hour of sleep). The prevalence has ranged from 27% in older community dwellers, 33% in the acute-care setting, to 42% in nursing home residents. Population-based studies noted the prevalence to be 3%, 33%, and 39% in 60-, 70-, and 80-year-olds, respectively (17). Duran et al. (19) reported that the prevalence of sleep apnea at age >71 years was 80% and increased with age with an odds ratio of 2.2 for each 10-year of increase. Epidemiologic studies also indicate that CSA per se is more prevalent in older adults relative to middle-aged individuals (12,13,15,16). In one of the earliest studies involving 40 older individuals (mean age 72.7 years), Carskadon and Dement (22) found that 37.5% of all subjects over the age of 62 had apneas or hypopneas and that most of these were central apneas. Large epidemiologic cohorts have also demonstrated a higher percentage of central apneas in the older population. Bixler et al. (12) noted that the prevalence of any type of sleep apnea (central and obstructive) was age related, with a prevalence of central apneas of 1.1% at age >65 years vs. 0.4% at 45 to 64 years. This large community-based epidemiologic study found that the prevalence of central sleep apnea (defined as central apnea index, CI ≥ 2.5) increased from 1.7% (0.8, 3.4) in the middle age group to 12.1% (6.5, 21.6) in the older age group (OR = 8.3) (12). Interestingly, no men in the youngest age group met the threshold of CI ≥ 2.5 and all the men who met a high CI ≥ 20 were in the ≥65-year age group. The age-specific prevalence of a CI ≥ 20 for males aged ≥ 65 years was 5.2%. The findings in women were different as the prevalence of central apnea (CI ≥ 2.5) in women was only 0.3%. In addition, the Wisconsin Sleep Cohort (20) study containing both cross-sectional and longitudinal data, confirmed an increase in the AHI from 2.5/hr at baseline to 5.1/hr at follow-up after eight years. Figure 1 summarizes an algorithm for the management of central sleep apnea based on pathogenesis. Similarly, the Cleveland Family Study (21) demonstrated that AHI increased from 2 to 6.2/hr over five years of follow-up. However, these cohort studies addressed age and not *aging*, and they did not include *older participants at the outset*. Another limitation of existing epidemiologic studies is the paucity of studies that have separated central apnea as a distinct term from the rubric "obstructive sleep apnea" (Table 1). CSA in older people may have important clinical implications as it has been associated with adverse clinical sequelae, including increased risk for heart disease and cardiovascular mortality (14,16). Further investigations with large longitudinal studies in older populations are needed to clarify the natural history and clinical outcomes of this disorder.

CENTRAL APNEA RISK FACTORS IN THE OLDER ADULT

Age: While CSA is more prevalent in older adults relative to middle-aged individuals, the effect of aging on sleep-related decrease in ventilatory drive in humans is unclear. We know that sleep eliminates the wakefulness drive to breathe (23), leading to reduced ventilatory motor output. Findings from a canine model suggest that aging is associated with decreased minute ventilation and increased $PaCO_2$ during slow wave sleep (24). However, the effect of aging on sleep-related decrease in ventilatory drive and on chemosensitivity during wakefulness in humans is uncertain. Available studies have reached conflicting conclusions regarding the effect of age on chemoresponsiveness. A few have shown a difference (25,26) or decreased responsiveness (27) to hypercapnia during wakefulness or sleep (28). The response to hypoxia is also variable. While one study (27) demonstrated a lower initial increase in minute ventilation in response to acute mild hypoxia in men >70 years, others (29–31) reported that the ventilatory response to sustained hypoxia declined in older men but was the same as in younger men.

The effect of age on susceptibility to periodic breathing is also unclear. The available limited evidence does not indicate a higher susceptibility to developing periodic breathing (32). In fact, a recent study (33) found no difference in loop gain in the older OSA group upon using proportional assist ventilation. However, the application of proportional assist ventilation may alter some of the components of the loop gain, namely, plant gain and mixing factors and hence obscure real differences among subjects (34). The hypocapnic apneic threshold (HAT) is a measure of a robust marker of susceptibility to post-hyperventilation apnea and possibly to periodic breathing. Nasal mechanical ventilation is used to induce hypocapnia and hence central apnea. It is sensitive to the changes in the background drive to breathe ("plant gain") (34–35) as well as to the slope of the reduction in ventilation below eupnea in response to induced hypocapnia ("controller gain") (35). The effect of aging on plant and controller gains is yet to be studied.

Aging also has an important influence on respiratory plasticity in animals. One example of respiratory plasticity is the long-term facilitation (LTF) phenomenon. LTF is a physiologic response noted in animal models and humans in response to episodic hypoxia (EH) (36–42) and is characterized by prolonged increase in ventilation up to hours, demonstrating a form of respiratory neuroplasticity. Although the physiologic relevance of LTF remains unclear, it reflects a general mechanism whereby intermittent serotonin receptor activation elicits respiratory plasticity, adapting system performance to the ever-changing requirements of life (43). Evidence from animal studies suggest that LTF exhibits an age-dependent expression, with decline in LTF with aging (44–46). In a study comparing phrenic and hypoglossal LTF in young (3–4 months) and aged (13 months) male rats, significant decrease in LTF was noted in the aged rats following EH (46). In addition, ventilatory LTF was greater in one-month- versus two-month-old rats, indicating that younger animals may have a greater capacity for EH-induced ventilatory plasticity. A decline in LTF in humans may attenuate a significant protective mechanism that maintains upper airway patency (43). A recent study reported a significant negative correlation between age and the genioglossus muscle LTF in normal humans (47). LTF of genioglossus was present in healthy non-flow-limited humans ($n = 12$) during NREM sleep, and this was inversely correlated with age. However, this study only investigated a narrow age range, and similar investigations in older age groups are lacking (47). Thus, further explorations of the basic mechanisms of an increased occurrence of central apneas in older people (in turn leading to obstructive apneas), examining the factors modulating ventilatory control stability with well-designed experiments, are needed.

In addition to age, several physiologic and pathologic factors may modulate the susceptibility of older people to developing central apnea. These include gender, sex hormones, sleep state, and medical conditions.

Gender is a significant modifier of the effects of age on the susceptibility to central apnea. There is epidemiologic and empiric evidence that central apnea is less common in premenopausal women relative to men or postmenopausal women. One large population study (12) demonstrated paucity of central apnea in premenopausal women. Likewise, there is experimental evidence that the hypocapnic central apnea sleep is higher in men relative to women. Using nasal mechanical ventilation during stable NREM sleep, Zhou et al. (48) have shown that the apneic threshold was −3.5 mmHg vs. −4.7 mmHg below room air level in men and women, respectively. This difference was not due to progesterone. Rowley et al. (49) explored the determinants of the apneic threshold in normal individuals. Interestingly, age, per se, was not an independent determinant of the apneic threshold in men or postmenopausal women. Only premenopausal women demonstrated narrowing between eupenic and apneic PCO_2 with aging, indicative ventilatory instability.

Sex hormones also influence the susceptibility to central apneas. Male sex hormones are important determinants of the apneic threshold. Administration of testosterone to healthy premenopausal women for 12 days elevates the apneic threshold closer to eupnea, narrowing the magnitude of hypocapnic required for induction of central apnea during NREM sleep (50). Conversely, suppression of testosterone with leuprolide acetate in healthy males decreases the hypocapnic apneic threshold (51). Finally, administration of hormone replacement therapy to postmenopausal women lowered their apneic threshold to the level of pre-menopausal women (49). The complex interactions between age, gender, sex hormones, and menopausal status render broad generalizations difficult to uphold. In addition, the proportion of participants in studies declines with advancing age, whether because of substantial comorbidity or as a survival effect.

Sleep state oscillations may precipitate central apnea in older adults (3,54). Transient breathing instability and central apnea often occurs during the transition from wakefulness to NREM sleep. As sleep state oscillates between wakefulness and light sleep (3,54–57), the level of $PaCO_2$ is at or below the hypocapnic level required to maintain rhythmic breathing during sleep (i.e., the "apneic threshold"), resulting in central apnea; recovery from apnea is associated with transient wakefulness and hyperventilation. The subsequent hypocapnia elicits apnea upon resumption of sleep. Consolidation of sleep alleviates the oscillation in sleep and respiration and stabilizes $PaCO_2$ at a higher set point above the apneic threshold. Interestingly, central apnea may occur without preceding hyperventilation at the transition from alpha to theta in normal subjects and is associated with prolongation of breath duration (58).

REM sleep: Post-hyperventilation CSA is uncommon during REM sleep, raising the possibility that breathing during REM sleep is impervious to chemical influences, possibly due to increased ventilatory motor output (59,60) relative to NREM sleep. This question is further confounded by the difficulty in conducting such experiments without disrupting REM sleep. Nevertheless, central apnea due to hypoventilation may be seen in REM sleep, triggered by the loss of intercostal muscle activity during phasic REM sleep and subsequent hypoventilation. This may manifest as apparent central apnea or hypopnea in patients with neuromuscular disease diaphragmatic dysfunction or compromised pulmonary mechanics. If severe impairment is present, nadir tidal volume may be negligible and the event may appear as central apnea. Thus, central apnea during REM sleep represents transient hypoventilation rather than post-hyperventilation hypocapnia.

Medical conditions may increase the propensity to central apnea. Congestive heart failure (CHF) is associated with a high prevalence of central apnea. Sleep apnea is common in patients with CHF (61–65). Javaheri et al. demonstrated that 51% of male patients with CHF had sleep-disordered breathing, (40% had CSA, and 11% obstructive apnea). Risk factors for CSA in this group of patients included age >60 years, male gender, atrial fibrillation, and daytime hypocapnia (PCO_2 < 38 mmHg) (66). However, risk factors for OSA differed by gender; the only independent determinant in men was body mass index (BMI), whereas age over 60 was the only independent determinant in women (66). Patients with central apnea and CHF demonstrate pulmonary vascular congestion leading to hyperventilation and hypocapnia; hence, there is an absence of a rise in PCO_2 from wakefulness to sleep (65).

Sleep apnea is common after a cerebrovascular accident (CVA) (70–72), with central apnea being the predominant type in 40% of patients of sleep apnea after a CVA (72). Likewise, central apnea occurs in 30% of patients on stable methadone maintenance treatment (73). Finally, several medical conditions, in addition to CHF and atrial fibrillation (74), predispose to the development of central apnea, including hypothyroidism (75), acromegaly (76,77), and renal failure (78). Notably, nocturnal hemodialysis has been associated with improvement in sleep apnea indices (78).

ETIOLOGIC CLASSIFICATION OF CSA IN THE OLDER ADULT

Primary CSA

By definition, primary CSA is of unknown etiology and involves five or more central apneas per hour of sleep associated with one or more of the following symptoms: daytime sleepiness, frequent awakenings with complaints of insomnia or awakening with shortness of breath, and the absence of another concurrent sleep disorder, medical or neurological disorders or medication/substance use (1). Thus, it is a diagnosis of exclusion. Typically these patients demonstrate increased chemoresponsiveness and sleep state instability (79,80). Frequent oscillation between wakefulness and stage 1 NREM sleep may cause sleep fragmentation and poor nocturnal sleep as the presenting symptoms. Other symptoms like snoring and witnessed apneas may be present. Patients with primary CSA have a high hypercapnic response (81). Hypocapnia leads to central apnea if end-tidal CO_2 ($P_{ET}CO_2$) is reduced below a threshold, the hypocapnic apneic threshold. These patients have significantly lower mean transcutaneous and $P_{ET}CO_2$ during sleep and lower arterial $PaCO_2$ levels while awake (typically a 2–3 mmHg difference from controls) and have increased wake ventilatory responses to CO_2 (79). The onset of central apnea may initiate several processes that perpetuate breathing instability, including inertia of the ventilatory control system, hypoxia, and transient arousal, as described above. These combined factors produce ventilatory overshoot, hypocapnia, and recurrent central apneas and perpetuate further breathing instability (80).

The prevalence of primary CSA in the older adult is not known. In addition, it is not clear whether gender, aging, or genetics modify the prevalence in this group. White et al. (82) and Bradley et al. (81) reported a strong male predominance, while Roehrs et al. (83) observed central apneas more commonly in women. While there are no prospective studies evaluating the course and long-term outcomes, it is believed that the chemoresponsiveness of the respiratory system is high, so that significant hypoxia and hypercapnia rarely develop during the course of the disease. It is distinguished from Cheynes–Stokes respiration (CSR) in that there is no crescendo–decrescendo pattern and the cycle times are shorter. In primary CSA, the apneas are terminated with an abrupt, large breath, not with a gradual increment in ventilation. Unlike sleep-related hypoventilation syndromes, the hypoxemia in primary CSA is less pronounced and there is absence of hypercapnia on waking arterial blood gases.

In primary CSA, daytime hypersomnolence is less common than with OSA, although such daytime sleepiness has been commonly described in patients with central apnea (81). As the proportion of obstructive or mixed events increases in these patients, hypersomnolence may become more frequent. The primary complaint of many patients with central apnea tends to be insomnia, restless sleep, or frequent awakenings during the night that may be accompanied by shortness of breath. Patients with these central apneas also tend to have a normal body habitus, unlike the characteristically obese patient with obstructive apnea. Arousals from apneas disrupt normal sleep architecture. There was a reduction in the normal percentage of stage 3 or 4 sleep and an increase in stage 1 or 2 sleep in a group of patients with about 50% central apneas (83). Frequent arousals and awakenings generally associated with the hypercapnia after an apnea can lead to disruption of the normal distribution of sleep stages (82).

Cheyne–Stokes Breathing Pattern in Heart Failure

On polysomnography, the Cheyne–Stokes breathing pattern is the presence of at least 10 central apneas and hypopneas per hour of sleep in which the hypopnea has a crescendo–decrescendo pattern of tidal volume accompanied by frequent arousals from asleep and occurs in association with a serious medical illness such as heart failure, stroke, or renal failure (1). In this section, CSR occurring in the context of heart failure is discussed. Patients with central apnea and CHF demonstrate pulmonary vascular congestion leading to hyperventilation and hypocapnia; hence, there is an absence of rise in $P_{ET}CO_2$ from wakefulness to sleep (65,88). Increased ventilation and reduced $P_{ET}CO_2$ indicate decreased plant gain (67,69), which should be stabilizing. In other words, steady-state reduction of $PaCO_2$ is potentially stabilizing rather than destabilizing, as is commonly thought. However, the apneic threshold in CHF patients with central apnea is precariously close to the eupneic $PaCO_2$, owing to increased controller gain. Those with CSA have a significantly larger ventilatory response to carbon dioxide than those without CSA (5.1±3.1 vs. 2.1±1.0 liters per minute per millimeter of mercury, $p = 0.007$) (63), with a significant positive correlation between ventilatory response and the number of episodes of apnea and hypopnea per hour during sleep ($r = 0.6$, $p = 0.01$). Consequently, small decrements in $PaCO_2$ cause central apnea.

Given that CHF is a major public health problem (84), the association between sleep-disordered breathing (SDB) and CHF has important clinical significance. CHF patients have a higher prevalence of SDB, ranging from 40% to 80% (61–64). The wide range is explained by varied definitions of AHI and differences in study designs. Both retrospective (66) and prospective analysis (61) have documented increased prevalence of SDB in CHF. As mentioned above, Javaheri et al. demonstrated that 51% of male patients with CHF had SDB, 40% had CSA, and 11% obstructive apnea. Risk factors for CSA (66) were male gender [odds ratio (OR) 3.50; 95% confidence interval (CI), 1.39–8.84), atrial fibrillation (OR 4.13; 95% CI 1.53–11.14), age >60 years (OR 2.37; 95% CI 1.35–4.15), and hypocapnia (PCO_2 < 38 mmHg during wakefulness) (OR 4.33; 95% CI 2.50–7.52). In women, those aged 60 years or older had six (95% CI 1.22–35.47) times the risk of CSA compared with those below this age cutoff, whereas in men the risk was increased by 2.2-fold (95%

CI 1.24–4.11). Similarly, those who were hypocapnic had over a sixfold (95% CI 1.42–29.08) increase in risk for CSA in women and a fourfold (95% CI 2.27 to 7.22) increase in men. The presence of atrial fibrillation was also an independent risk factor for CSA in both men and women. In CSA related to heart failure, concomitant symptoms of the underlying disorder may be present; these may include dyspnea and lower extremity edema (66).

Recent studies suggest that CSA is an independent predictor of a higher mortality rate (85) or higher combined mortality and heart transplantation rate (86). Treatments aimed specifically at alleviating CSA can improve left-ventricular ejection fraction (LVEF) and reduce atrial natriuretic peptide and sympathetic nervous system activity as well as increase ejection fraction of the left ventricle (87).

CSA in Stroke and Neurodegenerative Diseases

Central apneas and periodic breathing occur with increased frequency in subjects with neurologic disorders such as infarction, tumor, or diffuse encephalopathies. Patients with cerebrovascular disease (stroke, or transient ischemic attacks) have a high prevalence of SDB, mainly OSA (70–71). Whether stroke is a cause or a result of SDB is not clear. In one study (72) there was no change in the frequency of obstructive apneas three months after a stroke compared with apnea frequency at 48 hours after a stroke. However, in that study central apneas decreased at three months, leading the authors to conclude that the obstructive events probably occurred before the stroke and were a risk factor for stroke, whereas the CSAs developed after stroke (72). More recent data from a prospective series of first-ever stroke, suggest that central periodic breathing during sleep may develop in strokes involving autonomic (insula) and volitional (cingulated cortex, thalamus) respiratory networks and that this seems to resolve within three months (89).

CSAs may also be present in neurodegenerative disorders [e.g., Parkinson's disease and multisystem atrophy (MSA) (90)], where it may be the presenting feature or may develop in the late stages of the disorder. In CSA related to central degenerative disorder, concomitant symptoms of the underlying disorder may be present; these may include ataxia, dementia, cogwheel rigidity, or dysautonomia. MSA is a sporadic, progressive, adult-onset disorder characterized by autonomic dysfunction, parkinsonism, and ataxia in various combinations (90,91). Damage to the brainstem, particularly the medullary area, may lead to hypoventilation during wakefulness but more commonly affects ventilation during sleep early in the disease. The autonomic manifestations include orthostatic hypotension, impaired vagal regulation of heart rate (cardiovagal failure), anhidrosis, impotence, and urinary incontinence or retention, which may precede the motor symptoms (91). Respiratory dysfunction, including sleep-related breathing disorders, may be a serious manifestation of MSA (92,93). Although OSA is an important manifestation of this disorder, CSA may also occur as the presenting feature of MSA where CSA may develop prior to the onset of MSA [4 years in one study(94)] or develop in later stages of the disease (95). In a case series of six patients (95), sleep-disordered breathing was present as an early finding of MSA. Three of these patients presented with acute respiratory distress before the ultimate diagnosis of MSA was made; the other three had OSA due to bilateral vocal cord paralysis and presented with stridor.

Pathogenesis in neurodegenerative diseases: CSA may reflect impaired ventilatory chemosensitivity in MSA, as these patients have been shown to have impaired ventilatory responses to hypercapnia (96) or hypoxia (97). CSA associated with neurodegenerative disorders in the older adult may be the manifestation of an aging process and may arise because the neuropathologic changes of MSA are prominent in the brainstem regions where the respiratory centers are located. The central pathological process in MSA involves neuronal cell loss and gliosis throughout the CNS, especially in the putamen, caudate, substantia nigra, locus coerulus, pontine nucleus, inferior olivary nucleus purkinje cells, and the intermediolateral cell columns of the thoracic spinal cord (98). The pathologic hallmarks of MSA are argyrophyllic cellular inclusions in oligodendrocytes throughout the involved regions of the CNS (99). In MSA, oligodendrocyte apoptosis occurs in a distribution similar to the finding of these cellular inclusions (100). Specifically, there is loss of pre-Bötzinger complex neurons (preBötC) of the medulla, which are thought to be responsible for respiratory rhythmogenesis (98,99). In addition, the ventral medullary arcuate nucleus (ArcN) degenerates in MSA with severe depletion of putative chemosensitive glutamatergic and serotonergic neurons in the ArcN of the ventral medullary surface in MSA (98,100,101). It is postulated that involvement of any or both of these neurons may contribute to impaired ventilatory responses to hypercapnia and hypoxia in this disorder (101). In addition, the neurokinin 1-expressing (NK1R) neurons of the preBötC in the ventrolateral medulla are depleted by 60% in Parkinson's disease and by 89% in individuals with MSA, suggesting substantial damage to the preBötC. Similarly, preBot NK1R neuron ablation in adult rats leads to an ataxic breathing when 80% of the neurons were ablated (102), indicating the importance of this area in respiration. MSA should probably be considered in the differential diagnosis of the neurogenic causes of late-onset CSA and progressive alveolar hypoventilation. Case reports of CSA in Parkinson's disease have also been reported (103). Assessment of respiratory function, both when patients are awake and when they are asleep, may be diagnostically helpful in patients with atypical parkinsonism, ataxia, or dysautonomia. There is a need for longitudinal studies in larger populations to determine the frequency and spectrum of neurodegenerative diseases in the older population with CSA. Although an association between OSA and APOE epsilon-4 genotype (a marker of Alzheimer's disease) has been reported in individuals <65 years (134), it has specifically not been related to CSA.

Finally, chronic neuromuscular diseases, such as amyotrophic lateral sclerosis, muscular dystrophy, or myasthenia gravis, may lead to waking alveolar hypoventilation with further hypoventilation during sleep. These may occasionally be associated with central apneas, although hypoventilation is the more prominent disorder. The treatment of the nocturnal hypoventilation with noninvasive nasal ventilation may delay frank waking respiratory failure.

POLYSOMNOGRAPHY

Nocturnal polysomnography is the standard diagnostic method for CSA, including measurements of sleep and respiration (104). The latter includes detection of flow, measurement of oxyhemoglobin saturation, and detection of respiratory effort. Detection of respiratory effort is important to distinguish central from obstructive apnea. This requires measurement of esophageal pressure, as a reflection of pleural pressure changes (105). However, the complexity and invasiveness of the procedure have precluded widespread use. Instead, most clinical sleep laboratories utilize surface recording of effort to detect displacement of the abdominal and thoracic compartments and dysynchrony during episodes of upper airway obstruction. Respiratory inductive plethysmography (RIP), calibrated or uncalibrated, can adequately assess respiratory effort (104). A complete absence of thoracoabdominal motion (RIP or strain gauges) throughout an apnea suggests the event is central in origin (106). Measurement of the lapsed time for a pulse signal to reach the periphery, or pulse transit time (PTT), can also serve as a noninvasive index of respiratory effort (104). The technique measures the elapsed time between R wave on the ECG and the arrival of the pulse wave to the finger. The underlying physiologic principle is that blood pressure influences vessel stiffness and hence the speed of the pulse wave. When blood pressure increases during an apnea owing to increased intrathoracic pressure swings, the PTT displays parallel swings.

TREATMENT OF CENTRAL SLEEP APNEA

Despite the increased prevalence of this disorder in the older adult and its potential morbidity and mortality, a lack of knowledge about the specific underlying pathogenic mechanisms hinders the development of novel pharmacologic therapies for CSA. Current principal therapies remain limited to mechanical devices, while there have been rudimentary attempts at pharmacologic therapy with respiratory stimulant drugs and O_2 and CO_2 gas supplementation.

Positive Pressure Therapy

Central apnea may respond to nasal CPAP therapy, especially if in combination with episodes of obstructive or mixed apnea. Moreover, primary CSA may respond to nasal CPAP therapy by preventing pharyngeal narrowing during central apnea (7) and hence mitigating the ensuing ventilatory overshoot and perpetuation of ventilatory instability (135). Many patients with idiopathic CSA receive a trial of nasal CPAP, which has been shown to reverse CSA, even in the absence of obstructive respiratory events (107,108), especially supine-dependent CSA. The response may be due to prevention of upper airway occlusion during central apnea and subsequent ventilatory overshoot (109). Prevention of ventilatory overshoot may explain the reported increase PCO_2 after CPAP (110). Nasal CPAP for one month in patients with central apnea and CHF resulted in a decrease in the frequency of apneas and hypopneas, an increase in mean transcutaneous PCO_2, a reduction in mean minute ventilation, and an increase in mean oxyhemoglobin saturation (O_2 Sat) during sleep. The combination of increased PCO_2 and increased O_2 Sat readily explains the amelioration of central apnea. Hence, nasal CPAP is the initial option during a therapeutic titration study, despite the lack of systematic studies on nasal CPAP therapy in patients with primary CSA. Older individuals probably utilize CPAP as well as younger patients. CPAP should be used throughout the sleep duration.

Treatment of CSR usually consists of optimization of medical management for CHF. Nasal CPAP may have significant salutary effects in patients with CHF and CSA. Several lines of evidence, both theoretical and empiric, underpin the use of CPAP in this setting. For example, one study has demonstrated increased LVEF and a reduction of combined mortality–cardiac transplantation risk by 81%, but only in patients with CSA (111). However, the exuberance regarding nasal CPAP therapy in patients with central apnea and CHF did not withstand the rigors of controlled clinical trials. The Canadian Continuous Positive Airway Pressure trial, or CAN-PAP (87), tested the hypothesis that CPAP would improve the survival rate without heart transplantation in patients with heart failure and CSA. The study enrolled 258 patients who had heart failure and CSA; participants were randomly assigned to the nasal CPAP treatment group ($n = 128$) or no CPAP (130 patients). Duration of follow-up was for a mean of two years. There was greater improvement in the CPAP group at three months relative to the placebo group as evidenced by greater reductions in the AHI, ejection fraction, mean nocturnal oxyhemoglobin saturation, plasma norepinephrine levels, and the distance walked in six minutes. Nevertheless, there was no difference in the overall event rates (death and heart transplantation) between the two groups. Thus, nasal CPAP had no effect on survival, despite the effect on the "severity" of central apnea and several intermediate outcome variables. Therefore, current evidence does not support the use of CPAP to extend life in patients who have heart failure and CSA. In a post hoc analysis of the CANPAP (112), of the 258 heart failure patients with CSA in CANPAP, 110 of the 130 randomized to the control group and 100 of the 128 randomized to CPAP had sleep studies three months later. CPAP patients were divided post hoc into those whose AHI *was or was not* reduced below 15 at three months (CPAP-CSA suppressed, $n = 57$, and CPAP-CSA unsuppressed, $n = 43$, respectively). Despite similar CPAP pressure and hours of use in the two groups, CPAP-CSA–suppressed subjects experienced a greater increase in LVEF at three months ($p = 0.001$) and significantly better transplant-free survival [hazard ratio (95% CI) 0.371 (0.142–0.967), $p = 0.043$] than control subjects, whereas the CPAP-CSA–unsuppressed group did not [for LVEF, $p = 0.984$, and for transplant-free survival, hazard ratio 1.463 (95% CI 0.751–2.850), $p = 0.260$]. These results suggest that CPAP might improve both LVEF and heart transplant–free survival in heart failure patients if CSA is suppressed soon after its initiation (112,113).

Noninvasive positive pressure ventilation (NIPPV) using pressure support mode (bilevel nasal positive pressure) is effective in restoring alveolar ventilation during sleep (114). Clinical indications include nocturnal ventilatory failure and central apnea secondary to hypoventilation. There is evidence that NIPPV exerts a salutary effect on survival in patients with ventilatory failure secondary to amyotrophic lateral sclerosis (115,116). It is unclear whether NIPPV exerts a similar effect in other neuromuscular conditions associated with nocturnal ventilatory failure. However, the overall evidence supports the use of noninvasive positive pressure ventilation in a pressure support mode to treat CSA secondary to hypoventilation, such as neuromuscular or chest wall–related nocturnal hypoventilation. If the ventilatory motor output is insufficient to "trigger" the mechanical inspiration, adding a backup rate ensures adequate ventilation.

Most patients with ventilatory failure tolerate NIPPV well. However, there are a few specific drawbacks. The use of NIPPV in the controlled mode results in laryngeal aperture narrowing and may decrease the delivered tidal volume during NIPPV (117). Alleviating this problem is feasible with appropriate adjustments of volume, flow, and inspiratory time (118). The potential role of NIPPV in the treatment of nonhypercapnic, post-hyperventilation central apnea is uncertain. The addition of a backup rate renders NIPPV-controlled mechanical ventilation. However, NIPPV in the pressure support, bilevel mode augments tidal volume; the ensuing hyperventilation results in hypocapnia and possible worsening of central apnea and periodic breathing during sleep (119). Recent technological advances allowed for variations in the mode of delivering positive pressure ventilation. One such method is adaptive servo ventilation (ASV), which provides a small but varying amount of ventilatory support, against a background of low level of CPAP. Contrary to bilevel pressure support devices, with ASV changes in respiratory effort result in reciprocal changes in the magnitude of ventilatory support. Thus, ventilation remains slightly below the baseline, eupneic average. There is preliminary evidence that ASV may be more effective than CPAP, bi-level pressure support ventilation or increased dead space in alleviating CSA (120).

More research is needed on the use of positive airway pressure (PAP) treatment in the older adult. Evaluations of immediate and long-term benefits of PAP treatment, including evaluation for cardiovascular, cognitive, psychological, and functional outcomes, are required. Research also needs to investigate whether the response to treatment is similar between older and younger adults, determine which patients should receive treatment, and determine if there are complications to CPAP treatment that are unique to the older patient.

Pharmacologic Agents

Certain pharmacologic agents may influence the propensity to develop central apnea. Therapy of the underlying condition that is predisposing to CSA should be initiated. For example, the use of beta-blockers in patients with CSA and CHF is associated with reduced apnea index (133). Conversely, narcotics may worsen central apnea; so a change in the pain control regimen may ameliorate the severity of CSA (121). If a concomitant clinical condition is present, such as CHF, hypothyroidism, or acromegaly, optimization of medical therapy is also required and may ameliorate the severity of central apnea. However, the role of pharmacological therapy for primary central apnea is very modest, and there are no controlled clinical trials demarcating the outcomes. There is evidence derived from small studies, but no large clinical trials, to support the use of acetazolamide and theophylline in the treatment of central apnea (122). Acetazolamide is a carbonic anhydrase inhibitor and a weak diuretic that causes mild metabolic acidosis and enhances the respiratory drive. In a few studies, acetazolamide ameliorated CSA when administered as a single dose of 250 mg before bedtime (123). In a study by White et al. (124), there was a reduction in central apneas, an increase in O_2 saturation, and an improvement in symptoms with acetazolamide. However, in another study an improvement was not consistently observed (125). In patients with heart failure and Cheyne–Stokes breathing with an AHI of more than 15/hr, administration of a single dose of acetazolamide before sleep improved CSA and related daytime symptoms; the mean age of patients was 66 ± 6 years (126).

Theophylline ameliorates the severity of Cheyne–Stokes respiration in patients with CHF (122,127). The short-term administration of oral theophylline improved sleep-disordered breathing and reduced associated arterial blood oxyhemoglobin desaturation in patients with stable heart failure (127), without adverse effects on sleep architecture (mean age of the study participants was not reported). Nevertheless, theophylline is rarely used for the treatment of central apnea owing to the narrow therapeutic margin, interaction with other medications, and the risks of toxicity.

Supplemental O_2 and CO_2

Several studies have demonstrated a salutary effect of supplemental O_2 in patients with idiopathic CSA and patients with CHF-CSR (65,128). The mechanism of action is by ameliorating hypoxemia and minimizing the subsequent ventilatory overshoot. Thus, oxygen may improve CSA by the suppression of the hypercapnic and the hypoxic ventilatory drives. Conversely, supplemental O_2 may elevate cerebral PCO_2 by the Haldane effect. Likewise, supplemental CO_2 eliminates central apnea in patients with pure CSA. In one study of six patients with primary CSA (129), mild reduction of end-tidal CO_2 during sleep that was associated with uncontrollable mixed disease, a single night of increasing PCO_2 by 2 to 3 mmHg, to the low normal level, as an adjunct to CPAP or bilevel PAP therapy, resulted in complete abolition of central apneas. In this case series, only one patient was >65 years of age. The mechanism of action is by raising PCO_2 above the apneic threshold. However, this therapy is not practical given the need for a closed circuit to deliver supplemental CO_2 (129,130).

Subjects with CSA have enhanced CO_2 chemosensitivity. During arousals, enhanced CO_2 (and hypoxic) chemosensitivity above eucapnia will tend to lower the prevailing PCO_2 and increase the likelihood of the occurrence of apnea during subsequent sleep. One study reported that there was considerable reduction in the number of central apneas present in a patient with central alveolar hypoventilation after oxygen therapy was begun (131). Recently, the addition of low levels of CO_2 to the CPAP circuit has been reported as an effective treatment of refractory mixed or CSA (132) and is a promising solution for some older people. However, there are very few large-scale studies assessing treatment efficacy with either O_2 or CO_2 in older subjects with CSA who do not have CHF.

CONCLUSION

There is an increased prevalence of CSA with aging. However, whether the presence of increased numbers of central apneas during sleep is an epiphenomenon or portends harmful sequelae is not known. On the other hand, CSA in the older adult may be a clinical marker of underlying cardiac or neurologic disease, with resultant serious morbidity and mortality. Studies that investigate pathophysiology and long-term impact of CSA on health and mortality in the older adult are absent. Lack of understanding of the underlying pathophysiology limits development of new therapeutic strategies. Further research in this field will allow us to clarify the pathophysiologic determinants of breathing instability with aging, as a prerequisite to the development of novel therapeutic interventions for CSA.

REFERENCES

1. American Academy of Sleep Medicine. International Classification of Sleep Disorders. 2nd ed.: Diagnostic and Coding Manual. Westchester, IL: American Academy of Sleep Medicine, 2005:35–37.
2. Bradley TD, Phillipson EA 1992. Central sleep apnea. Clin.Chest Med 13:493–505.
3. Pack A.I., Cola MF, Goldszmidt A, et al. Correlation between oscillations in ventilation and frequency content of the electroencephalogram. J. Appl. Physiol 1992; 72:985–992.

4. Hudgel DW, Chapman KR, Faulks C, et al. Changes in inspiratory muscle electrical activity and upper airway resistance during periodic breathing induced by hypoxia during sleep. Am Rev Respir Dis 1987; 135:899–906.
5. Onal E., Burrows DL, Hart RH,et al. Induction of periodic breathing during sleep causes upper airway obstruction in humans. J Appl Physiol 1986; 61:1438–1443.
6. Warner G, Skatrud JB, and Dempsey JA. Effect of hypoxia-induced periodic breathing on upper airway obstruction during sleep. J Appl Physiol 1987; 62:2201–2211.
7. Badr MS, Toiber F, Skatrud JB, et al. Pharyngeal narrowing or occlusion during central sleep apnea. J Appl Physiol 1995; 78(5):1806–1815.
8. Younes M, Ostrowski M, Thompson W, et al. Chemical control stability in patients with obstructive sleep apnea. Am J Respir Crit Care Med 2001; 163:1181–1190.
9. Younes M. Contributions of upper airway mechanics and control mechanisms to severity of obstructive apnea. Am J Respir Crit Care Med 2003; 168(6):645–658.
10. Mezon BL, West P, Israels J, et al. Sleep breathing abnormalities in kyphoscoliosis. Am Rev Respir Dis 1980; 122:617–621.
11. Ancoli-Israel S, Kripke DF, Klauber MR, et al. Sleep-disordered breathing in community-dwelling elderly. Sleep 1991; 14:486–495.
12. Bixler EO, Vgontzas AN, Lin HM, et al. Prevalence of sleep-disordered breathing in women: effects of gender. Am J Respir Crit Care Med 2001; 163:608–613.
13. Mason WJ, Ancoli-Israel S, Kripke DF. Apnea revisited: a longitudinal follow-up. Sleep 1989; 12(5):423–429.
14. Ancoli-Israel S, Kripke DF, Klauber MR, et al. Morbidity, mortality and sleep-disordered breathing in community dwelling elderly Sleep 1996; 19:277–282.
15. Bliwise DL, Bliwise NG, Partinen M, et al. Sleep apnea and mortality in an aged cohort. Am J Public Health 1988; 78(5):544–547.
16. Ancoli-Israel S, DuHamel ER, Stepnowsky C, et al. The relationship between congestive heart failure, sleep apnea, and mortality in older men. Chest. 2003; 124(4):1400–1405.
17. Hoch CC, Reynolds CFIII, Monk TH, et al. Comparison of sleep-disordered breathing among healthy elderly in the seventh, eighth, and ninth decades of life. Sleep 1990; 13(6):502–511.
18. Phillips BA, Berry DT, Schmitt FA, et al. Sleep-disordered breathing in the healthy elderly. Chest 1992; 101(2):345–349.
19. Duran J, Esnaola S, Rubio R, et al. Obstructive sleep apnea-hypopnea and related clinical features in a population-based sample of subjects aged 30 to 70 yr. Am J Respir Crit Care Med 2001; 163(3 pt 1):685–689.
20. Young T, Palta M, Dempsey J, et al. The occurrence of sleep-disordered breathing among middle-aged adults. NEJM 1993; 328(17):1230–1235.
21. Redline S, Schluchter MD, Larkin EK, et al. Predictors of longitudinal change in sleep-disordered breathing in a nonclinic population. Sleep 2003; 26(6):703–709.
22. Carskadon M, Dement W. Respiration during sleep in the aged human. J Gerontol 1981; 36:420–425.
23. Colrain IM, Trinder J, Fraser G. Ventilation during sleep onset in young adult females. Sleep 1990; 13:491–501.
24. Phillipson EA, Kumar LF. Effect of aging on metabolic respiratory control in sleeping dogs. Am Rev Respir Dis 1993; 147:1521–1525.
25. Nishimura M, Yamamoto M, Yoshioka A, et al. Longitudinal analyses of respiratory chemo sensitivity in normal subjects. Am Rev Respir Dis 1991; 143(6):1278–1281.
26. Chapman KR, Cherniak NS. Aging effects on the interaction of hypercapnia and hypoxia as ventilatory stimuli. J Gerontol 1987; 42:202–209.
27. Poulin MJ, Cunningham DA, Paterson DH. Dynamics of the ventilatory response to step changes in end-tidal PCO_2 in older humans. Can J Appl Physiol 1997; 22:368–383.
28. Browne HA, Adams L, Symonds AK, et al. Ageing does not influence the sleep-related decrease in the hypercapnic ventilatory response. Eur Respir J 2003; 21:523–529.
29. Smith WD, Poulin MJ, Paterson DH, et al. Dynamic ventilator response to acute isocapnic hypoxia in septuagenarians. Exp Physiol 2001; 86:117–126.

30. Ahmed M, Giesbrecht GG, Serrette C, et al. Ventilatory response to hypoxia in elderly humans. Respir Physiol 1991; 83(3):343–351.
31. Vovk A, Smith WD, Paterson ND, et al. Peripheral chemoreceptor control of ventilation following sustained hypoxia in young and older adult humans. Exp Physiol 2004; 89:647–656.
32. Younes M, Ostrowski M, Thompson W, et al. Chemical control stability in patients with obstructive sleep apnea. Am J Respir Crit Care Med 2001; 163:1181–1190.
33. Wellman A, Malhotra A, Jordan AS, et al. Chemical control stability in the elderly. J Physiol 2007; 58:291–298.
34. Dempsey JA Crossing the apnoeic threshold: causes and consequences. Exp Physiol 2005; 90:13–24.
35. Nakayama H, Smith CA, Rodman JR, et al. Carotid body denervation eliminates apnea in response to transient hypocapnia. J Appl Physiol 2003; 94,155–164.
36. Mateika JH, Fregosi RF. Long-term facilitation of upper airway muscle activities in vagotomized and vagally intact cats. J Appl Physiol 1997; 82:419–425.
37. Bach KB and Mitchell GS. Hypoxia-induced long-term facilitation of respiratory activity is serotonin dependent. Respir Physiol 1996; 104:251–260.
38. Babcock MA and Badr MS. Long-term facilitation of ventilation in humans during NREM sleep. Sleep 1998; 21:709–716.
39. Babcock M, Shkoukani M, Aboubakr SE, et al. Determinants of long-term facilitation in humans during NREM sleep. J Appl Physiol 2003; 94:53–59.
40. Aboubakr SE, Taylor A, Ford R, et al. Long-term facilitation in obstructive sleep apnea patients during NREM sleep. J Appl Physiol 2001; 91(6):2751–2757.
41. Gozal E and Gozal D. Respiratory plasticity following intermittent hypoxia: developmental interactions. J. Appl. Physiol 2001; 90:1995–1999.
42. Shkoukani M, Babcock MA, and Badr MS. Effect of episodic hypoxia on upper airway mechanics in humans during NREM sleep. J Appl Physiol 2002; 92:2565–2570.
43. Mahamed S, Mitchell G. Is there a link between intermittent hypoxia-induced respiratory plasticity and obstructive sleep apnoea? Exp Physiol 2007; 92:27–37.
44. Zabka AG, Mitchell GS, Behan M. Ageing and gonadectomy have similar effects on hypoglossal long-term facilitation in male Fischer rats. J Physiol 2005; 563:557–568.
45. Zabka AG, Mitchell GS, Behan M. Selected contribution: Time-dependent hypoxic respiratory responses in female rats are influenced by age and by the estrus cycle. J Appl Physiol 2001; 91:2831–2838.
46. Zabka AG, Mitchell GS, Behan M. Long term facilitation of respiratory motor output decreases with age in male rats. J Physiol 2001; 531:509–514.
47. Chowdhuri S, Pierchala L, Aboubakr SE, et al. Long-term facilitation of genioglossus activity is present in normal humans during NREM sleep. Respir Physiol Neurobiol 2007; Aug 25 [epub].
48. Zhou XS, Shahabuddin S, Zahn BK, et al. Effect of gender on the development of hypocapnic apnea/hypopnea during NREM sleep. J Appl Physiol 2000; 89:192–199.
49. Rowley JA, Deebajah I, Parikh S, et al. The influence of episodic hypoxia on upper airway collapsibility in subjects with obstructive sleep apnea. J Appl Physiol 2007; 103(3):911–916.
50. Zhou XS, Rowley JA, Demirovic F, et al. Effect of testosterone on the apneic threshold in women during NREM sleep. J Appl Physiol 2003; 94:101–107.
51. Mateika JH, Omran Q, Rowley JA, et al. Treatment with leuprolide acetate decreases the threshold of the ventilatory response to carbon dioxide in healthy males. J Physiol 2004; 561:637–646.
52. Phillips B, Cook Y, Schmitt F, et al. Sleep apnea: prevalence of risk factor in a general population. South Med J 1989; 82:1090–1092.
53. Phillips BA, Berry DT, Schmitt FA, et al. Sleep-disordered breathing in the healthy elderly. Clinically significant? Chest 1992; 101:345–349.
54. Pack AI, Silage DA, Millman RP, et al. Spectral analysis of ventilation in elderly subjects awake and asleep. J Appl Physiol 1988; 64:1257–1267.

55. Trinder J, Whitworth F, Kay A, et al. Respiratory instability during sleep onset. J Appl Physiol 1992; 73:2462–2469.
56. Dunai J, Wilkinson M, and Trinder J. Interaction of chemical and state effects on ventilation during sleep onset. J Appl. Physiol 1996; 81:2235–2243.
57. Dunai J, Kleiman J, and Trinder J. Ventilatory instability during sleep onset in individuals with high peripheral chemosensitivity. J Appl Physiol 1999; 87:661–672.
58. Thomson S, Morrell MJ, Cordingley JJ, et al. Ventilation is unstable during drowsiness before sleep onset. J Appl Physiol 2005; 99:2036–2044.
59. Orem J. Neuronal mechanisms of respiration in REM sleep. Sleep 1980; 3:251–267.
60. Orem J, Lovering AT, Dunin-Barkowski W, et al. Tonic activity in the respiratory system in wakefulness, NREM and REM sleep. Sleep 2002; 25:488–496.
61. Javaheri S, Parker TJ, Liming JD, et al. Sleep apnea in 81 ambulatory male patients with stable heart failure. Types and their prevalences, consequences, and presentations. Circulation 1998; 97:2154–2159.
62. Javaheri S, Parker TJ, Wexler L, et al. Occult sleep-disordered breathing in stable congestive heart failure. Ann Intern Med 1995; 122:487–492.
63. Javaheri S. A mechanism of central sleep apnea in patients with heart failure. N Engl J Med 1999; 341(13):949–954.
64. Javaheri S, Parker TJ, Liming JD, et al. Sleep apnea in 81 ambulatory male patients with stable heart failure. Types and their prevalences, consequences, and presentations. Circulation 1998; 97:2154–2159.
65. Bradley TD and Floras JS. Sleep apnea and heart failure. Part II: central sleep apnea. Circulation 2003; 107:1822–1826.
66. Sin DD, Fitzgerald F, Parker JD, et al. Risk factors for central and obstructive sleep apnea in 450 men and women with congestive heart failure. Am J Respir Crit Care Med 1999; 160:1101–1106.
67. Xie A, Skatrud JB, Puleo DS, et al. Apnea-hypopnea threshold for CO_2 in patients with congestive heart failure. Am J Respir Crit Care Med 2002; 165:1245–1250.
68. Dempsey JA, Sheel AW, Haverkamp HC, et al. [The John Sutton Lecture: CSEP, 2002]. Pulmonary system limitations to exercise in health. Can J Appl Physiol 2003; 28(suppl):S2–S24; 165;1245–1250.
69. Dempsey JA, Smith CA, Przybylowski T, et al. The ventilatory responsiveness to CO2 below eupnoea as a determinant of ventilatory stability in sleep. J. Physiol 2004; 560:1–11.
70. Bassetti C and Aldrich MS. Sleep apnea in acute cerebrovascular diseases: final report on 128 patients. Sleep 1999; 22:217–223.
71. Bassetti C, Aldrich MS, Chervin RD, et al. Sleep apnea in patients with transient ischemic attack and stroke: a prospective study of 59 patients. Neurology 1996; 47:1167–1173.
72. Parra O, Arbiox A, Bechich S, et al. Time course of sleep-related breathing disorders in first-ever stroke or transient ischemic attack. Am J Respir Crit Care Med 2000; 161:375–380.
73. Wang D, Teichtahl H, Drummer O, et al. Central sleep apnea in stable methadone maintenance treatment patients. Chest 2005; 128:1348–1356.
74. Leung RS, Huber MA, Rogge T, et al. Association between atrial fibrillation and central sleep apnea. Sleep 2005; 28:1543–1546.
75. Kapur VK, Koepsell TD, deMaine J, et al. Association of hypothyroidism and obstructive sleep apnea. Am J Respir Crit Care Med 1998; 158:1379–1383.
76. Grunstein RR, Ho KY, Berthon-Jones M, et al. Central sleep apnea is associated with increased ventilatory response to carbon dioxide and hypersecretion of growth hormone in patients with acromegaly. Am J Respir Crit Care Med 1994; 150:496–502.
77. Grunstein RR, Ho KY, and Sullivan CE. Sleep apnea in acromegaly. Ann Intern Med 1991; 115:527–532.
78. Hanly PJ and Pierratos A. Improvement of sleep apnea in patients with chronic renal failure who undergo nocturnal hemodialysis. New Engl J Med 2001; 344:102–107.

79. Xie A, Rutherford R, Rankin F, et al. Hypocapnia and increased ventilatory responsiveness in patients with idiopathic central sleep apnea. Am J Respir Crit Care Med 1995; 152:1950–1955.
80. Xie A, Wong B, Phillipson EA, et al. Interaction of hyperventilation and arousal in the pathogenesis of idiopathic central sleep apnea. Am J Respir Crit Care Med 1994; 150:489–495.
81. Bradley TD, McNicholas WT, Rutherford R, et al. Clinical and physiological heterogeneity of the central sleep apnea syndrome. Am Rev Respir Dis 1986; 134:217–221.
82. White D, Zwillich C, Pickett C, et al. Central sleep apnea: improvement with acetazolamide[Rx] therapy Arch Intern Med 1982; 142:1816–1819.
83. Roehrs T, Conway W, Wittig R, et al. Sleep complaints in patients with sleep-related respiratory disturbances. Am Rev Respir Dis 1985; 132:520–523.
84. Hunt SA, Baker DW, Chin MH, et al. ACC/AHA Guidelines for the Evaluation and Management of Chronic Heart Failure in the Adult: Executive Summary A Report of the American College of Cardiology/American Heart Association Task Force on Practice Guidelines (Committee to Revise the 1995 Guidelines for the Evaluation and Management of Heart Failure). Circulation 2001; 104:2996–3007.
85. Lanfranchi PA, Braghiroli A, Bosimini E, et al. Prognostic value of nocturnal Cheyne-Stokes respiration in chronic heart failure. Circulation 1999; 99: 1435–1440.
86. Hanly P, and Zuberi-Khokhar N. Increased mortality associated with Cheyne-Stokes respiration in patients with congestive heart failure. Am J Respir Crit Care Med 1996; 153:272–276.
87. Bradley TD, Logan AG, Kimoff RJ, et al. Continuous positive airway pressure for central sleep apnea and heart failure. N Engl J Med 2005; 353:2025–2033.
88. Javaheri S. A mechanism of central sleep apnea in patients with heart failure. N Engl J Med 1999; 341,949–954.
89. Hermann DM, Siccoli M, Kirov P, et al. Central periodic breathing during sleep in acute ischemic stroke. Stroke 2007; 38(3):1082–1084.
90. Gilman S, Low PA, Quinn N, et al. Consensus statement on the diagnosis of multiple system atrophy. J Neurol Sci. 1999;163(1):94–8.
91. Wenning GK, Colosimo C, Geser F, et al. Multiple system atrophy. Lancet Neurol 2004; 3:93–103.
92. Silber MH, Levine S. Stridor and death in multiple system atrophy. Mov Disord 2000; 5:699–704.
93. Ghorayeb I, Bioulac B, Tison F. Sleep disorders in multiple system atrophy. J Neural Transm 2005; 112:1669–1675
94. Cormican LJ, Higgins S, Davidson AC, et al. Multiple system atrophy presenting as central sleep apnoea. Eur Respir J 2004; 24:323–325.
95. Glass GA, Josephs KA, Ahlskog JE. Respiratory insufficiency as the primary presenting symptom of multiple-system atrophy. Arch Neurol 2006; 63; 978–981.
96. Chokroverty S, Sharp JT, Barron KD. Periodic respiration in erect posture in Shy-Drager syndrome. J Neurol Neurosurg Psychiatry 1978; 41:980–986.
97. Tsuda T, Onodera H, Okabe S, et al. Impaired chemosensitivity to hypoxia is a marker of multiple system atrophy. Ann Neurol 2002; 52(3):367–371.
98. Benarroch EE, Schmeichel AM, Parisi JE. Depletion of cholinergic neurons of the medullary arcuate nucleus in multiple system atrophy. Auton Neurosci 2001; 87:293–299.
99. Benarroch EE, Schmeichel AM, Low PA, et al. Depletion of ventromedullary NK-1 receptor–immunoreactive neurons in multiple system atrophy. Brain 2003; 126:2183–2190.
100. Noda K, Katayama S, Watanabe C, et al. Decrease of neurons in the medullary arcuate nucleus of multiple system atrophy: quantitative comparison with Parkinson's disease and amyotrophic lateral sclerosis. J Neurol Sci 1997; 151:89–91.
101. Benarroch EE, Schmeichel AM, Low PA, et al. Depletion of putative chemosensitive respiratory neurons in the ventral medullary surface in multiple system atrophy. Brain 2007; 130:469–475.

102. McKay LC, Janczewski WA, Feldman JL. Sleep-disordered breathing after targeted ablation of preBotzinger complex neurons. Nat Neurosci 2005; 8(9):1142–1144.
103. Maria B, Sophia S, Michalis M, et al. Sleep breathing disorders in patients with idiopathic Parkinson's disease. Respir Med 2003; 97(10):1151–1157.
104. Farre R, Montserrat JM, Navajas D. Noninvasive monitoring of respiratory mechanics during sleep. Eur Respir J 2004; 24:1052–1060.
105. Boudewyns A, Willemen M, Wagemans M, et al. Assessment of respiratory effort by means of strain gauge and esophageal pressure swings: a comparative study. Sleep 1997; 20:168–170.
106. Staats BA, Bonekat HW, Harris CD, et al. Chest wall motion in sleep apnea. Am Rev Respir Dis 1984; 130:59–63.
107. Issa FG, Sullivan CE. Reversal of central sleep apnea using nasal CPAP. Chest 1986; 90:165–171.
108. Hoffstein V, Slutsky AS. Central sleep apnea reversed by continuous positive airway pressure. Am Rev Respir Dis 1987; 135:1210–1212.
109. Badr MS, Toiber F, Skatrud JB, et al. Pharyngeal narrowing/occlusion during central sleep apnea. J Appl Physiol 1995; 78:1806–1815.
110. Naughton MT, Benard DC, Rutherford R, et al. Effect of continuous positive airway pressure on central sleep apnea and nocturnal PCO_2 in heart failure. Am J Respir Crit Care Med 1994; 150:1598–1604.
111. Sin DD, Logan AG, Fitzgerald FS, et al. Effects of continuous positive airway pressure on cardiovascular outcomes in heart failure patients with and without Cheyne-Stokes respiration. Circulation 2000; 102:61–66.
112. Arzt M, Floras JS, Logan AG, et al. Suppression of central sleep apnea by continuous positive airway pressure and transplant-free survival in heart failure: a post hoc analysis of the Canadian Continuous Positive Airway Pressure for Patients With Central Sleep Apnea and Heart Failure Trial (CANPAP). Circulation 2007; 115:3173–3180.
113. Olson LJ, Somers VK. Treating central sleep apnea in heart failure: outcomes revisited. Circulation 2007; 115:3140–3142.
114. Guilleminault C, Stoohs R, Schnieder H, et al. Central alveolar hypoventilation and sleep: treatment by intermittent positive-pressure ventilation through nasal mask in an adult. Chest 1989; 96:1210–1212.
115. Aboussouan LS, Khan SU, Banerjee M, et al. Objective measures of the efficacy of noninvasive positive-pressure ventilation in amyotrophic lateral sclerosis. Muscle Nerve 2001; 24:403–409.
116. Aboussouan LS, Khan SU, Meeker DP, et al. Effect of noninvasive positive-pressure ventilation on survival in amyotrophic lateral sclerosis. Ann. Intern Med 1997; 127:450–453.
117. Jounieaux V, Aubert G, Dury M, et al. Effects of nasal positive-pressure hyperventilation on the glottis in normal sleeping subjects. J Appl Physiol 1995; 79:186–193.
118. Parreira VF, Jounieaux V, Delguste P, et al. Determinants of effective ventilation during nasal intermittent positive pressure ventilation. Eur Respir J 1997; 10:1975–1982.
119. Johnson KG and Johnson DC. Bilevel positive airway pressure worsens central apneas during sleep. Chest 2005; 128:2141–2150.
120. Teschler H, Dohring J, Wang YM, et al. Adaptive pressure support servo-ventilation: a novel treatment for Cheyne-Stokes respiration in heart failure. Am J Respir Crit Care Med 2001; 164:614–619.
121. Wang D, Teichtahl H, Drummer O, et al. Central sleep apnea in stable methadone maintenance treatment patients. Chest 2005; 128:1348–1356.
122. Hudgel DW, Thanakitcharu S. Pharmacologic treatment of sleep-disordered breathing. Am J Respir Crit Care Med 1998; 158:691–699.
123. DeBacker WA, Verbraecken J, Willemen M, et al. Central apnea index decreases after prolonged treatment with acetazolamide. Am J Respir Crit Care Med 1995; 151:87–91.
124. White DP, Zwillich CW, Pickett C, et al. Central sleep apnea: improvement with acetazolamide therapy. Arch Intern Med 1982; 142:1816–1819.

125. Sakamoto T, Nakazawa Y, Hashizume Y, et al. Effects of acetazolamide on the sleep apnea syndrome and its therapeutic mechanism. Psychiatry Clin Neurosci 1995; 49:59–64.
126. Javaheri S. Acetazolamide improves central sleep apnea in heart failure: a double-blind, prospective study. Am J Respir Crit Care Med 2006; 173:234–237.
127. Javaheri S, Parker TJ, Wexler L, et al. Effect of theophylline on sleep-disordered breathing in heart failure. N Engl J Med 1996; 335:562–567.
128. Javaheri S, Ahmed M, Parker TJ, et al. Effects of nasal O_2 on sleep-related disordered breathing in ambulatory patients with stable heart failure. Sleep 1999; 22:1101–1106.
129. Xie A, Rankin F, Rutherford R, et al. Effects of inhaled CO_2 and added dead space on idiopathic central sleep apnea. J Appl Physiol 1997; 82:918–926.
130. Lorenzi-Filho G, Rankin F, Bies I, et al. Effects of inhaled carbon dioxide and oxygen on Cheyne-Stokes respiration in patients with heart failure. Am J Respir Crit Care Med 1999; 159:1490–1498.
131. McNicholas W, Carter J, Rutherford R, et al. Beneficial effect of oxygen in primary alveolar hypoventilation with central sleep apnea. Am Rev Respir Dis 1982; 125:773–775.
132. Thomas RJ, Daly RW, Weiss JW. Low-concentration carbon dioxide is an effective adjunct to positive airway pressure in the treatment of refractory mixed central and obstructive sleep-disordered breathing. Sleep 2005; 28:69–77.
133. Tamura A, Kawano Y, Naono S, et al. Relationship between beta-blocker treatment and the severity of central sleep apnea in chronic heart failure. Chest 2007; 131:130–135.
134. Gottlieb DJ, DeStefano AL, Foley DJ, et al. APOE epsilon4 is associated with obstructive sleep apnea/hypopnea: the Sleep Heart Health Study. Neurology 2004; 63(4):664–668.
135. Issa FG, Sullivan CE. Reversal of central sleep apnea using nasal CPAP. Chest 1986; 90:165–171.

10 Circadian Rhythm Sleep Disorders in Aging

Erik Naylor and Phyllis C. Zee

Department of Neurology, Northwestern University Medical School, Chicago, Illinois, U.S.A.

INTRODUCTION

Significant changes in both sleep and circadian regulation occur with aging. A recent National Sleep Foundation survey found that 36% of respondents over the age of 65 experienced sleep disturbances (1). Commonly reported complaints include habitually earlier bedtimes and wake times, inability to maintain sleep through the night, undesired early morning awakening, and frequent daytime sleepiness (2–5). A combination of age-related changes in sleep and circadian rhythm regulation, paired with decreased levels of light exposure and activity, contributes to the development of the circadian rhythm–based sleep disorders in older adults. Thus, the prevalence of circadian rhythm sleep disorders (CRSDs), such as advanced sleep phase disorder and irregular sleep-wake rhythm, are increasingly more common among older adults (6). This chapter reviews our current understanding of the pathophysiology, evaluation, and treatment of the more common age-related CRSDs.

CIRCADIAN SYSTEMS: AN OVERVIEW

Sleep and wake are governed by two major interacting factors: a homeostatic drive for sleep, which increases with time spent awake, and a daily circadian oscillation. The homeostatic need for sleep builds the longer we remain awake and is dissipated during sleep, whereas the circadian process both produces an alerting signal during the day to oppose the homeostatic sleep buildup and provides temporal organization (7–10). Although both the homeostatic and circadian processes function independently, their interaction results in consolidated sleep during the night and wakefulness during the day.

Most physiological, hormonal, and behavioral processes, including the sleep–wake cycle, exhibit near-24-hour (circadian) rhythms. These endogenous circadian rhythms are generated by the suprachiasmatic nucleus (SCN), a paired nuclei in the hypothalamus of the brain (11–13). In humans this endogenous circadian rhythm has a frequency of oscillation that is slightly longer than 24 hours (14). Because the period of the circadian clock is not exactly 24 hours, synchronizing signals (zeitgebers), such as light and social and physical activities, are needed to ensure correct synchronization between internal physiological processes with the external 24-hour light–dark cycle. Light has been demonstrated as the strongest entraining agent for the circadian clock (15). However, nonphotic agents such as physical activity (16) and pineal melatonin (17) have been demonstrated to affect circadian function.

In addition to timing, the circadian clock plays an important role in the regulation of sleep and wakefulness. Evidence for a circadian regulatory process

179

regulating sleep initiation and duration was first obtained in the temporal isolation studies conducted by Aschoff et al. (18). On the basis of the results of these and subsequent studies, it has been suggested that a primary role of the human circadian pacemaker is to facilitate the consolidation of sleep and wakefulness (8,14,19–21). The duration of sleep episodes and architecture, including the distribution of rapid eye movement (REM) sleep and sleep spindles, are all influenced by the circadian system (22).

AGE-RELATED CHANGES IN THE CIRCADIAN SYSTEM

Age-related physical degeneration of the SCN such as decreased cell numbers (23,24) and decreased vasopressin neuronal activity (25,26) have been shown in older adults, particularly in association with dementia. Evidence of breakdown of the central circadian oscillator itself had also been shown in animal studies. For example, old animals have a reduced temperature rhythm and fragmented activity patterns (27) that are similar to changes observed in young animals with SCN lesions. Zhang et al. (28) demonstrated a reduction in the expression of the immediate early gene c-fos in response to a light pulse in the hamster SCN. Similar experiments in rats have shown a deficit in cyclic AMP response element-binding protein phosphorylation (29) and decreased expression of Per1 and Per2, genes important for circadian clock control, following light exposure in rats (30). Two other clock-related genes, *Clock* and *Bmal1*, have also found to be altered in aged mice (31). On the basis of the results of these studies, it is feasible that neuronal breakdown associated with aging may be directly affecting the circadian clock mechanisms and contributing to sleep disturbances noted in aging.

Changes in circadian amplitude and entrainment seen in aging may also be due to a decreased responsiveness to light within the circadian system. In the retinal ganglion cells (RGCs) of the eye, melanopsin-containing photoreceptors provide the primary photic input to the circadian clock, transmitting it to the neurons of the SCN (32). Light information is then integrated with other time cues, and the resulting regulatory signals are transmitted to sleep–wake centers in the ventrolateral preoptic nucleus and lateral hypothalamic area via connections through the dorsomedial hypothalamus (for review see Ref. 33). Light transmission may be decreased in advanced age by cataracts or yellowing of the lens, which has been demonstrated to reduce blue light transmittance by as much as 80% in primates (34). Yellowing of the lens may be particularly detrimental as melanopsin-containing RGCs respond chiefly to blue wavelength light (35).

Age-related reductions in the circadian amplitude of body temperature rhythms have been observed in numerous animal studies. McDonald et al. (27) reported that the amplitude of the temperature rhythm in old rats was significantly less than that of young rats. In another study, Satinoff (36) noted, "In almost all old rats there is a clear decrease in the amplitude of the circadian temperature rhythm." In studies of aging humans, decreased amplitudes of body temperature rhythms have been noted under both entrained (37,38) and free-running (39–41) conditions.

Melatonin, a circadian-regulated and sleep-promoting hormone, has also been shown to decline with aging (42–44). Thus, it has been postulated that decreased levels of melatonin may play a role in the decline of sleep quality in older adults. Although melatonin is released from the pineal gland, its output is regulated by the SCN via a series of neuronal connections (45). The timing of melatonin release by the

SCN, paired with the strong suppressing effects of light, results in melatonin levels that are highest during the nighttime and nearly undetectable during the day (46). It is likely that melatonin acts at the level of the SCN to promote sleep. Melatonin has been shown to decrease the firing rate of SCN neurons (47). It has been proposed that by its inhibition of SCN firing, the increase of melatonin in the evening creates a sleep-permissive state. These lower evening melatonin levels in the elderly may be contributing to sleep difficulties during the night (48).

Interestingly, age-related changes are not universally seen in older adults. Other studies have failed to demonstrate a difference in the amplitude of core body temperature (49–51) or melatonin rhythms in the healthiest older adults. Zeitzer et al. (52) found no difference in the endogenous amplitude of the plasma mela-tonin rhythm between a group of young men and a cohort of healthy, drug-free men and women over 65 years of age. Another study reported that approximately 25% of the population over 65 reported no sleep complaints (53). These results suggest that factors other than chronological age, such as comorbid disorders, level of light exposure, or physical activity, are also likely to play a role in the observed circadian rhythm alterations.

One consistent finding of most circadian aging studies is a phase advance in the timing of circadian rhythms under entrained and constant conditions (40,49,54,55). Similar to the core body temperature rhythm, earlier onset of corti-sol, TSH, and melatonin rhythms have been reported in the elderly compared with young subjects (43,56,57).

Aging of the circadian system may also alter the circadian pacemaker's response to zeitgebers such as light or exercise. A study by Zee at al. (58) demon-strated that 16-month-old hamsters took longer to re-entrain to an 8-hour phase delay of the light–dark cycle than young hamsters. Van Reeth et al. (59,60) inves-tigated the effects of two nonphotic stimuli (benzodiazepines and dark pulses), known to cause phase shifts in young hamsters, on aged hamsters. Their results showed an expected increase in locomotor activity; however, no concurrent phase shifting effect was seen. Examination of glucose utilization within the SCN by Wise et al. (61 62) showed that aged rats use less glucose in response to light–dark transi-tions than younger rats.

Laboratory experiments examining phase-shifting ability in older subjects provide further support for the idea that the elderly may have greater difficulty adapting. When Monk et al. (63) induced a 6-hour phase advance or delay on 15 elderly subjects living in time isolation, they found that "circadian rectal tempera-ture rhythms confirmed that phase adjustment was slow in both directions" and that significantly more sleep and circadian rhythm disruption was present after the phase advance than after the phase delay. It was concluded that sleep disrup-tion (and daytime sleepiness) appeared to be longer lived in the elderly, showing little of the recovery over time observed in younger subjects (64). Another study looking at phase shifts in response to ocular light exposure reported that the mag-nitude of phase advances was significantly attenuated in the older group (65). However, the response of the circadian clock to moderately bright light was not significantly different between young and older subjects (66), but phase advance response was not tested in this study. Finally, Baehr et al. (67) concluded that the phase shifts in response to exercise, as measured by dim light melatonin onset (DLMO), is preserved in older adults. Altogether, it appears that the cir-cadian system of older adults retains the ability to respond to light and activity, but the level or intensity of these time givers may need to be increased in older adults.

Exposure to external cues that are known to entrain and enhance the amplitude of circadian rhythms are vital for maintaining correct alignment of the internal clock with the outside environment. In the elderly, exposure to these cues can be severely attenuated, further limiting the stability of circadian rhythms. Bright light exposure is the primary synchronizer for the circadian clock (15). However, in the elderly, overall light exposure has been found to be significantly reduced (68,69). Older adults also have more sedentary lifestyles (70), resulting in lower mean activity levels (71). Furthermore, this group are much more likely to be socially disengaged and participate in fewer social interactions (72). Both light and sociopsychological clues such as daily contact with other individuals and structured schedules of activity are thought to act as zeitgebers for the circadian system (20,73). Therefore, it is likely that both the reduction in external zeitgeber exposure and a decline in circadian clock function contribute to the common age-related circadian rhythm sleep disorders.

CIRCADIAN RHYTHM SLEEP DISORDERS IN AGING

Optimal sleep quality is achieved when the desired sleep time coincides with the timing of the endogenous circadian rhythm of sleep and wake propensity. CRSDs arise from alterations of the central circadian clock or a misalignment between the endogenous circadian timing and the external 24-hour social and physical environment. While the primary pathophysiology of CRSDs is due to a disruption of circadian timing, the actual clinical presentation of CRSD is often influenced by a combination of physiological, behavioral, and environmental factors. This section will discuss CRSDs with an emphasis on those that are prevalent in the elderly: advanced sleep phase type and irregular sleep wake type.

Diagnostic Evaluation of CRSDs

For diagnosis CRSDs, an accurate clinical history, sleep diary, and/or actigraphy for at least seven days should be obtained. Other physiological markers of the circadian phase, such as dim light melatonin onset (DLMO) and nadir core body temperature, may be used as adjunctive tools to confirm the phase or amplitude of circadian rhythms. Polysomnography is not routinely indicated; however, because of the age-related increase in the prevalence of other sleep disorders, such as sleep apnea and REM sleep behavior disorder, a careful assessment for these conditions should be performed in all patients with CRSD (74). Furthermore, psychiatric conditions, including depression and anxiety disorders, are often comorbid with CRSDs and must be considered in the evaluation and differential diagnosis.

CRSDs and Their Treatments

Advanced Sleep Phase Type (Also Known as Advanced Sleep Phase Syndrome and Advanced Sleep Phase Disorder)

Clinical Presentation

The defining characteristics of the advanced sleep phase type (ASPT) are earlier than desired or conventional sleep and wake times (Fig. 1). Sleep times of 6:00 to 9:00 PM, coupled with wake times between 2:00 AM to 5 AM occur, even if the patient attempts to delay his or her sleep times, resulting in excessive sleepiness and sleep

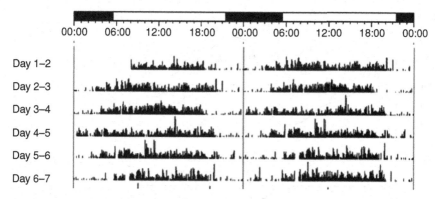

FIGURE 1 Actigraphy record of a patient exhibiting advanced sleep–wake disorder. Data are double plotted with clock time indicated across the top and the height of the black bars corresponding to activity level.

maintenance insomnia (75,76). Sleep is otherwise normal when subjects are permitted to sleep on their typical sleep–wake schedule. Diagnostic criteria require verification of the advanced sleep–wake phase through the use of at least 1 week of actigraphy or sleep log. Additionally, the sleep disturbance should not be better explained by other sleep, medical, mental, or substance use disorders or medication use (74). As to be expected, an earlier onset of melatonin and core body temperature minimum are seen, which can be used to confirm the diagnosis (77). It is, however, important to note that not all individuals with an advanced sleep phase have ASPT. In fact, many older people are not particularly bothered by their sleep phase and have no consequent impairment in functioning characteristic of the CRSDs. As such, these individuals can be considered "morning types" or "larks" rather than ASPT patients.

Epidemiology
The prevalence of ASPT in the general population is not well defined. In middle- to old-aged adults, a prevalence of 1% to 7% has been estimated (78,79). Within the general population, ASPT may be much less common, with only a few cases of non-age-related ASPT (80–82) Thus, the prevalence of ASPT increases with advancing age.

Pathophysiology
The pathogenesis of ASPT is likely to reflect a combination of behavioral and genetic factors. For example, early sleep times and opthalmological conditions such as cataracts may decrease light exposure at a time that would delay their sleep phase, perpetuating the advanced sleep phase. Intrinsic factors, such as a shortened endogenous circadian period (<24 hours) (80) or alterations in the relationship of circadian timing and sleep homeostatic regulation (83), have been suggested to play a role in the development of ASPT. Furthermore, familial forms of ASPT have been reported in which the phenotype segregates with an autosomal dominant mode of inheritance (80,82,84) and mutations in the circadian clock *hPer2* and CK1 delta genes have been identified and linked to familial ASPT (85,86). Therefore, decreased

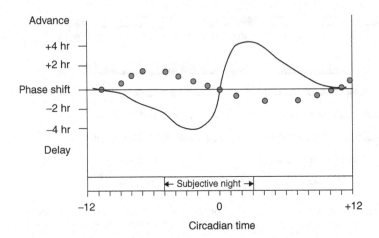

FIGURE 2 Phase response curves to both light (black line) and melatonin (gray dots) plotted on a representative time scale. Circadian time 0 corresponds to the normal time of body temperature nadir.

exposure or weakened responses to entrainment agents such as light and physical activity, together with intrinsic changes in circadian and sleep regulation, may contribute to the development of ASPT in older adults (87,88).

Treatment
The major goal of treatment of ASPT is to delay the timing of sleep and wake. Although chronotherapy has been shown in small studies to be effective, its use may be limited in clinical practice. Therefore, use of evening light within the phase delay portion of the light phase response curve (PRC) (Fig. 2) represents an effective therapeutic approach. In addition to light, sleep hygiene and other behavioral adjustments are central to the effective treatment of the disorder.

Light
Bright light therapy used in the delay portion (i.e., the evening, between 7 PM and 9 PM or before CT 0 in Fig. 2) of the light PRC may help normalize circadian rhythms in patients with ASPT. Successful phase delay with the use of evening light therapy has been reported in several studies, and light in these patients may additionally improve sleep efficiency and total sleep time (89,90). In older adults, tolerance of bright light may be problematic, and close follow-up is advised. Unfortunately, light at lower intensities may not be effective in delaying sleep phase (69). Additionally, relative to their younger counterparts, older subjects appear to have a reduced response to the generally superior phase-shifting properties of short-wavelength light, raising the question of the usefulness of light within this spectrum in the treatment of older subjects with ASPT (91). Light boxes can be expensive, with usual costs of at least $200 and many models being considerably more expensive. If light therapy is to be used for a finite period of time, rental units are available. Ultraviolet rays are filtered by light boxes, and they are typically thought of as safe. However, side effects of hypomania, mild headache, nausea and vomiting, and self-limited visual problems have all been reported (92). Patients with ophthalmological disease

should be evaluated by an ophthalmologist before beginning light therapy in order to determine appropriateness for therapy. Additional caution is advised in subjects with preexisting mania, retinal photosensitivity, and migraine. In sum, although the exact length of treatment and dosing needed have yet to be clearly established, light therapy represents a potentially important instrument in the manipulation of circadian phase. The American Academy of Sleep Medicine also has confirmed the potential usefulness of light therapy on the basis of current level II and level III evidence (93).

Melatonin

Melatonin delivered in the morning should result in a delay in sleep phase based on the melatonin PRC (17), so theoretically it could be a useful. However, data supporting the efficacy of melatonin in ASPT are lacking. Additionally, melatonin may contain soporific effects, which may result in residual morning sleepiness.

Other therapeutic approaches

Chronotherapy has also been used successfully in ASPT when sleep times are advanced by 3 hours every 2 days until the desired sleep–wake time has been achieved. However, the need for rigorous compliance, the length of the treatment, and the necessity for close follow-up again limit its overall clinical practicality. As mentioned earlier, behavioral strategies, such as bed time restriction, good sleep hygiene practices, and increased exposure to bright light, and social and physical activities during the day are important considerations in the treatment of ASPT.

Delayed Sleep Phase Type (Also Known as Delayed Sleep Phase Syndrome and Delayed Sleep Phase Disorder)

Clinical Presentation

In contrast to ASPT, delayed sleep phase type (DSPT) is characterized by sleep and wake times that are 3 to 6 hours later than desired (94). DSPT patients typically report difficulty falling asleep before 2 AM and prefer wake times between 10 AM and 1 PM. Adherence to socially enforced sleep–wake times results in classical symptoms of chronic sleep-onset insomnia and difficulty waking up in the morning for work, school, or social obligations (95). DSPT patients rate as "evening types" when classified using the Horne–Ostberg questionnaire (96) and demonstrate preferences for being more alert during late evening hours. The occurrence of DSPT in the general population is between 0.13% and 0.17% (97), with a more common prevalence (7–16%) in adolescents (94). Although DSPT can occur in older individuals, it is most common among younger adults and adolescents. Therefore, the discussion of this disorder in this chapter will be limited.

As with ASPT, the exact pathophysiological mechanisms of DSPT remain incompletely understood and are likely due to both internal (circadian) and external factors. A genetic basis for DSPT is supported by a report of one large family in which the DSPT phenotype was shown to segregate as an autosomal dominant trait (98), and recent evidence of polymorphisms in the circadian rhythm genes, such as *hPer3*, arylalkylamine *N*-acetyltransferase, HLA, and *Clock*, in individuals with DSPT (99–101).

Treatment

Approaches to the treatment of DSPT are directed at advancing the circadian phase to a more conventional time. Circadian-based therapeutic options include timed exposure to morning light and evening administration of melatonin (6). In addition, as with ASPT, sleep hygiene and other behavioral approaches are essential for the successful management of DSPT.

Light

The ability of light to advance the timing of circadian rhythms is now well established (65,102,103). In clinical practice, light is typically delivered through the use of a light box using 2,000 to 10,000 lux light in the morning (93). Perhaps, just as important as light therapy, the avoidance of bright light in the evening, either through behavioral strategies or through the use of dark glasses, should also be recommended. Both for convenience and in order to avoid the phase delay portion of the PRC (Fig. 2), light should be delivered upon habitual wake time for 1 to 3 hours (104,105).

Melatonin

Exogenous melatonin has also been used for the treatment of DSPT. Although the optimal dosing and timing have yet to be established, doses between 0.3 and 3 mg when given at 5 to 7 hours before habitual bed time have been used in several studies (106,107). Melatonin may represent a useful adjunct to light therapy as the combination of the treatments appears to be more effective relative to light therapy used in isolation (6). It is important to note that melatonin is not approved for the treatment of DSPT or other circadian rhythm sleep disorders by the U. S. Food and Drug Administration, and the treatment thus represents "off label" use. From a safety standpoint, melatonin may have vasoconstrictive properties and should be prescribed with caution in those with cardiovascular disease (108). It may also interact with medications such as some anticonsulvants and warfarin (109).

Other therapeutic approaches

Chronotherapy involves a progressive further delay of bed and wake times until the desired sleep–wake times are reached. A patient is instructed to delay his or her sleep and wake times by 3 hours every 2 days. The length of time required for successful treatment and the need for rigid compliance may preclude the use of this treatment modality in subjects who have occupational or social demands.

Behavioral strategies are also important components of the overall treatment approach. The maintenance of a regular sleep wake schedule and good sleep hygiene are critical. Even in the absence of formal phototherapy, subjects should be advised to avoid bright light in the evening and to maximize exposure to light in the morning upon awakening.

Free-Running Type (Also Known as Nonentrained Type)

Clinical Presentation

The free-running type is characterized by sleep and wake times that are not stably entrained to the 24-hour day. As the circadian period is generally longer than 24 hours, patients with free-running type experience progressive delay of their sleep and wake times. The sleep and wake times may, for a brief time, be aligned with that of the 24-hour light–dark cycle, before inevitably delaying further. Therefore, a key feature of the disorder is symptoms of excessive daytime sleepiness, insomnia, and daytime impairment, which wax and wane as a patient's sleep–wake schedule moves in and out of phase with the physically and socially desired sleep–wake schedule.

Free-running type is common in totally blind individuals. It has been estimated that about 50% of totally blind people have nonentrained circadian rhythms (110). Although rare, nonentrained sleep and wake patterns have also been reported in sighted individuals (111). Decrease or lack of photic reception is the most likely cause of nonentrained circadian rhythms in blind people. In sighted individuals, it has been suggested that an underlying cause may be an unusually long endogenous circadian period beyond entrainment to a 24-hour day (112). In older adults, reduced exposure to bright light, social and physical activities, and a weakened circadian system are also likely causes for this condition.

Treatment
In blind people, the use of light in the treatment of the disorder is generally not feasible, and as such, alternative means of entrainment must be sought. This is typically accomplished with the use of exogenous melatonin. A starting dose of 10 mg administered 1 hour before desired bedtime, followed by maintenance of just 0.5 mg, has been shown to be effective (113–115). Additionally, the concurrent use of behavioral entraining agents including structured and timed social and physical activities is also important. In sighted individuals, increased exposure to bright light during the day (particularly in the morning) and enforcement of regularly timed physical and social activities is usually recommended (88). Regular melatonin administration can also be used to maintain a 24-hour schedule in sighted individuals (116).

Other therapeutic approaches
The establishment of regular exercise and social cues, as well as proper sleep hygiene, is an important step in effective treatment of the disorder. Another pharmacological option that has been reported in the literature is vitamin B12. When given both with and without a concurrent hypnotic, vitamin B12 has been reported effective in non-24-hour sleep–wake cycles (117,118).

Irregular Sleep–Wake Type (Also Known as Irregular Sleep Wake Rhythm)
Clinical Features
Irregular sleep–wake type is characterized by the lack of a clearly identifiable circadian pattern of consolidated sleep and wake times. Although the total amount of sleep obtained over a 24-hour period is generally normal, sleep is broken into at least three different variable sleep periods (Fig. 3). Daytime is often composed of erratic napping, whereas nighttime sleep is severely fragmented and shortened. Consequent symptoms of chronic insomnia and/or daytime sleepiness ensue. The ICSD-2 also requires the exclusion of other disorders, which may better explain the patient's irregular sleep, as well as at least 1 week of actigraphy or the use of a sleep log demonstrating three or more sleep bouts within the 24-hour day (74).

Epidemiology
The disorder is most commonly in seen patients with dementia, particularly those who are institutionalized, but other disorders of the central nervous system,

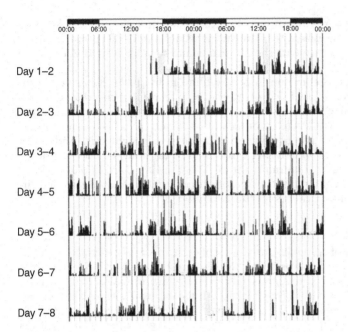

FIGURE 3 Actigraphy record of a patient exhibiting irregular sleep–wake rhythm. Data are double plotted with clock time indicated across the top and the height of the black bars corresponding to activity level.

including traumatic brain injury and mental retardation, can also lead to an irregular sleep–wake pattern (119–122).

Pathophysiology

It has been suggested that both dysfunction of the central processes responsible for the generation of the circadian rhythm and decreased exposure to external synchronizing agents such as light and social activities play a role in the development and maintenance of the irregular sleep–wake rhythm. The pathogenesis of the disease may be related to a loss of neurons or other deleterious changes within the SCN (23). A few studies have demonstrated a decrease in the number of neurons present within the SCN in patients with Alzheimer's disease (123,124). Older people in long-term care facilities often lack exposure to appropriate light or daytime activities, which may further contribute to a decrease in the amplitude of circadian rhythms. In fact, lower daytime light levels are associated with an increase in nighttime awakenings, even after controlling for the level of dementia (125).

Treatment

The primary goal of treatment of an irregular sleep–wake rhythm is to consolidate the sleep–wake cycle. To this end, measures aimed at restoring or enhancing exposure to the various zeitgebers are critical. Patients should be exposed to bright light during the day, and bright light should be avoided in the evening (126,127). Daytime physical and social activities should also be strongly encouraged (88,128–130).

A multicomponent approach using a variety of behavioral treatment options is recommended.

Light
The overall approach to light therapy for the treatment of the irregular sleep–wake type is to increase both the duration and intensity of light exposure throughout the daytime and avoid exposure to bright light in the evening. Bright light exposure delivered for 2 hours in the morning at 3000 to 5000 lux over the course of 4 weeks has been found to decrease daytime napping and increase nighttime sleep in demented subjects (131). Light may further help consolidate nighttime sleep, decrease agitated behavior, and result in stronger amplitudes of the circadian rhythm (126,127,131).

Melatonin
When compared with the effects of bright light, studies evaluating the use of melatonin in irregular sleep–wake type have yielded inconsistent results. One large scale trial of 157 patients with Alzheimer's disease found no statistically significant differences in actigraphy-derived sleep measures between a control group and those taking 2.5 mg melatonin (132), although a trend toward improvement was seen with a 10 mg dose of melatonin. Overall, the efficacy of melatonin treatment for circadian and sleep disorders remains undetermined (for review see Ref. 133). However, melatonin has been suggested to be effective in patients with known melatonin deficiency (42).

Other therapeutic approaches
Structured physical activity and social activity may help provide temporal cues to increase the regularity of the sleep–wake schedule. Allowing for a favorable sleep environment by reducing nighttime light and noise and improving incontinence care can reduce awakenings in nursing home residents (134). Furthermore, Alessi et al. (135) documented that elderly subjects reported decreased daytime sleep and increased participation in social and physical activities and social conversation by following a routine of reduced time in bed during the day, structured bedtime routine at night, 30 minutes or more of sunlight exposure a day, and increased physical activity. The use of a multidimensional, nonpharmacological approach including an increase in sunlight exposure and social activity during the day and a decrease in daytime in-bed time and nighttime noise may be particularly effective.

SUMMARY
Sleep disturbances, specifically early-morning awakenings, insomnia, and increased daytime napping, show higher prevalence with advanced age. Age-related circadian changes are seen at all levels, from molecular and cellular within the SCN to physiological, hormonal, and behavioral outputs of the circadian clock. Recent advances in our understanding of the molecular and cellular basis of some of advanced sleep phase and delayed sleep phase disorders should lead to improved and targeted behavioral and pharmacological therapies. It is being increasingly recognized that in addition to these age-related changes in circadian biology, health status, medications, social structure, and physical environment also play important roles in the development of circadian-based sleep disturbances.

Therefore, behavioral and environmental modifications during early and midlife may be key to the prevention of CRSDs in late life.

REFERENCES

1. Foley D, Ancoli-Israel S, Britz P, et al. Sleep disturbances and chronic disease in older adults: results of the 2003 National Sleep Foundation Sleep in America Survey. J Psychosom Res 2004; 56(5):497–502.
2. Dement WC, Miles LE, Carskadon MA. "White paper" on sleep and aging. J Am Geriatr Soc 1982; 30(1):25–50.
3. Mellinger GD, Balter MB, Uhlenhuth EH. Insomnia and its treatment. Prevalence and correlates. Arch Gen Psychiatry 1985; 42(3):225–232.
4. Middelkoop HA, Smilde-van den Doel DA, Neven AK, et al. Subjective sleep characteristics of 1,485 males and females aged 50–93: effects of sex and age, and factors related to self-evaluated quality of sleep. J Gerontol A Biol Sci Med Sci 1996; 51(3):M108–M115.
5. Prinz PN. Sleep and sleep disorders in older adults. J Clin Neurophysiol 1995; 12(2):139–146.
6. Reid KJ, Chang AM, Zee PC. Circadian rhythm sleep disorders. Med Clin North Am 2004; 88(3):631–651, viii.
7. Borbely AA. Sleep: circadian rhythm vs. recovery process. In: Koukkou M, Loehmann D, Angst J, eds. Functional States of the Brain: Their Determinants. Amsterdam: Elsevier/North Holland; 1980:151–161.
8. Dijk DJ, Czeisler CA. Paradoxical timing of the circadian rhythm of sleep propensity serves to consolidate sleep and wakefulness in humans. Neurosci Lett 1994; 166(1):63–68.
9. Daan S, Beersma DG, Borbely AA. Timing of human sleep: recovery process gated by a circadian pacemaker. Am J Physiol 1984; 246(2 pt 2):R161–R183.
10. Kronauer RE, Czeisler CA, Pilato SF, et al. Mathematical model of the human circadian system with two interacting oscillators. The American journal of physiology 1982; 242(1):R3–R17.
11. Moore RY, Eichler VB. Loss of a circadian adrenal corticosterone rhythm following suprachiasmatic lesions in the rat. Brain Res 1972; 42(1):201–206.
12. Pittendrigh CS. Circadian oscillations in cells and the circadian organization of multicellular systems. In: Schmitt FC, Worden FG, eds. The Neurosciences Third Study Program. Cambridge: MIT press; 1974:437–458.
13. Mouret J, Coindet J, Debilly G, et al. Suprachiasmatic nuclei lesions in the rat: alterations in sleep circadian rhythms. Electroencephalogr Clin Neurophysiol 1978; 45(3):402–408.
14. Czeisler CA, Duffy JF, Shanahan TL, et al. Stability, precision, and near-24-hour period of the human circadian pacemaker. Science 1999; 284(5423):2177–2181.
15. Czeisler CA, Allan JS, Strogatz SH, et al. Bright light resets the human circadian pacemaker independent of the timing of the sleep-wake cycle. Science 1986; 233(4764):667–671.
16. Buxton OM, Lee CW, L'Hermite-Baleriaux M, Turek FW, Van Cauter E. Exercise elicits phase shifts and acute alterations of melatonin that vary with circadian phase. Am J Physiol Regul Integr Comp Physiol 2003; 284(3):R714–R724.
17. Lewy AJ, Ahmed S, Jackson JM, et al. Melatonin shifts human circadian rhythms according to a phase-response curve. Chronobiol Int 1992; 9(5):380–392.
18. Aschoff J. Circadian rhythms in man. Science 1965; 148:1427–1432.
19. Akerstedt T, Gillberg M. The circadian variation of experimentally displaced sleep. Sleep 1981; 4(2):159–169.
20. Wever RA. Influence of physical workload on freerunning circadian rhythms of man. Pflugers Archiv: European journal of physiology 1979; 381(2):119–126.
21. Zulley J, Wever R, Aschoff J. The dependence of onset and duration of sleep on the circadian rhythm of rectal temperature. Pflugers Archiv 1981; 391(4):314–318.

22. Czeisler CA, Weitzman E, Moore-Ede MC, Zimmerman JC, Knauer RS. Human sleep: its duration and organization depend on its circadian phase. Science 1980; 210(4475):1264–1267.
23. Swaab DF, Fliers E, Partiman TS. The suprachiasmatic nucleus of the human brain in relation to sex, age and senile dementia. Brain Res 1985; 342(1):37–44.
24. Swaab DF, Van Someren EJ, Zhou JN, Hofman MA. Biological rhythms in the human life cycle and their relationship to functional changes in the suprachiasmatic nucleus. Prog Brain Res 1996; 111:349–368.
25. Hofman MA. The human circadian clock and aging. Chronobiol Int 2000; 17(3):245–259.
26. Hofman MA, Swaab DF. Alterations in circadian rhythmicity of the vasopressin-producing neurons of the human suprachiasmatic nucleus (SCN) with aging. Brain Res 1994; 651(1–2):134–142.
27. McDonald RB, Hoban-Higgins TM, Ruhe RC, et al. Alterations in endogenous circadian rhythm of core temperature in senescent Fischer 344 rats. Am J Physiol 1999; 276(3 pt 2):R824–R830.
28. Zhang Y, Kornhauser JM, Zee PC, et al. Effects of aging on light-induced phase-shifting of circadian behavioral rhythms, fos expression and CREB phosphorylation in the hamster suprachiasmatic nucleus. Neuroscience 1996; 70(4):951–961.
29. Sutin EL, Dement WC, Heller HC, et al. Light-induced gene expression in the suprachiasmatic nucleus of young and aging rats. Neurobiol Aging 1993; 14(5):441–446.
30. Asai M, Yoshinobu Y, Kaneko S, et al. Circadian profile of Per gene mRNA expression in the suprachiasmatic nucleus, paraventricular nucleus, and pineal body of aged rats. J Neurosci Res 2001; 66(6):1133–1139.
31. Kolker DE, Fukuyama H, Huang DS, et al. Aging alters circadian and light-induced expression of clock genes in golden hamsters. J Biol Rhythms 2003; 18(2):159–169.
32. Rollag MD, Berson DM, Provencio I. Melanopsin, ganglion-cell photoreceptors, and mammalian photoentrainment. J Biol Rhythms 2003; 18(3):227–234.
33. Saper CB, Scammell TE, Lu J. Hypothalamic regulation of sleep and circadian rhythms. Nature 2005; 437(7063):1257–1263.
34. Dillon J, Zheng L, Merriam JC, et al. Transmission of light to the aging human retina: possible implications for age related macular degeneration. Exp Eye Res 2004; 79(6):753–759.
35. Hattar S, Liao HW, Takao M, et al. Melanopsin-containing retinal ganglion cells: architecture, projections, and intrinsic photosensitivity. Science 2002; 295(5557):1065–1070.
36. Satinoff E. Patterns of circadian body temperature rhythms in aged rats. Clin Exp Pharmacol Physiol 1998; 25(2):135–140.
37. Touitou Y, Reinberg A, Bogdan A, et al. Age-related changes in both circadian and seasonal rhythms of rectal temperature with special reference to senile dementia of Alzheimer type. Gerontology 1986; 32(2):110–118.
38. Richardson GS, Carskadon MA, Orav EJ, et al. Circadian variation of sleep tendency in elderly and young adult subjects. Sleep 1982; 5:S82–S94.
39. Weitzman ED, Moline ML, Czeisler CA, et al. Chronobiology of aging: temperature, sleep-wake rhythms and entrainment. Neurobiol Aging 1982; 3(4):299–309.
40. Czeisler CA, Dumont M, Duffy JF, et al. Association of sleep-wake habits in older people with changes in output of circadian pacemaker. Lancet 1992; 340(8825):933–936.
41. Vitiello MV, Smallwood RG, Avery DH, et al. Circadian temperature rhythms in young adult and aged men. Neurobiol Aging 1986; 7(2):97–100.
42. Pandi-Perumal SR, Zisapel N, Srinivasan V, et al. Melatonin and sleep in aging population. Exp Gerontol 2005; 40(12):911–925.
43. van Coevorden A, Mockel J, Laurent E, et al. Neuroendocrine rhythms and sleep in aging men. Am J Physiol 1991; 260(4 pt 1):E651–E661.
44. Skene DJ, Swaab DF. Melatonin rhythmicity: effect of age and Alzheimer's disease. Exp Gerontol 2003; 38(1–2):199–206.
45. Murphy PJ, Campbell SS. Physiology of the circadian system in animals and humans. J Clin Neurophysiol 1996; 13(1):2–16.

46. Dijk DJ, Beersma DG, Daan S, et al. Bright morning light advances the human circadian system without affecting NREM sleep homeostasis. Am J Physiol 1989; 256(1 pt 2):R106–R111.

47. Liu C, Weaver DR, Jin X, et al. Molecular dissection of two distinct actions of melatonin on the suprachiasmatic circadian clock. Neuron 1997; 19(1):91–102.

48. Richardson GS. Circadian Rhythms and Aging. In: Schneider EL, Rowe JW, eds. Handbook of the Biology of Aging. San Diego: Academic Press; 1990.

49. Monk TH, Buysse DJ, Reynolds CF III, et al. Circadian temperature rhythms of older people. Exp Gerontol 1995; 30(5):455–474.

50. Monk TH, Buysse DJ, Reynolds CF, et al. Rhythmic vs homeostatic influences on mood, activation, and performance in young and old men. Journal of Gerontology 1992; 47(4):P221–P227.

51. Buysse DJ, Monk TH, Reynolds CF III,et al. Patterns of sleep episodes in young and elderly adults during a 36-hour constant routine. Sleep 1993; 16(7):632–637.

52. Zeitzer JM, Daniels JE, Duffy JF, et al. Do plasma melatonin concentrations decline with age? Am J Med 1999; 107(5):432–436.

53. Maggi S, Langlois JA, Minicuci N, et al. Sleep complaints in community-dwelling older persons: prevalence, associated factors, and reported causes. J Am Geriatr Soc 1998; 46(2):161–168.

54. Dijk DJ, Duffy JF, Riel E, et al. Ageing and the circadian and homeostatic regulation of human sleep during forced desynchrony of rest, melatonin and temperature rhythms. The Journal of physiology 1999; 516:611–627.

55. Duffy JF, Dijk DJ, Hall EF, et al. Relationship of endogenous circadian melatonin and temperature rhythms to self-reported preference for morning or evening activity in young and older people. J Investig Med 1999; 47(3):141–150.

56. Van Cauter E, Leproult R, Kupfer DJ. Effects of gender and age on the levels and circadian rhythmicity of plasma cortisol. J Clin Endocrinol Metab 1996; 81(7):2468–2473.

57. Van Cauter E, Leproult R, Plat L. Age-related changes in slow wave sleep and REM sleep and relationship with growth hormone and cortisol levels in healthy men. JAMA 2000; 284(7):861–868.

58. Zee PC, Rosenberg RS, Turek FW. Effects of aging on entrainment and rate of resynchronization of circadian locomotor activity. Am J Physiol 1992; 263(5 pt 2):R1099–R1103.

59. Van Reeth O, Zhang Y, Reddy A, et al. Aging alters the entraining effects of an activity-inducing stimulus on the circadian clock. Brain Res 1993; 607(1–2):286–292.

60. Van Reeth O, Zhang Y, Zee PC, et al. Aging alters feedback effects of the activity-rest cycle on the circadian clock. Am J Physiol 1992; 263(4 pt 2):R981–R986.

61. Wise PM, Cohen IR, Weiland NG, et al. Aging alters the circadian rhythm of glucose utilization in the suprachiasmatic nucleus. Proc Natl Acad Sci U S A 1988; 85(14):5305–5309.

62. Wise PM, Walovitch RC, Cohen IR, et al. Diurnal rhythmicity and hypothalamic deficits in glucose utilization in aged ovariectomized rats. J Neurosci 1987; 7(11):3469–3473.

63. Monk TH, Buysse DJ, Carrier J, et al. Inducing jet-lag in older people: directional asymmetry. J Sleep Res 2000; 9(2):101–116.

64. Monk TH, Buysse DJ, Reynolds CF III,et al. Inducing jet lag in older people: adjusting to a 6-hour phase advance in routine. Exp Gerontol 1993; 28(2):119–133.

65. Klerman EB, Duffy JF, Dijk DJ, et al. Circadian phase resetting in older people by ocular bright light exposure. J Investig Med 2001; 49(1):30–40.

66. Benloucif S, Green K, L'Hermite-Baleriaux M, et al. Responsiveness of the aging circadian clock to light. Neurobiol Aging 2005. In press.

67. Baehr EK, Eastman CI, Revelle W, et al. Circadian phase-shifting effects of nocturnal exercise in older compared with young adults. Am J Physiol Regul Integr Comp Physiol 2003; 284(6):R1542–1550.

68. Campbell SS, Kripke DF, Gillin JC, et al. Exposure to light in healthy elderly subjects and Alzheimer's patients. Physiol Behav 1988; 42(2):141–144.

69. Shochat T, Martin J, Marler M, et al. Illumination levels in nursing home patients: effects on sleep and activity rhythms. J Sleep Res 2000; 9(4):373–379.

70. Bortz WM, 2nd. Disuse and aging. JAMA 1982; 248(10):1203–1208.
71. Harper DG, Volicer L, Stopa EG, et al. Disturbance of endogenous circadian rhythm in aging and Alzheimer disease. Am J Geriatr Psychiatry 2005; 13(5):359–368.
72. Bassuk SS, Glass TA, Berkman LF. Social disengagement and incident cognitive decline in community-dwelling elderly persons. Ann Intern Med 1999; 131(3):165–173.
73. Aschoff J, Fatranska M, Giedke H, et al. Human circadian rhythms in continuous darkness: Entrainment by social cues. Science 1971; 171:213–215.
74. Diagnostic Classification Steering Committee. International Classification of Sleep Disorders: Diagnostic and Coding Manual. Rev. ed. Rochester, MN: American Sleep Disorders Association; 2001.
75. Kamei Y, Urata J, Uchiyaya M, et al. Clinical characteristics of circadian rhythm sleep disorders. Psychiatry Clin Neurosci 1998; 52(2):234–235.
76. Ondze B, Espa F, Ming LC, et al. [Advanced sleep phase syndrome]. Rev Neurol (Paris) 2001; 157(11 pt 2):S130–134.
77. Reid KJ, Chang AM, Turek FW, et al. Identification and characterization of familial advanced sleep phase. Sleep Research Online 1999; 2(suppl 1):424.
78. Ando K, Kripke DF, Ancoli-Israel S. Estimated prevalence of delayed and advanced sleep phase syndromes. Sleep Res 1995; 24:509.
79. Ando K, Kripke DF, Ancoli-Israel S. Delayed and advanced sleep phase symptoms. Isr J Psychiatry Relat Sci 2002; 39(1):11–18.
80. Jones CR, Campbell SS, Zone SE, et al. Familial advanced sleep-phase syndrome: A short-period circadian rhythm variant in humans. Nat Med 1999; 5(9):1062–1065.
81. Moldofsky H, Musisi S, Phillipson EA. Treatment of a case of advanced sleep phase syndrome by phase advance chronotherapy. Sleep 1986; 9(1):61–65.
82. Reid KJ, Chang AM, Dubocovich ML, et al. Familial advanced sleep phase syndrome. Arch Neurol 2001; 58(7):1089–1094.
83. Duffy JF, Czeisler CA. Age-related change in the relationship between circadian period, circadian phase, and diurnal preference in humans. Neurosci Lett 2002; 318(3):117–120.
84. Satoh K, Mishima K, Inoue Y, et al. Two pedigrees of familial advanced sleep phase syndrome in Japan. Sleep 2003; 26(4):416–417.
85. Toh KL, Jones CR, He Y, et al. An hPer2 phosphorylation site mutation in familial advanced sleep phase syndrome. Science 2001; 291(5506):1040–1043.
86. Xu Y, Padiath QS, Shapiro RE, et al. Functional consequences of a CKIdelta mutation causing familial advanced sleep phase syndrome. Nature 2005; 434(7033):640–644.
87. Ancoli-Israel S, Kripke DF. Prevalent sleep problems in the aged. Biofeedback and self-regulation 1991; 16(4):349–359.
88. Naylor E, Penev PD, Orbeta L, et al. Daily social and physical activity increases slow-wave sleep and daytime neuropsychological performance in the elderly. Sleep 2000; 23(1):87–95.
89. Campbell SS, Dawson D, Anderson MW. Alleviation of sleep maintenance insomnia with timed exposure to bright light. J Am Geriatr Soc 1993; 41(8):829–836.
90. Lack L, Wright H, Kemp K, et al. The treatment of early-morning awakening insomnia with 2 evenings of bright light. Sleep 2005; 28(5):616–623.
91. Herljevic M, Middleton B, Thapan K, et al. Light-induced melatonin suppression: age-related reduction in response to short wavelength light. Exp Gerontol 2005; 40(3):237–242.
92. Terman M, Terman JS. Bright light therapy: side effects and benefits across the symptom spectrum. J Clin Psychiatry 1999; 60(11):799–808; quiz 9.
93. Chesson AL, Jr., Littner M, Davila D, et al. Practice parameters for the use of light therapy in the treatment of sleep disorders. Standards of Practice Committee, American Academy of Sleep Medicine. Sleep 1999; 22(5):641–660.
94. Weitzman ED, Czeisler CA, Coleman RM, et al. Delayed sleep phase syndrome. A chronobiological disorder with sleep-onset insomnia. Arch Gen Psychiatry 1981; 38(7):737–746.
95. Regestein QR, Monk TH. Delayed sleep phase syndrome: a review of its clinical aspects. Am J Psychiatry 1995; 152(4):602–608.

96. Horne JA, Ostberg O.A self-assessment questionnaire to determine morningness-eveningness in human circadian rhythms. International Journal of Chronobiology 1976; 4(2):97–110.

97. Schrader H, Bovim G, Sand T. The prevalence of delayed and advanced sleep phase syndromes. J Sleep Res 1993; 2(1):51–55.

98. Ancoli-Israel S, Schnierow B, Kelsoe J, et al. A pedigree of one family with delayed sleep phase syndrome. Chronobiol Int 2001; 18(5):831–840.

99. Archer SN, Robilliard DL, Skene DJ, et al. A length polymorphism in the circadian clock gene Per3 is linked to delayed sleep phase syndrome and extreme diurnal preference. Sleep 2003; 26(4):413–415.

100. Ebisawa T, Uchiyama M, Kajimura N, et al. Association of structural polymorphisms in the human period3 gene with delayed sleep phase syndrome. EMBO Rep 2001; 2(4):342–346.

101. Iwase T, Kajimura N, Uchiyama M, et al. Mutation screening of the human Clock gene in circadian rhythm sleep disorders. Psychiatry Res 2002; 109(2):121–128.

102. Van Cauter E, Sturis J, Byrne MM, et al. Demonstration of rapid light-induced advances and delays of the human circadian clock using hormonal phase markers. Am J Physiol 1994; 266(6 pt 1):E953–E963.

103. Czeisler CA, Kronauer RE, Allan JS, et al. Bright light induction of strong (type 0) resetting of the human circadian pacemaker. Science 1989; 244(4910):1328–1333.

104. Boivin DB, James FO. Circadian adaptation to night-shift work by judicious light and darkness exposure.J Biol Rhythms 2002; 17(6):556–567.

105. Reid KJ, Burgess HJ. Circadian rhythm sleep disorders. Prim Care 2005; 32(2):449–473.

106. Kamei Y, Hayakawa T, Urata J, et al. Melatonin treatment for circadian rhythm sleep disorders. Psychiatry Clin Neurosci 2000; 54(3):381–382.

107. Mundey K, Benloucif S, Harsanyi K, et al. Phase-dependent treatment of delayed sleep phase syndrome with melatonin. Sleep 2005; 28(10):1271–1278.

108. Cavallo AO, Zee PC. Melatonin: Prototype monograph summary. In: Schneeman B, ed. Dietary Supplements: A Framework for Evaluating Safety. Washington, DC: The National Academies Press; 2005:367–371.

109. Herxheimer A, Waterhouse J. The prevention and treatment of jet lag.Br Med J 2003; 326(7384):296–297.

110. Sack RL, Lewy AJ, Blood ML, et al. Circadian rhythm abnormalities in totally blind people: incidence and clinical significance.J Clin Endocrinol Metab 1992; 75(1):127–134.

111. McArthur AJ, Lewy AJ, Sack RL. Non-24-hour sleep-wake syndrome in a sighted man: circadian rhythm studies and efficacy of melatonin treatment. Sleep 1996; 19(7):544–553.

112. Uchiyama M, Okawa M, Ozaki S, et al. Delayed phase jumps of sleep onset in a patient with non-24-hour sleep-wake syndrome. Sleep 1996; 19(8):637–640.

113. Hack LM, Lockley SW, Arendt J, et al. The effects of low-dose 0.5-mg melatonin on the free-running circadian rhythms of blind subjects. J Biol Rhythms 2003; 18(5):420–429.

114. Lewy AJ, Bauer VK, Hasler BP, et al. Capturing the circadian rhythms of free-running blind people with 0.5 mg melatonin. Brain Res 2001; 918(1–2):96–100.

115. Sack RL, Brandes RW, Kendall AR, et al. Entrainment of free-running circadian rhythms by melatonin in blind people. N Engl J Med 2000; 343(15):1070–1077.

116. Lewy AJ, Emens JS, Bernert RA, et al. Eventual entrainment of the human circadian pacemaker by melatonin is independent of the circadian phase of treatment initiation: clinical implications.J Biol Rhythms 2004; 19(1):68–75.

117. Kamgar-Parsi B, Wehr TA, Gillin JC. Successful treatment of human non-24-hour sleep-wake syndrome. Sleep 1983; 6(3):257–264.

118. Okawa M, Mishima K, Hishikawa Y. Vitamin B12 treatment for sleep-wake rhythm disorders. The Japanese journal of psychiatry and neurology 1991; 45(1):165–166.

119. Hoogendijk WJ, van Someren EJ, Mirmiran M, et al. Circadian rhythm-related behavioral disturbances and structural hypothalamic changes in Alzheimer's disease. Int Psychogeriatr 1996; 8(suppl 3):245–252; discussion 69–72.

120. Wagner DR. Disorders of the circadian sleep-wake cycle. Neurol Clin 1996; 14(3):651–670.

121. Wagner DR. Circadian rhythm sleep disorders. Curr Treat Options Neurol 1999; 1(4):299–308.
122. Witting W, Kwa IH, Eikelenboom P, et al. Alterations in the circadian rest-activity rhythm in aging and Alzheimer's disease. Biol Psychiatry 1990; 27(6):563–572.
123. Swaab DF. Ageing of the human hypothalamus. Horm Res 1995; 43(1–3):8–11.
124. Zhou JN, Hofman MA, Swaab DF. VIP neurons in the human SCN in relation to sex, age, and Alzheimer's disease. Neurobiol Aging 1995; 16(4):571–576.
125. Ancoli-Israel S, Klauber MR, Jones DW, et al. Variations in circadian rhythms of activity, sleep, and light exposure related to dementia in nursing-home patients. Sleep 1997; 20(1):18–23.
126. Ancoli-Israel S, Gehrman P, Martin JL, et al. Increased light exposure consolidates sleep and strengthens circadian rhythms in severe Alzheimer's disease patients. Behav Sleep Med 2003; 1(1):22–36.
127. Ancoli-Israel S, Martin JL, Kripke DF, et al. Effect of light treatment on sleep and circadian rhythms in demented nursing home patients. J Am Geriatr Soc 2002; 50(2):282–289.
128. Benloucif S, Orbeta L, Ortiz R, et al. Morning or evening activity improves neuropsychological performance and subjective sleep quality in older adults. Sleep 2004; 27(8):1542–1551.
129. Niggemyer KA, Begley A, Monk T, et al. Circadian and homeostatic modulation of sleep in older adults during a 90-minute day study. Sleep 2004; 27(8):1535–1541.
130. Vitiello MV, Prinz PN, Schwartz RS. Slow wave sleep but not overall sleep quality of healthy older men and women is improved by increased aerobic fitness. Sleep Res 1994; 23:149.
131. Mishima K, Okawa M, Hishikawa Y, et al. Morning bright light therapy for sleep and behavior disorders in elderly patients with dementia. Acta Psychiatr Scand 1994; 89(1):1–7.
132. Singer C, Tractenberg RE, Kaye J, et al. A multicenter, placebo-controlled trial of melatonin for sleep disturbance in Alzheimer's disease. Sleep 2003; 26(7):893–901.
133. Brzezinski A, Vangel MG, Wurtman RJ, et al. Effects of exogenous melatonin on sleep: a meta-analysis. Sleep Med Rev 2005; 9(1):41–50.
134. Schnelle JF, Alessi CA, Al-Samarrai NR, et al. The nursing home at night: effects of an intervention on noise, light, and sleep. J Am Geriatr Soc 1999; 47(4):430–438.
135. Alessi CA, Martin JL, Webber AP, et al. Randomized, controlled trial of a nonpharmacological intervention to improve abnormal sleep/wake patterns in nursing home residents. J Am Geriatr Soc 2005; 53(5):803–810.

11 Restless Legs Syndrome: Manifestations in Aging and Dementia

Donald L. Bliwise

Program in Sleep, Aging and Chronobiology, Department of Neurology, Emory University Medical School, Atlanta, Georgia, U.S.A.

Restless legs syndrome (RLS) is a condition involving an uncontrollable urge to move one's legs at night, usually accompanied by an uncomfortable and unpleasant sensation of the legs, which worsens with inactivity and improves with movement. The diagnosis is based on the patient's description of symptoms. The differential diagnosis for RLS and other conditions that may be confused with this problem are listed in Table 1. Of note, the possibility that RLS could have a unique presentation in dementia was implicit within the summary statement of the 2002 National Institutes of Health (NIH) Diagnosis and Workshop Conference on RLS (1). The focus of the current review will be on factors associated with RLS in older people, and how RLS might be a component of the behavioral disturbance seen in some patients with dementia.

RLS: PREVALENCE AND ASSOCIATED FACTORS

Despite a large number of population-based studies (2–20), data conflict to some degree as to whether RLS shows an age-dependent increased prevalence in older adults. The varying upper age limit across these studies complicates this issue, since in some studies the oldest participants were 50 to 59 years old (9) whereas in other studies the upper age limit was 90 to 99 years (19). Additionally, the ways of defining RLS differed substantially among studies, with some studies relying upon in-person or telephone interviews, whereas others used simple questionnaires, some of which followed International Restless Legs Syndrome Study Group guidelines (1). The reported prevalence across these studies is quite large and ranges from 1.0% in women (aged 70–79 years) and 0.5% in men (aged 80 + years) in the study by Van de Vijver et al. (7) in the United Kingdom, to 16.3 % in women (aged 60–69 years) and 7.8% in men (aged 50–59 years) in the northern Italian (Tyrol) study of Hogl et al. (14), and to 19.4% in women (aged 50–59) and 13.2% in men (aged 60–69 years) in the German study of Berger et al. (12). Studies in Asian populations (15,16) suggest lower prevalences in these populations. Generally speaking, studies from Northern European populations [Germany (10,12), Scandinavian countries (2,3), and the Netherlands (19)] tend to have relatively higher prevalences, although some studies of North American populations are compatible with a high prevalence as well (4,5,11). Most studies that have included both women and men and presented data separately for each gender suggest higher prevalence in women

TABLE 1 Differential Diagnosis of Restless Legs Syndrome

Restless legs syndrome	Awake symptom diagnosis made by clinical history, uncomfortable deep creepy crawling sensation brought on at time of inactivity or rest (sitting and lying) immediate relief either complete or partial with movement, symptomatic relief is persistent as long as movement continues, presence of circadian pattern
Periodic limb movement disorder	Sleep phenomenon, diagnosis made by sleep study, no sensory symptoms like an urge to move or paresthesias while awake. May have sleep disturbance and complaint of daytime fatigue and sleepiness, must exclude other causes of PLMS, including sleep disorder breathing
Nocturnal leg cramps	Leg cramps or "Charlie horse cramps" are a common experience. Despite starting at night and being relieved with stretching, cramps are experienced as a usually painful muscular contraction, unlike RLS sensations.
Painful peripheral neuropathy	Sensory symptoms commonly reported as numbness, burning, and pain; these descriptors are not as common in RLS. Although the sensory symptoms can increase at night, they usually present throughout the day, while complete and persistent relief is not obtained while walking or during sustained movement.
Hypotensive akathisias	Feeling of restlessness, which may be localized in legs, brought on by sitting still. Should not occur while lying down, but might be relieved with movement. Occurs in individuals with orthostatic hypotension
Arthritis of the lower limbs	Discomfort centered more in joints does not usually have prominent circadian pattern as seen in RLS
Volitional movements, foot tapping, leg rocking	Occurs in individuals who fidget, especially when bored or anxious, but usually do not experience associated sensory symptoms, discomfort, or conscious urge to move. Usually lacks a circadian pattern.
Positional discomfort	Often starts with prolonged sitting or lying in the same position but usually relieved by a simple change in position, unlike RLS which often returns when change of position, movement, or walking is not continued.
Neuroleptic-induced akathisia	Usually whole body sensation rather than centered only in limbs with no pronounced circadian pattern, less associated sensations, and often no relieve with movement. Should have history of specific medication exposure.
Burning or painful feet and moving toes	Feet involved more, no circadian pattern. Usually have continuous slow writhing or repetitive movements of toes.

(2,4,6–12,14,16,18,19), regardless of absolute prevalence in the total sample. An interesting issue is whether these aging effects represent age dependence (i.e., prevalence increases purely as a function of age) versus whether these effects represent an age-related phenomenon (i.e., encompassing a particular window of age vulnerability) (21). This problem is similar to the problem which arises when discussing sleep disordered breathing in older persons. Until more is understood regarding the mechanisms underlying RLS, such questions are likely to remain unaddressed in epidemiologic studies of prevalence.

Although observational epidemiologic studies are limited in some degree to evaluating age dependence, these studies can offer insights as to other relevant risk factors for RLS within populations of older individuals. For example, cardiovascular disease and diabetes with or without peripheral neuropathy are both common in older people. RLS may be associated with broadly defined cardiovascular conditions (including hypertension) in various populations (3,6,12,22), although not uniformly in all studies (2,14,17,18). Similarly, conflicting data exist for links between RLS and diabetes/neuropathy (5–7,10,12,17,18,22,23). Arthritis is also common in older people, and some (6,22) but not all (7) studies show relationships between RLS and this condition. Other conditions possibly associated with RLS having relevance for the aging population include hypothyroidism (7,12), renal disease (7,14,17), gastroesophageal reflux (22), and daytime sweating (24).

Because the population tends to become more sedentary with advancing years, lack of physical activity could represent another risk factor for RLS in older persons. Compatible with this are data to suggest that lack of physical activity confers risk for RLS (5), although some opposing data (i.e., exercise increases risk) exist (6). Other studies show no relationship between physical activity and RLS (14,18). The relationship between smoking and increased risk of RLS appears less equivocal (5,6,10,12,17,18,22). Other risks may include alcohol and caffeine (6), although, curiously, use of alcohol may be associated with reduced risk for RLS (5,18) or have no influence whatsoever (17). Because these associations were all derived from cross-sectional data collected at a single point in time, considerable ambiguity exists as to whether any of these inferred risk factors truly represent a true, prospective risk for RLS. Longitudinal collection of data would be required to determine whether incident RLS (new cases) were portended by the presence of any putative risk factor in initially unaffected individuals. We must also stress that none of the cross-sectional studies to date have insinuated that the higher prevalence in older age groups reflected any risk factor singly or in combination. Such attempts would need to show that mere chronologic age was no longer a risk when other competing risk factors were controlled. Determining causality becomes particularly difficult when discussing relationships between depression and RLS (25). Generally speaking, the geriatric population endorses items suggestive of depression at higher rates than younger populations. Epidemiologic studies have shown that RLS may be related to symptoms of depressed mood (2,3,7,10,13,17,22,26,27) or overall indices of poorer mental health (5,6). Perhaps it is most reasonable to assume that RLS symptoms, if untreated, may be associated with depression rather than vice versa (i.e., depression causing RLS). On the other hand, because these reports have not controlled for concurrent use of psychoactive medications, including tricyclic antidepressants, selective serotonin reuptake inhibitors, or neuroleptics which may increase likelihood of RLS (6,7,10) and/or periodic limb movements of sleep (PLMS) (28), the relationships observed could reflect usage of such drugs.

Given the high prevalence of anemia in older populations, altered iron metabolism associated with RLS and aging requires special consideration, and several surveys have noted such associations (17,22). O'Keeffe (29) was the first to note that elderly individuals with RLS were likely to show low serum ferritin levels. Although overt anemia and reduced serum iron may not always co-occur with RLS, neuroimaging and cerebrospinal fluid (CSF) studies have suggested that total brain iron concentrations are lowered in RLS, findings that are compatible with modified blood/brain transport (30,31). Because anemia is highly prevalent in older people, it is well within the range of possibility that iron metabolism moderates the high prevalence of RLS in the aged. A surprisingly small number of studies have assessed this in older populations. O'Keeffe (32) replicated the original finding with a small additional case series suggesting that serum ferritin levels <50 ng/mL were significantly more likely in older patients with recent onset RLS, but other population-based studies demonstrate a more complicated situation. One study demonstrated that RLS was not accompanied by low levels of serum ferritin or by higher levels of soluble transferrin receptor, but mid-range levels of serum iron and transferrin saturation appeared protective for RLS (33). Neither serum ferritin nor hemoglobin levels less than 2 standard deviations below gender-expected values were significant risk factors for RLS in a German study across the age range 20 to 79 years (12). In a northern Italian older population (South Tyrol), however, higher soluble transferrin receptor levels (often seen in early stage anemia) and lower serum iron were correlated with RLS (14). Another study showed that CSF ferritin levels in older, late onset RLS patients were not related to onset of RLS symptoms (34). That study also showed that older patients had higher levels of CSF ferritin than younger patients (34). Taken together, these studies imply that iron deficiency may not be a relevant risk factor for RLS presenting in older populations, unless the RLS also is of early onset.

RLS AND PERIODIC LIMB MOVEMENTS OF SLEEP (FIG. 1)

Although there is an association between PLMS (i.e., repetitive, stereotypic leg movements that generally occur in non-REM (non-Rapid Eye Movement) sleep) and RLS, it is important to bear in mind that PLMS can occur in many older persons without accompanying RLS symptoms. In older populations, the prevalence of PLMS (without reference to RLS) has been reported to be as high as 45% (35), and more than 85% of older individuals had a PLMS Index (i.e., average number of movements per hour at night) more than 5.0 across 5 nights of recordings (36). Complaints of poor and/or altered sleep architecture were unrelated to PLMS in many studies (37–39). One study (35) found that PLMS were related to nocturnal leg kicking and breathing symptoms, but were unrelated to many aspects of sleep disruption (e.g., lower total sleep time, prolonged sleep onset latency); the best correlate of PLMS was the estimated number of awakenings on the recording night. Other studies of older subjects found a relationship between difficulty falling asleep and PLMS (40), or a relationship with lower total sleep times and wake after sleep onset (41). By contrast, other studies have suggested no relationships between PLMS and symptoms. For example, Mendelson (42) could find no relationships between PLMS arousals and symptoms of sleep disturbance. Montplaisir et al. (43) compared controls, individuals with insomnia and individuals with hypersomnia and found no differences in PLMS among groups. Karadeniz et al (44) were unable to show changes in macrosleep or microsleep architecture in conjunction with PLMS in insomnia patients aged 40 to 64 years. Hornyak et al (45) found no relationship between PLMS and sleep quality in insomniac patients without RLS. In another study, PLMS were unrelated to polysomnographically defined sleep quality in 70 normal subjects aged 40 to 60 years, although in men a small but significant effect was reported for lower sleep quality in relation to PLMS Index greater than 10 (46). When viewed in their totality, these results present a very mixed picture as to the correlates of PLMS in old age in the absence of frank RLS.

Of final note, there is some evidence that polysomnographic features may distinguish PLMS in older people. For example, night-to-night variability has been reported in older individuals with PLMS who do not have apparent RLS (36,47–49), and the number of PLMS with arousals or awakenings have been reported to be higher in older age groups (42,50,51). Finally, reduced magnitude of heart rate

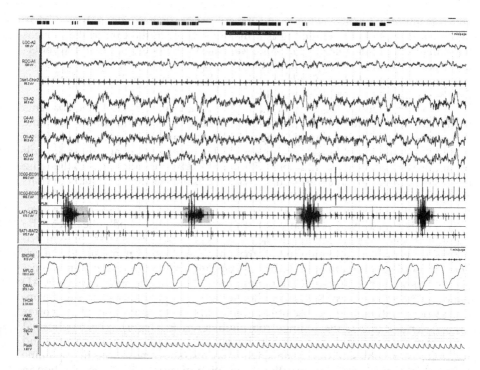

FIGURE 1   This is a one minute sleep epoch from a diagnostic polysomnogram of a 71-year-old man with difficulties maintaining asleep, excessive daytime sleepiness, and uncomfortable sensations in his legs associated with an irresistible urge to move his legs. His wife described nighttime kicking and jerking movements which disrupted his sleep. Illustrated in this figure is a succession of five periodic limb movements occurring in the anterior tibialis muscles (*labeled* LAT1-LAT2). Channels (*from top to bottom*) are as follows: electrooculogram (*left*: LOC-A2, *right*: ROC-A1), chin electromyogram (Chin-Chin), electroencephalogram [Left central (C3-A2), right central (C4-A1), left occipital (O1-A2), right occipital (O2-A1)], electrocardiogram (ECG), limb EMG [left leg (LAT), right leg (RAT)], patient position, snoring (SNORE), nasal-oral airflow (N/O), respiratory effort [Thoracic (THOR), Abdominal (ABD)], nasal pressure (NPRE), and oxygen saturation (SpO2) and plethysmography channel.

variability accompanying PLMS in older, relative to younger, subjects has also been reported (52).

RLS IN DEMENTIA

It is a formidable task to recognize RLS in a patient with dementia. In the non-dementia patient, the clinician relies heavily on the verbal reports of the patient's symptoms. In dementia patients, one is forced to employ indirect indicators, including kneading of the legs, motor signs such as wandering, and other suggestions of resting leg discomfort that are ameliorated by movement. The presence of such indicators at particular times of day, (i.e., late afternoon and/or early evening) may also allow inference of an RLS diagnosis.

Although not directly discussed at the 2002 NIH Diagnosis and Workshop Conference on RLS (1), wandering, itself a major issue in the behavioral management of dementia patients and the subject of several monographs (53,54), may be a form of RLS. Wandering is a major problem in the care of the dementia patient (54,55).Of note, pharmacological interventions employed for wandering behaviors often use dopaminergic blocking agents, which might worsen, rather than improve, wandering, if indeed the underlying condition being expressed is RLS (see Treatment Considerations later).

Emergency service personnel and police may become involved when patients with dementia wander outside their home, and even wandering within the home environment may be fraught with danger (56). Alzheimer's Disease (AD) caregivers typically note nocturnal wandering as one of the least tolerated and most difficult behaviors with which they must deal (55,57). The study of wandering is challenging to research. Most data are descriptive, and emphasize vectors and maps to characterize the behavior (58), or otherwise focus on what is attributed as "escape-like" behaviors that are associated with the ambulation (59). A more neurologically sophisticated interpretation has been offered by Duffy and colleagues who present clinical and basic science studies that suggest such behaviors represent primary deficits in visual attention circuits that engender confusion in visuospatial orientation (60,61). Neuroimaging studies, specifically those involving positron emission tomography, found reduced dopamine uptake in caudate and putamen in AD patients who wandered versus those who did not wander. These findings were confined to lowered cerebral glucose utilization in both the temporal and frontal cortex (62, 63). A replication of the findings from another research team has been published (64). There are undeniable parallels here between these findings in AD patients and neuroimaging studies in RLS patients, who may also show reductions in dopamine terminal storage (65,66); however the assumption of nigrostriatal degeneration in RLS patients may be unfounded, (see section on Parkinsonism later).

The temporal dimension of RLS also bears some similarity to wandering in dementia. An intriguing, real-time video monitoring study that focused on so-called "travel behavior" in institutionalized patients looked at time in when these behaviors occurred as an independent variable (67). "Travel behavior" was most likely to occur between 19:00 and 21:00, an interval that would match the peak occurrence of RLS symptoms in the nondemented population.

The importance of a careful family history in establishing a diagnosis of RLS in dementia cannot be overstated. As one example, demented patients who wandered were reported by caregivers and/or family members as demonstrating life-long walking behavior whenever under duress (58). If other conditions associated with RLS in the nondemented population (e.g., musculoskeletal diseases, neuropathy, anemia, diabetes) are also present in the wandering dementia patient, the astute clinician should consider RLS in the differential diagnosis. Unfortunately, little evidence is available to evaluate this hypothesis. AD patients were no more likely to have RLS symptoms or leg twitches (per caregiver report) when compared to older controls (68). In another study with possible implications for this topic, individuals with RLS demonstrated prefrontal cognitive deficits resembling those seen under sleep loss (69). At least in principle, these data imply that RLS symptoms could be related to cognitive dyscontrol, possibly of the magnitude seen in dementia.

Perhaps the neurodegenerative disease common in the aged offering the most immediate intuitive parallels with RLS is Parkinsonism. Both RLS and Parkinsonism are dopamine deficient conditions. This leads to the prediction that RLS should be more likely to occur in Parkinsonian conditions, such as idiopathic Parkinson's disease and related conditions, such as dementia with Lewy bodies and multisystem atrophy. Only one study to date has supported this hypothesis (70) and numerous other studies have shown mixed evidence (71,72) or no relationship (7,9,33,73). One study reported that low serum ferritin levels may account for some RLS in Parkinsonism (71), but another study has suggested that iron metabolism may be less of a factor in RLS with later onset (34). If RLS and Parkinsonism are largely independent conditions, a more thorough understanding of their lack of overlap may be informative mechanistically. Because neuroimaging studies consistently have revealed presynaptic dysfunction in Parkinson's disease (74), the independence of RLS may suggest the importance of postsynaptic or, possibly diencephalospinal dysfunction in RLS (75). Features occasionally accompanying RLS, such as flexor reflex or sensory abnormalities are consistent with dysfunction of dopaminergic efferents and afferents within the dorsal horn of the spinal cord that are atypical for Parkinsonism (75). Neuroimaging single photon emission computed tomography (SPECT) visualizing the dopamine transporter in age-matched RLS and Parkinson's disease patients indicated binding preservation in the RLS patients (76), also arguing for the independence of the two conditions. Finally, a postmortem series of RLS patients failed to demonstrate Lewy bodies or alpha-synuclein deposits, which represent defining features of all forms of Parkinsonism (77).

TREATMENT CONSIDERATIONS FOR THE DEMENTIA PATIENT WITH POSSIBLE RLS

In the dementia patient who wanders where there is corroborative informant history of RLS and/or a medical comorbidity related to RLS, an empirical trial of a low-dose dopaminergic agonist (e.g., 0.25–0.5 mg ropinirole; 0.125–0.25 mg pramipexole) could be used. The clinician, however, must bear in mind that because of possible dopamine-induced psychosis in a potentially vulnerable patient population, rapid dose escalation of such medications is ill advised, as might be entertained in a customary adult patient with RLS. A reasonable first step would be to consider carefully all ongoing medications to determine the potential of any of these to exacerbate RLS, before implementing any new treatment regimen. Studies in nondemented populations showing that selective serotonin-reuptake inhibitors (6,28), and antidepressants such as venlafaxine (28), and mirtazapine (78,79) can be associated with PLMS and/or RLS, suggest that these medications be discontinued as an initial intervention, although one recent study presented conflicting data (80).

Perhaps even more relevant for the dementia population are several case reports suggesting that atypical antipsychotics (e.g., olanzapine, quetiapine, risperidone) that exert partial blockade at specific dopaminergic receptors (e.g., olanzapine at D1-D4, quetiapine at D1/D2, risperidone at D2) may aggravate RLS or PLMS (81–83). Such medications are often used to decrease nocturnal agitation (including wandering) in dementia patients, and, curiously, at least one case series reported successful treatment of nocturnal wandering in AD patients (84) using risperidone. Nonetheless, neuroleptic use was a risk factor for RLS in population-based studies of nondemented populations (7,10), and such medication would be hypothesized only to aggravate, rather than improve, wandering behavior in a demented patient. Some perspective on this was also offered by secondary analyses from a double-blind, placebo-controlled trial of risperidone in dementia (85). In those analyses, wandering at baseline predicted higher rates of falls at 2.0 mg/day but

TABLE 2 Pharmacological treatment of restless legs syndrome

Drug class	Drug	Initial Dose	Risks
Iron	Ferrous sulfate (recommended if serum ferritin level is < 50 mcg)	325 mg once a day; can increase to 2 to 3 times a day; take with orange juice or other mildly acidic drink	Constipation
Dopaminergic agents	Levodopa/cardidopa	25/100 carbidopa/levodopa thirty minutes before bed; increase up to 3 tablets slowly as needed	Nausea, daytime sleepiness, occasionally insomnia; high sustained dosages may cause augmentation
Dopamine agonists	Pramipexole	0.125 mg one hour before bed; can increase slowly to.25–.50 mg as needed	Impulsive behaviors have been reported with all dopamine agonists; severe daytime sleepiness, nausea; high sustained disease may cause augmentation
	Ropinirole	0.25 mg one hour before bed; can increase slowly to 3 mg as needed	
Anticonvulsants	Gabapentin	300–600 mg one hour before bed; can increase slowly with divided doses up to 2400 mg daily	Daytime sleepiness, nausea
Benzodiazepines	Clonazepam	0.125 mg thirty minutes before bedtime; can increase up to 0.5 mg in needed	Oversedation, falls, dizziness
Opioids	Codeine	15 mg at bedtime; can increase to 30 mg as needed	Nausea, vomiting, restlessness, constipation, skin rash, drug dependence/tolerance

appeared protective at 1.0 mg. Because this study was not specifically focused on identification of RLS, it remains unclear whether any of these patients might have met NIH Workshop Guidelines criteria for RLS, although that is certainly possible. Additional, possibly, relevant data derive from a study of normal adults administered quetiapine (25 mg and 100 mg) (86). In that study, both dosages of quetiapine improved polysomnographically defined sleep architecture, but there was a significant increase in PLMS with the quetiapine 100-mg dose.When viewed in aggregate, these studies imply that usage of atypical antipsychotics for wandering in the dementia patient (itself constituting an off-label use) should be entertained only after full consideration of premorbid likelihood of RLS. Indeed a recent meta-analysis (87) has suggested that sudden cardiac death is as possible with the atypical antipsychotics as with older generation antipsychotics (88), which also exert dopaminergic blockade. Thus, judicious use of these medications in the wandering dementia patient is indicated. A summary of treatments available for RLS is offered in Table 2.

ACKNOWLEDGEMENTS
Supported by AG-020269, AG-025688, NS-35345, NS-050595, AT-00011 and a grant from the Alzheimer's Association.

REFERENCES

1. Allen RP, Picchietti D, Hening WA, et al. Restless legs syndrome: Diagnostic criteria, special considerations, and epidemiology. A report from the restless legs syndrome diagnosis and epidemiology workshop at the National Institutes of Health. Sleep Med 2003; 4(2):101–119.
2. Bjorvatn B, Leissner L, Ulfberg J, et al. Prevalence, severity and risk factors of restless legs syndrome in the general adult population in two Scandinavian countries. Sleep Med 2005; 6(4):307–312.
3. Ulfberg J, Nystrom B, Carter N, et al. Prevalence of restless legs syndrome among men aged 18 to 64 years: An association with somatic disease and neuropsychiatric symptoms. Mov Disord 2001; 16(6):1159–1163.
4. Lavigne GJ, Montplaisir JY. Restless legs syndrome and sleep bruxism: Prevalence and association among Canadians. Sleep 1994; 17(8):739–743.
5. Phillips B, Young T, Finn L, et al. Epidemiology of restless legs symptoms in adults. Arch Intern Med 2000; 160(14):2137–2141.
6. Ohayon MM, Roth T. Prevalence of restless legs syndrome and periodic limb movement disorder in the general population. J Psychosom Res 2002; 53(1):547–554.
7. Van De Vijver DA, Walley T, Petri H. Epidemiology of restless legs syndrome as diagnosed in UK primary care. Sleep Med 2004; 5(5):435–440.
8. Tison F, Crochard A, Leger D, et al. Epidemiology of restless legs syndrome in French adults: A nationwide survey: The INSTANT Study. Neurology 2005; 65(2):239–246.
9. Wenning GK, Kiechl S, Seppi K, et al. Prevalence of movement disorders in men and women aged 50–89 years (Bruneck Study cohort): A population-based study. Lancet Neurol 2005; 4(12):815–820.
10. Rothdach AJ, Trenkwalder C, Haberstock J, et al. Prevalence and risk factors of RLS in an elderly population: The MEMO study. Memory and Morbidity in Augsburg Elderly. Neurology 2000; 54(5):1064–1068.
11. Nichols DA, Allen RP, Grauke JH, et al. Restless legs syndrome symptoms in primary care: A prevalence study. Arch Intern Med 2003; 163(19):2323–2329.
12. Berger K, Luedemann J, Trenkwalder C, et al. Sex and the risk of restless legs syndrome in the general population. Arch Intern Med 2004; 164(2):196–202.
13. Allen RP, Walters AS, Montplaisir J, et al. Restless legs syndrome prevalence and impact: REST general population study. Arch Intern Med 2005; 165(11):1286–1292.
14. Hogl B, Kiechl S, Willeit J, et al. Restless legs syndrome: A community-based study of prevalence, severity, and risk factors. Neurology 2005; 64(11):1920–1924.
15. Tan EK, Seah A, See SJ, et al. Restless legs syndrome in an Asian population: A study in Singapore. Mov Disord 2001; 16(3):577–579.
16. Mizuno S, Miyaoka T, Inagaki T, et al. Prevalence of restless legs syndrome in non-institutionalized Japanese elderly. Psychiatry Clin Neurosci 2005; 59(4):461–465.
17. Sevim S, Dogu O, Camdeviren H, et al. Unexpectedly low prevalence and unusual characteristics of RLS in Mersin, Turkey. Neurology 2003; 61(11):1562–1569.
18. Kim J, Choi C, Shin K, et al. Prevalence of restless legs syndrome and associated factors in the Korean adult population: The Korean Health and Genome Study. Psychiatry Clin Neurosci 2005; 59(3):350–353.
19. Rijsman R, Neven AK, Graffelman W, et al. Epidemiology of restless legs in The Netherlands. Eur J Neurol 2004; 11(9):607–611.
20. Kageyama T, Kabuto M, Nitta H, et al. Prevalences of periodic limb movement-like and restless legs-like symptoms among Japanese adults. Psychiatry Clin Neurosci 2000; 54(3):296–298.

21. Brody JA, Schneider EL. Diseases and disorders of aging: An hypothesis. J Chronic Dis 1986; 39(11):871–876.
22. Phillips B, Hening W, Britz P, et al. Prevalence and correlates of restless legs syndrome: Results from the 2005 National Sleep Foundation Poll. Chest 2006; 129(1):76–80.
23. Mold JW, Vesely SK, Keyl BA, et al. The prevalence, predictors, and consequences of peripheral sensory neuropathy in older patients. J Am Board Fam Pract 2004; 17(5):309–318.
24. Mold JW, Roberts M, Aboshady HM. Prevalence and predictors of night sweats, day sweats, and hot flashes in older primary care patients: an OKPRN study. Ann Fam Med 2004; 2(5):391–397.
25. Picchietti D, Winkelman JW. Restless legs syndrome, periodic limb movements in sleep, and depression. Sleep 2005; 28(7):891–898.
26. Sukegawa T, Itoga M, Seno H, et al. Sleep disturbances and depression in the elderly in Japan. Psychiatry Clin Neurosci 2003; 57(3):265–270.
27. Hornyak M, Kopasz M, Berger M, et al. Impact of sleep-related complaints on depressive symptoms in patients with restless legs syndrome. J Clin Psychiatry 2005; 66(9):1139–1145.
28. Yang C, White DP, Winkelman JW. Antidepressants and periodic leg movements of sleep. Biol Psychiatry 2005; 58(6):510–514.
29. O'Keeffe ST, Gavin K, Lavan JN. Iron status and restless legs syndrome in the elderly. Age Ageing 1994; 23(3):200–203.
30. Earley CJ, Connor JR, Beard JL, et al. Abnormalities in CSF concentrations of ferritin and transferrin in restless legs syndrome. Neurology 2000; 54(8):1698–1700.
31. Allen RP, Barker PB, Wehrl F, et al. MRI measurement of brain iron in patients with restless legs syndrome. Neurology 2001; 56(2):263–265.
32. O'Keeffe ST. Secondary causes of restless legs syndrome in older people. Age Ageing 2005; 34(4):349–352.
33. Berger K, von Eckardstein A, Trenkwalder C, et al. Iron metabolism and the risk of restless legs syndrome in an elderly general population—the MEMO-Study. J Neurol 2002; 249(9):1195–1199.
34. Earley CJ, Connor JR, Beard JL, et al. Ferritin levels in the cerebrospinal fluid and restless legs syndrome: Effects of different clinical phenotypes. Sleep 2005; 28(9):1069–1075.
35. Ancoli-Israel S, Kripke DF, Klauber MR, et al. Periodic limb movements in sleep in community-dwelling elderly. Sleep 1991; 14(6):496–500.
36. Youngstedt SD, Kripke DF, Klauber MR, et al. Periodic leg movements during sleep and sleep disturbances in elders. J Gerontol A Biol Sci Med Sci 1998; 53(5):M391–M394.
37. Bixler EO, Kales A, Vela-Bueno A, et al. Nocturnal myoclonus and nocturnal myoclonic activity in the normal population. Res Commun Chem Pathol Pharmacol 1982; 36(1):129–140.
38. Kales A, Bixler EO, Soldatos CR, et al. Biopsychobehavioral correlates of insomnia, part 1: Role of sleep apnea and nocturnal myoclonus. Psychosomatics 1982; 23(6):589–600.
39. Mosko SS, Dickel MJ, Paul T, et al. Sleep apnea and sleep-related periodic leg movements in community resident seniors. J Am Geriatr Soc 1988; 36(6):502–508.
40. Bliwise D, Petta D, Seidel W, et al. Periodic leg movements during sleep in the elderly. Arch Gerontol Geriatr 1985; 4(3):273–281.
41. Youngstedt SD, Kripke DF, Elliott JA, et al. Circadian abnormalities in older adults. J Pineal Res 2001; 31(3):264–272.
42. Mendelson WB. Are periodic leg movements associated with clinical sleep disturbance? Sleep 1996; 19(3):219–223.
43. Montplaisir J, Michaud M, Denesle R, et al. Periodic leg movements are not more prevalent in insomnia or hypersomnia but are specifically associated with sleep disorders involving a dopaminergic impairment. Sleep Med 2000; 1(2):163–167.
44. Karadeniz D, Ondze B, Besset A, et al. Are periodic leg movements during sleep (PLMS) responsible for sleep disruption in insomnia patients? Eur J Neurol 2000; 7(3):331–336.
45. Hornyak M, Trenkwalder C. Restless legs syndrome and periodic limb movement disorder in the elderly. J Psychosom Res 2004; 56(5):543–548.

46. Carrier J, Frenette S, Montplaisir J, et al. Effects of periodic leg movements during sleep in middle-aged subjects without sleep complaints. Mov Disord 2005; 20(9):1127–1132.
47. Bliwise DL, Carskadon MA, Dement WC. Nightly variation of periodic leg movements in sleep in middle aged and elderly individuals. Arch Gerontol Geriatr 1988; 7(4):273–279.
48. Edinger JD, McCall WV, Marsh GR, et al. Periodic limb movement variability in older DIMS patients across consecutive nights of home monitoring. Sleep 1992; 15(2):156–161.
49. Mosko SS, Dickel MJ, Ashurst J. Night-to-night variability in sleep apnea and sleep-related periodic leg movements in the elderly. Sleep 1988; 11(4):340–348.
50. Coleman RM, Miles LE, Guilleminault CC, et al. Sleep-wake disorders in the elderly: Polysomnographic analysis. J Am Geriatr Soc 1981; 29(7):289–296.
51. Chabli A, Michaud M, Montplaisir J. Periodic arm movements in patients with the restless legs syndrome. Eur Neurol. 2000; 44(3):133–138.
52. Gosselin N, Lanfranchi P, Michaud M, et al. Age and gender effects on heart rate activation associated with periodic leg movements in patients with restless legs syndrome. Clin Neurophysiol 2003; 114(11):2188–2195.
53. Algase DL. Wandering in dementia. Annu Rev Nurs Res. 1999; 17:185–217.
54. Silverstein NM, Flaherty G, Tobin TS. Dementia and Wandering Behavior: Concern for the Lost Elder. New York: Springer Publishing Company, 2002.
55. Logsdon RG, Teri L, McCurry SM, et al. Wandering: A significant problem among community-residing individuals with Alzheimer's disease. J Gerontol B Psychol Sci Soc Sci 1998; 53(5):P294–P299.
56. Rowe MA, Glover JC. Antecedents, descriptions and consequences of wandering in cognitively-impaired adults and the Safe Return (SR) program. Am J Alzheimers Dis Other Demen 2001; 16(6):344–352.
57. Tractenberg RE, Singer CM, Cummings JL, et al. The Sleep Disorders Inventory: An instrument for studies of sleep disturbance in persons with Alzheimer's disease. J Sleep Res 2003; 12(4):331–337.
58. Snyder LH, Rupprecht P, Pyrek J, et al. Wandering. Gerontologist 1978; 18:272–280.
59. Nasman B, Bucht G, Eriksson S, et al. Behavioural symptoms in the institutionalized elderly: Relationship to dementia. Inter J Geriatr Psych. 1993; 8(843–849).
60. Kavcic V, Duffy CJ. Attentional dynamics and visual perception: Mechanisms of spatial disorientation in Alzheimer's disease. Brain 2003; 126(Pt 5):1173–1181.
61. Tetewsky SJ, Duffy CJ. Visual loss and getting lost in Alzheimer's disease. Neurology 1999; 52(5):958–965.
62. Meguro K, Yamaguchi S, Itoh M, et al. Striatal dopamine metabolism correlated with frontotemporal glucose utilization in Alzheimer's disease: A double-tracer PET study. Neurology 1997; 49(4):941–945.
63. Tanaka Y, Meguro K, Yamaguchi S, et al. Decreased striatal D2 receptor density associated with severe behavioral abnormality in Alzheimer's disease. Ann Nucl Med 2003; 17(7):567–573.
64. Rolland Y, Payoux P, Lauwers-Cances V, et al. A SPECT study of wandering behavior in Alzheimer's disease. Int J Geriatr Psychiatry 2005; 20(9):816–820.
65. Turjanski N, Lees AJ, Brooks DJ. Striatal dopaminergic function in restless legs syndrome: 18F-dopa and 11C-raclopride PET studies. Neurology 1999; 52(5):932–937.
66. Garcia-Borreguero D, Odin P, Serrano C. Restless legs syndrome and PD: A review of the evidence for a possible association. Neurology 2003; 61(6 suppl 3):S49–S55.
67. Martino-Saltzman D, Blasch BB, Morris RD, et al. Travel behavior of nursing home residents perceived as wanderers and nonwanderers. Gerontologist 1991; 31(5):666–672.
68. Tractenberg RE, Singer CM, Kaye JA. Characterizing sleep problems in persons with Alzheimer's disease and normal elderly. J Sleep Res. 2006; 15:97–103.
69. Pearson VE, Allen RP, Dean T, et al. Cognitive deficits associated with restless legs syndrome (RLS). Sleep Med 2006; 7(1):25–30.
70. Krishnan PR, Bhatia M, Behari M. Restless legs syndrome in Parkinson's disease: A case-controlled study. Mov Disord 2003; 18(2):181–185.
71. Ondo WG, Vuong KD, Jankovic J. Exploring the relationship between Parkinson's disease and restless legs syndrome. Arch Neurol 2002; 59(3):421–424.

72. Nomura T, Inoue Y, Miyake M, et al. Prevalence and clinical characteristics of restless legs syndrome in Japanese patients with Parkinson's disease. Mov Disord 2005.
73. Tan EK, Lum SY, Wong MC. Restless legs syndrome in Parkinson's disease. J Neurol Sci 2002; 196(1–2):33–36.
74. Micheli F, Cersosimo MG, Wooten GF. Neurochemistry and neuropharmacology of Parkinson's disease. In: Watts RL, Koeller WC, eds. Movement Disorders: Neurologic Principles and Practice, 2nd ed. New York: McGraw-Hill, 2004:197–207.
75. Rye DB. Parkinson's disease and RLS: The dopaminergic bridge. Sleep Med 2004; 5(3):317–328.
76. Linke R, Eisensehr I, Wetter TC, et al. Presynaptic dopaminergic function in patients with restless legs syndrome: Are there common features with early Parkinson's disease? Mov Disord 2004; 19(10):1158–1162.
77. Pittock SJ, Parrett T, Adler CH, et al. Neuropathology of primary restless leg syndrome: Absence of specific tau- and alpha-synuclein pathology. Mov Disord 2004; 19(6):695–699.
78. Agargun MY, Kara H, Ozbek H, et al. Restless legs syndrome induced by mirtazapine. J Clin Psychiatry 2002; 63(12):1179.
79. Bahk WM, Pae CU, Chae JH, et al. Mirtazapine may have the propensity for developing a restless legs syndrome? A case report. Psychiatry Clin Neurosci 2002; 56(2):209–210.
80. Brown LK, Dedrick DL, Doggett JW, et al. Antidepressant medication use and restless legs syndrome in patients presenting with insomnia. Sleep Med 2005; 6(5):443–450.
81. Pinninti NR, Mago R, Townsend J, et al. Periodic restless legs syndrome associated with quetiapine use: A case report. J Clin Psychopharmacol 2005; 25(6):617–618.
82. Kraus T, Schuld A, Pollmacher T. Periodic leg movements in sleep and restless legs syndrome probably caused by olanzapine. J Clin Psychopharmacol 1999; 19(5):478–479.
83. Wetter TC, Brunner J, Bronisch T. Restless legs syndrome probably induced by risperidone treatment. Pharmacopsychiatry 2002; 35(3):109–111.
84. Meguro K, Meguro M, Tanaka Y, et al. Risperidone is effective for wandering and disturbed sleep/wake patterns in Alzheimer's disease. J Geriatr Psychiatry Neurol 2004; 17(2):61–67.
85. Katz IR, Rupnow M, Kozma C, et al. Risperidone and falls in ambulatory nursing home residents with dementia and psychosis or agitation: Secondary analysis of a double-blind, placebo-controlled trial. Am J Geriatr Psychiatry 2004; 12(5):499–508.
86. Cohrs S, Rodenbeck A, Guan Z, et al. Sleep-promoting properties of quetiapine in healthy subjects. Psychopharmacology (Berl) 2004; 174(3):421–429.
87. Schneider LS, Dagerman KS, Insel P. Risk of death with atypical antipsychotic drug treatment for dementia: Meta-analysis of randomized placebo-controlled trials. JAMA 2005; 294(15):1934–1943.
88. Ray WA, Meredith S, Thapa PB, et al. Antipsychotics and the risk of sudden cardiac death. Arch Gen Psychiatry 2001; 58(12):1161–1167.

Jennifer L. Martin and Cathy A. Alessi
Veterans Administration Greater Los Angeles Healthcare System, Geriatric Research, Education and Clinical Center and David Geffen School of Medicine at UCLA, Department of Medicine, University of California, Los Angeles, California, U.S.A.

OVERVIEW

A growing number of older adults reside in nursing homes. Residents of nursing homes commonly suffer from nighttime sleep disruption, which is often accompanied by daytime sleepiness and may be caused by a multitude of factors. In the nursing home setting, sleep disturbance is associated with negative health outcomes, including higher risk of falling and elevated mortality risk. Factors contributing to sleep disturbance in the nursing home setting include medical and psychiatric illnesses and medications, sleep-disordered breathing (SDB), and other primary sleep disorders, circadian rhythm abnormalities, environmental conditions (e.g., nighttime noise), and lifestyle habits. Based on research with older adults in the community and work conducted within nursing home settings, pharmacotherapy cannot be universally recommended and some nonpharmacological treatments are shown to be effective. Further research on the implementation of practices that promote healthy sleep patterns within the nursing home setting is still needed.

CHARACTERISTICS OF NURSING HOME RESIDENTS

As the number of older adults continues to increase worldwide, and the long-term care needs of this growing segment of the population are often met in nursing homes, understanding and managing health conditions within the nursing home setting becomes increasingly important. As of 1999, there were over 18,000 nursing homes with approximately 1.6 million residents in the United States, with an average length of stay of 2.4 years (1). Based on projections of an increasing aged population, one can assume that the number may now exceed 2 million residents. National statistics also show that the typical nursing home resident is white (88%), widowed (63%), female (75%), and over age 75 (86%). Nearly all residents require some assistance with basic activities of daily living (e.g., toileting, bathing, dressing). Only 29% of residents are discharged because they recover or are sufficiently stabilized to return home. More commonly, residents die (27%) or are sent to acute care hospitals (28%) due to deteriorating health or acute medical emergency (2).

SLEEP/WAKE PATTERNS IN NURSING HOME RESIDENTS

Research suggests that sleep patterns of nursing home residents are commonly extremely fragmented. This is manifested not only as disrupted nighttime sleep but also as frequent daytime sleeping. Among nursing home residents, self-reported

TABLE 1 Prevalence of Sleep Disturbance in Four Representative Samples of Nursing Home Residents

Reference	Sample	Methods	Findings
Fetveit et al. (3)	$N = 29$ (1 facility)	Actigraphy; nurse observations	Sleep latency = 1 hr; WASO = 2.1 hr; sleep efficiency = 75%; napping on 87% of days; time in bed (bedtime to rise time) = 13:02 hr
Avidan et al. (4)	$N = 34,163$	MDS 2.0	6.3% of residents had insomnia item endorsed
Martin et al. (5)	$N = 492$ (4 facilities)	Research staff observations; actigraphy	% daytime sleep = 21.5%; % daytime time in bed = 27%; % with nighttime sleep <80% = 72% (among those with >15% daytime sleep)
Voyer et al. (6)	$N = 2332$ (28 facilities)	Nurse interviews	6.2% residents met criteria for insomnia; 17% had ≥ 1 insomnia symptom

Abbreviations: WASO, wake after sleep onset; MDS, Minimum Data Set.

difficulties with sleep are even more common and more severe than among older adults living at home in the community. Four studies have examined sleep disturbance among representative samples of nursing home residents (3–6). These studies (summarized in Table 1) show that while nursing staff recognize sleep disturbance in a small percentage of residents, other methods (e.g., research staff observation, wrist actigraphy) show that disrupted sleep is nearly universal.

A critical aspect of sleep disturbance in the nursing home is that residents are often asleep intermittently at all hours of the day and the typical nursing home resident shows a pattern of wakefulness that is frequently interrupted by brief periods of sleep. This is different from what has been seen in community-dwelling older adults, who may sleep in the form of a consolidated nap at a specified time of day. In the nursing home, daytime "wake fragmentation" is oftentimes accompanied by nighttime "sleep fragmentation." It is difficult to determine which is causal and which is symptomatic. Likely, this is a circular pattern where nighttime wakefulness contributes to daytime sleeping and vice versa. This perpetuates abnormal sleep/wake patterns in these residents over the long term. An extensive literature using either behavioral observations of sleep or wrist actigraphy (an objective estimate of sleep, measured using wrist movements) has shown that the sleep of nursing home residents is generally distributed across the 24-hour day rather than being consolidated to the nighttime hours. Residents rarely are asleep or awake for a continuous hour during the day or night (7,8).

An additional factor that must be considered is the role of neurodegenerative processes in the regulation of sleep and wakefulness. Some symptoms of dementia, such as irritability, poor concentration and memory, slower reaction time, and decreased overall cognitive performance may be exacerbated by sleep problems, particularly those that lead to daytime sleepiness. Among community-dwelling older women, recent findings suggest that short sleep at night, poor sleep efficiency (percent of the night spent asleep), and increased napping during the day are all associated with increased risk of falls (9), as well as increased risk of shorter survival (10,11). Sleep has also been associated with negative outcomes in the nursing home setting, including decreased survival (12).

Although the specific causes of sleep pattern disruption vary from person to person, there are several common causes of sleep difficulties in the nursing home setting. These include medical conditions, psychiatric disorders, medications/polypharmacy, circadian rhythm disruption, and primary sleep disorders. Environmental factors (e.g., noise and light during the night, low daytime indoor illumination, little time spent outdoors) and behavioral factors (e.g., physical inactivity, extended time spent in bed) also appear to contribute to the disruption of sleep/wake patterns among residents of nursing homes.

MEDICATIONS, MEDICAL ILLNESSES, AND PSYCHIATRIC DISORDERS

Nursing home residents are frequently in poor physical health. Examples of medical conditions among long-term residents that may contribute to sleep difficulty include pain (e.g., from arthritis), paresthesias, nighttime cough, dyspnea (from cardiac or pulmonary illness), gastroesophageal reflux, and incontinence/frequent nighttime urination. Management of these conditions should include consideration of effects on both daytime functioning and nighttime sleep quality.

There is increasing evidence of sleep abnormalities with neurological illnesses (e.g., Alzheimer's disease, Parkinson's disease) as well. Residents of nursing homes are often in the late stages of these disorders, where occurrence of sleep disturbance is common. For example, research suggests that demented patients generally have more sleep disruption [including lower sleep efficiency, more light sleep, less deep sleep, and perhaps less rapid eye movement (REM) sleep] compared with nondemented older people (13). "Sundowning," the term used to describe a worsening of confusion and behavior problems in the evening or night in people with dementia, may have an underlying neurological basis and is associated with circadian rhythm disruption (14). Sleep abnormalities such as excessive daytime sleepiness and parasomnias [e.g., REM sleep behavior disorder (RBD)] are commonly associated with Parkinson's disease and may be related to the pathology of the disorder and/or to its medication treatment. Problems may be even more common among nursing home residents with advanced Parkinson's disease (15).

In addition to these health conditions and dementing illnesses, nearly all nursing home residents take multiple medications. On average, residents of nursing homes take five to eight different medications and many take more than 10 different medications daily (8,14). It is very likely that one or more of these medications impact nighttime sleep, daytime alertness, or both. Some medications can be particularly problematic when taken near bedtime. For example, diuretics or stimulating agents (e.g., sympathomimetics, bronchodilators) can directly disrupt sleep at night. In addition, the use of sedating medications during the daytime (e.g., antihistamines, anticholinergics, sedating antidepressants) can contribute to daytime drowsiness, leading to daytime sleeping and further disruption of nighttime sleep. Some medications used in the treatment of depression, Parkinson's disease, and hypertension can impair sleep or cause nightmares. While medications may be necessary for medical reasons, changing the timing of administration of a medication can ameliorate sleep difficulties in some cases, particularly if sleep difficulties started or were exacerbated when the medication was first administered.

CIRCADIAN RHYTHM DISRUPTION

Circadian rhythm disruption contributes to sleep problems in nursing home residents as well. Among older adults in general, circadian rhythms may be blunted in amplitude and can be shifted to abnormal times. Research also shows that circadian rhythms are commonly altered among individuals with dementia and that the type of disruption depends upon the type of dementia. In one study, nursing home residents had less stable circadian rhythms of activity compared with older people living at home, regardless of the cognitive status (16). Other studies have found a relationship between circadian rhythm disturbance and degree of dementia in the nursing home setting (17) and circadian activity rhythm abnormalities have been associated with shorter survival (18,19).

The often-cited advance (i.e., shift to an earlier time) of circadian rhythms commonly seen in older adults can be exacerbated by environmental factors in the nursing home. In particular, exposure to bright light, the strongest synchronizer and stabilizer of circadian rhythms, is quite limited among nursing home residents. Typically, nursing home residents are exposed to even less bright light than older adults living in the community—only a few minutes per day—which is likely insufficient for entrainment of circadian rhythms (20). Since light exposure is the strongest known *zeitgeber* (time cue) in humans, this lack of daytime light may contribute to circadian dysregulation. Nursing home residents also spend extended periods in bed and are physically inactive during the daytime. While physical activity is likely less important than light exposure in circadian entrainment, lack of physical activity contributes to further circadian rhythm disturbance. This disruption of circadian rhythms likely underlies the chronicity of fragmentation of sleep and wakefulness. This is because circadian rhythms exert a strong influence on the timing of sleep, and weak circadian rhythms or rhythms that are shifted to inappropriate times are likely to cause sleep problems. Circadian rhythm disturbances are best treated with timed exposure to bright light. Several studies have found that exposure to bright light strengthens and stabilizes circadian rhythms (21–23). Although the optimal timing of bright light exposure among nursing home residents remains somewhat unclear, these studies suggest that daytime bright light exposure (via bright light boxes or sunlight) may improve circadian rest–activity rhythms and consolidate sleep/wake patterns among nursing home residents, particularly those with dementia and an irregular sleep/wake pattern.

PRIMARY SLEEP DISORDERS IN NURSING HOME RESIDENTS

To our knowledge, no large-scale epidemiological studies have been conducted to examine the prevalence of primary sleep disorders in nursing homes. One could assume, however, that sleep disorders that increase in prevalence with advancing age [e.g., SDB, restless legs syndrome (RLS), periodic limb movement disorder (PLMD), RBD] are at least as common (if not more common) among nursing home residents as in similarly aged older adults in community settings. In addition, some sleep disorders (such as SDB) are even more common among individuals with certain dementing illnesses (e.g., Alzheimer's disease, vascular dementia, Parkinson's disease with dementia) than among older adults without dementia. The absence of true prevalence information of primary sleep disorders in the nursing home setting is, in part, due to the difficulty in conducting polysomnographic sleep recordings with nursing home residents, especially among individuals with dementia or extreme frailty.

SDB may be a particularly important condition among nursing home residents. The limited studies that are available suggest that, depending upon the precise criteria for SDB and the study design used, at least half of nursing home residents have at least mild SDB. Negative consequences of SDB include increased risk for cardiovascular and cerebrovascular disease, depression, and other health problems. The literature suggests that, among nursing home residents, SDB is also associated with cognitive impairment, agitated behaviors, and increased mortality risk (24,25).

The use of positive airway pressure (PAP) for treatment of SDB has not been well-evaluated in the nursing home setting, but recent findings suggest that Alzheimer's disease patients living at home with a caregiver have the same level of compliance with PAP as general sleep disorder clinic patients (26). This finding suggests that PAP should still be considered the treatment of choice among individuals in the nursing home who suffer from SDB, and residing in a nursing home should not necessarily preclude treatment of SDB with PAP (27).

RLS increases in prevalence with age, and individuals with RLS sometimes report that their symptoms grow worse with age. This condition has not been studied in nursing homes; however, it may be a possible cause of motor restlessness and perhaps wandering among residents with coexisting dementia and (perhaps undiagnosed) RLS, particularly if these residents lack the cognitive ability to report the typical symptoms of RLS. Research in this area is needed since unrecognized RLS could potentially present as pacing and wandering at night, which may place the resident at risk for falls or may be misdiagnosed and treated as agitation, potentially exposing the resident to inappropriate medications. Likewise, the prevalence of periodic limb movement disorder (PLMD) among nursing home residents is unknown.

RBD is most common in old age (particularly among older men) and is more prevalent with certain neurodegenerative disorders (e.g., Lewy body disease, Parkinson's disease). The main risk associated with RBD is that individuals can fall out of bed or engage in dangerous behavior during the night as a result of acting out dream-related behaviors during sleep.

To date, no studies we are aware of have systematically examined treatment of SDB, RLS, PLMD, or RBD in nursing homes residents. The safety and efficacy of standard treatments for these conditions in nursing home residents is also unknown. In general, treatment of primary sleep disorders in nursing home residents should closely parallel the treatment of frail older adults in the community. The risk/benefit ratio of each treatment should be considered, including potential drug interactions and focusing on improvements in functional status, cognition, and quality of life as key outcomes. Further research on the treatment of primary sleep disorders in nursing home residents is needed.

ENVIRONMENTAL CONDITIONS AND SLEEP

The nighttime nursing home environment typically resembles an inpatient hospital setting more than a home sleep environment. Residents usually share rooms with one or more roommates, and frequent noise and light interruptions, which occur several times per hour on average (28), likely impact residents' ability to obtain sufficient consolidated sleep. Much of the noise produced in the facility is caused by staff, often while they provide incontinence care and other personal care to residents at night (28,29). In addition to noise, nighttime exposure to room-level light has the potential to suppress endogenous melatonin, disrupt sleep, and shift circadian rhythms (30). Lights are commonly left on at night in patient rooms, often by well-intended staff members who provide nighttime care to patients.

USE OF MEDICATIONS IN THE TREATMENT OF SLEEP PROBLEMS

Extensive long-term care reforms enacted with the Omnibus Budget Reconciliation Act (OBRA) of 1987 (which became effective in 1991) included limits on the use of psychoactive medications in the nursing home setting. While OBRA regulations specifically target antipsychotic medications, the interpretive guidelines that accompany these regulations also limit the use of anxiolytic agents and sedative-hypnotics (but not antidepressants). Use of regulated psychoactive medications must be documented in the medical record as necessary to treat a specific condition, with daily dose limits, requirements for monitoring treatment and adverse reactions, and attempts at dose reductions and discontinuation whenever possible. The guidelines also provide options for using psychoactive medications outside of the stated limits when such use is clearly clinically indicated. Since the OBRA guidelines were implemented, research has shown substantial decreases in the use of antipsychotics among nursing home residents, but studies generally report that the use of sedative-hypnotics and anxiolytics is unchanged, and the use of antidepressants has increased (31).

Evidence for the use of sleeping medication in nursing home residents has been limited, so clinicians must often make treatment decisions based on research performed in younger or typically healthier populations. There are a number of FDA-approved agents for the treatment of insomnia, and a number of additional medications that are commonly used "off-label" to manage sleep problems. Off-label use may be particularly common in the nursing home setting. Nationwide, trazodone (a sedating antidepressant) has been reported to be the most commonly used agent for treating sleep complaints (32). However, the National Institutes of Health (NIH) State-of-the-Science Conference on Insomnia (in 2005) concluded that the newer shorter acting nonbenzodiazepine hypnotics were more effective and safer than older, longer acting benzodiazepines; and antidepressants have potentially significant adverse effects raising concerns about the risk–benefit ratio when antidepressant medications are used to treat sleep problems in the absence of depression. In addition, barbiturates and antipsychotics have significant risks, and thus their use in the treatment of chronic insomnia was not recommended. Finally, there is no systematic evidence of efficacy and there are significant concerns about the risks of sedating antihistamines when used to treat sleep disturbances (25). The conclusions of the NIH insomnia panel were based primarily on studies conducted in younger adults and older adults in the community, and not in older adults with dementia or those living in nursing homes. While there are published reports on the efficacy and safety of the shorter acting nonbenzodiazepines in older adults in the community (33,34), research is still needed in the nursing home setting to establish the safety and efficacy of these newer medications.

When considering pharmacological therapy for sleep problems in the nursing home setting, it is important to consider the possibility that these medications can increase risk of some adverse outcomes, particularly falls (35–37). There has been some concern raised that at least part of the relationship between hypnotic medications and falls may be accounted for by the underlying sleep problems that precipitate the hypnotic use to begin with. One recent study using administrative nursing home data (the Minimum Data Set, MDS) found that an MDS item indicating insomnia, but not an item indicating hypnotic use, was associated with increased fall risk after controlling for many (but not all) fall risk factors documented in the MDS (4). These findings must be interpreted with caution, since there are no data to support the accuracy of the insomnia or hypnotic use items in the MDS and there is evidence that documentation of falls using this method is substandard (38). Another important consideration is that nearly all of this work included use of benzodiazepine medications, with less common use of newer nonbenzodiazepine agents. Research is needed in the nursing home setting to examine the safety and efficacy of the newer nonbenzodiazepines, and in particular, to examine the relationship between insomnia and risk of falls relative to use of newer medications to treat insomnia.

A second critical consideration is that, given the large number of medications nursing home residents already use, there is a potential for drug interactions and/or altered drug metabolism when a hypnotic agent is added to the medication list. The addition of a sedating medication to this potentially lengthy list in these frail, older people should not be taken lightly. Finally, use of pharmacological agents for sleep problems should not be viewed as a substitute for addressing other underlying causes of sleep disturbance such as sleep apnea, nighttime noise, inadequate control of pain or circadian rhythm disturbances.

NONPHARMACOLOGICAL TREATMENTS

The NIH State-of-the-Science Conference on Insomnia also concluded that cognitive-behavioral therapy (CBT) is as effective as prescription medications for treatment of chronic insomnia, with research showing that the beneficial effects of CBT may last well beyond the termination of the treatment (in contrast to medications) (39). While CBT would be difficult to perform with dementia patients due to cognitive limitations, investigators have studied the effectiveness of nonpharmacological interventions targeting some of the core components of CBT to improve sleep in the nursing home setting and have found some modest success.

Multiple studies have tested the effects of timed exposure to bright light as a means of improving circadian rhythms and sleep/wake patterns. Bright light exposure impacts circadian rhythms and can also increase alertness levels during and immediately after exposure. In randomized-controlled trials, nursing home residents exposed to bright light showed improved sleep relative to participants who received placebo interventions (22,23,40,41). Researchers have also examined the effectiveness of supplemental melatonin (a hormone, typically secreted at night, that is closely linked to sleep), but results are mixed and optimal administration timing, dose, and preparation (acute vs. sustained release) are not clear. A few studies have attempted to increase daytime activity levels, and results are, again, mixed. Some studies show that sleep improves, while others show minimal or no changes in sleep with increased daytime physical activity (42). Studies have also attempted to reduce nighttime noise and light in resident rooms. These studies have shown that it is extremely difficult to change the nursing home environment, and despite considerable efforts by researchers, the environment remains quite noisy at night (40,42,43). The efficacy of noise reduction in improving sleep therefore has not been adequately evaluated.

An alternative approach in the nursing home setting has been to use multicomponent interventions to address both internal physiological causes of sleep disturbance and external environmental factors. One such study tested a short-term (5-day) intervention combining daytime light exposure and physical activity, a structured and regularly timed bedtime routine, reduced time in bed during the day, plus provision of nighttime nursing care in a manner that minimizes disruption to sleep (40). This intervention was successful in reducing daytime sleepiness, and residents who received the intervention were more socially engaged and physically active during the day than residents receiving usual care; however, nighttime noise and light were not significantly reduced, and the intervention had a minimal effect on nighttime sleep. There were also improvements in rest–activity rhythms with this intervention (21). These results suggest that significant improvements in sleep in the nursing home setting likely require that multiple factors be addressed simultaneously, perhaps for long periods of time for substantial improvements to be achieved and maintained.

One final area for intervention, which has largely been overlooked by the research community, is working at the facility level to change staff training, policies, and caregiving practices that impact resident sleep. In our own qualitative work, we have found that nightshift staff are well aware of the difficulties associated with disrupting residents' nighttime sleep for caregiving activities; however, they feel they must check on residents regularly (often with lights on) in addition to providing required nighttime care. The addition of sleep-promoting practices and the removal of unnecessary sleep-disruptive activities by staff may lead to meaningful changes for all residents in a facility. Real change will require administrators and other staff to buy into the notion that sleep is important and that encouraging better quality sleep/wake patterns is beneficial to both residents and staff over the long term.

SUMMARY

In summary, nighttime sleep disruption and daytime sleepiness are characteristic of nursing home residents. This sleep disturbance is often caused by a multitude of factors, including medical and psychiatric illness, medications, circadian rhythm abnormalities, SDB, and other primary sleep disorders, environmental factors, and lifestyle habits. While data to support the use of pharmacotherapy for sleep in the nursing home are limited, there is some suggestion that these factors are amenable to nonpharmacological treatments. Further research on the implementation of these treatments within the nursing home setting is needed. Specifically, further research is needed to determine whether treating SDB and other primary sleep disorders is feasible and results in functional or quality of life improvements among nursing home residents. Additional work is also needed to understand the facility-level factors that might lead to systemic changes in how sleep is viewed and sleep problems are addressed in nursing home settings.

REFERENCES

1. Centers for Disease Control and Prevention. The National Nursing Home Survey: 1999 Summary (accessed 2/19/08). http://www.cdc.gov/nchs/data/series/sr_13/sr13_152.pdf, 2008. Ref type: electronic citation.
2. National Center for Health Statistics, Gabrel CS. Characteristics of elderly nursing home current residents and discharges: data from the 1997 national nursing home survey. Vital Health Stat 2000;312.

3. Fetveit A, Bjorvatn B. Sleep disturbances among nursing home residents. Int J Geriatr Psychiatry 2002;17:604–609.
4. Avidan AY, Fries BE, James ML, et al. Insomnia and hypnotic use, recorded in the Minimum Data Set, as predictors of falls and hip fractures in Michigan nursing homes. J Am Geriatr Soc 2005;53:955–962.
5. Martin JL, Webber AP, Alam T, et al. Daytime sleeping, sleep disturbance and circadian rhythms in nursing home residents. Am J Geriatr Psychiatry. 2006;14:121–129.
6. Voyer P, Verreault R, Mengue PN, et al. Prevalence of insomnia and its associated factors in elderly long-term care residents. Arch Gerontol Geriatr 2006;42:1–20.
7. Bliwise DL, Bevier WC, Bliwise NG, et al. Systemic 24-hour behavior observations of sleep and wakefulness in a skilled-care nursing facility. Psychol Aging 1990;15:16–24.
8. Jacobs D, Ancoli-Israel S, Parker L, et al. Twenty-four hour sleep–wake patterns in a nursing home population. Psychol Aging 1989;4(3):352–356.
9. Stone KL, Schneider JL, Blackwell T, et al. Impaired sleep increases the risk of falls in older women: a prospective actigraphy study. Sleep 2004;27:A125.
10. Stone KL, Blackwell T, Cummings SR, et al. Rest–activity rhythms predict risk of mortality in older women. Sleep abstract suppl.[29] 2006:A54.
11. Dew MA, Hoch CC, Buysse DJ, et al. Healthy older adults' sleep predicts all-cause mortality at 4 to 19 years of follow-up. Psychosom Med 2003;65:63–73.
12. Dale MC, Burns A, Panter L, et al. Factors affecting survival of elderly nursing home residents. Int J Geriatr Psychiatry 2001;16:70–76.
13. Bliwise DL. Review: sleep in normal aging and dementia. Sleep 1993;16:40–81.
14. Martin J, Marler MR, Shochat T, et al. Circadian rhythms of agitation in institutionalized patients with Alzheimer's disease. Chronobiol Int 2000;17:405–418.
15. Friedman JH, Chou KL. Sleep and fatigue in Parkinson's disease. Parkinsonism Relat Disord 2004;10:S27–S35.
16. Van Someren EJW, Hagebeuk EEO, Lijzenga C, et al. Circadian rest activity rhythm disturbances in Alzheimer's disease. Biol Psychiatry 1996;40:259–270.
17. Gehrman PR, Marler M, Martin JL, et al. The relationship between dementia severity and rest/activity circadian rhythms. Neuropsychiatr Dis Treatment 2005;1:155–163.
18. Gehrman PR, Marler M, Martin JL, et al. The timing of activity rhythms in patients with dementia is related to survival. J Gerontol Med Sci 2004;59A:1050–1055.
19. Bliwise DL, Hughes ML, Carroll JS, et al. Mortality predicted by timing of temperature nadir in nursing home patients. Sleep Res 1995; 24:510. Ref type: abstract.
20. Shochat T, Martin J, Marler M, et al. Illumination levels in nursing home patients: effects on sleep and activity rhythms. J Sleep Res 2000;9:373–380.
21. Martin JL, Marler MR, Harker JO, et al. A multicomponent nonpharmacological intervention improves activity rhythms among nursing home residents with disrupted sleep/wake patterns. J Gerontol Med Sci 2007;62A:67–72.
22. Ancoli-Israel S, Martin JL, Kripke DF, et al. Effect of light treatment on sleep and circadian rhythms in demented nursing home patients. J Am Geriatr Soc 2002;50:282–289.
23. Ancoli-Israel S, Gehrman PR, Martin JL, et al. Increased light exposure consolidates sleep and strengthens circadian rhythms in severe Alzheimer's disease patients. Behav Sleep Med 2003;1:22–36.
24. Ancoli-Israel S, Klauber MR, Kripke DF, et al. Sleep apnea in female patients in a nursing home: increased risk of mortality. Chest 1989;96(5):1054–1058.
25. Cohen-Zion M, Stepnowsky C, Marler M, et al. Changes in cognitive function associated with sleep disordered breathing in older people. J Am Geriatr Soc 2001;49:1622–1627.
26. Ayalon L, Ancoli-Israel S, Stepnowsky C, et al. Treatment adherence in patients with Alzheimer's disease and obstructive sleep apnea. Am J Geriatr Psychiatry 2006;14:176–180.
27. Gehrman PR, Martin JL, Shochat T, et al. Sleep disordered breathing and agitation in institutionalized adults with Alzheimer's disease. Am J Geriatr Psychiatry 2003;11:426–433.
28. Schnelle JF, Ouslander JG, Simmons SF, et al. The nighttime environment, incontinence care, and sleep disruption in nursing homes. J Am Geriatr Soc 1993;41:910–914.

29. Schnelle JF, Cruise PA, Alessi CA, et al. Sleep hygiene in physically dependent nursing home residents. Sleep 1998;21:515–523.
30. Boivin DB, James FO. Phase-dependent effect of room light exposure in a 5-h advance of sleep–wake cycle: implications for jet lag. J Biol Rhythms 2002;17:266–276.
31. Lantz MS, Giambanco V, Buchalter EN. A ten-year review of the effect of OBRA-87 on psychotropic prescribing practices in an academic nursing home. Psychiatr Services 1996;47:951–955.
32. Morlock RJ, An M, Itchell DY. Patient characteristics and patterns of drug use for sleep complaints in the United States: analysis of national ambulatory medical survey data, 1997–2002. Clin Ther 2006;28:1044–1053.
33. Ancoli-Israel S, Richardson GS, Mangano RM, et al. Long-term use of sedative hypnotics in older patients with insomnia. Sleep Med 2005;6:107–113.
34. Contronco A, Gareri P, Lacava R, et al. Use of zolpidem in over 75-year-old patients with sleep disorders and comorbidities. Arch Gerontol Geriatr 2004;9:93–96.
35. Campbell AJ, Borrie MJ, Spears GF. Risk factors for falls in a community-based prospective study of people 70 years and older. J Gerontol 1989;44(4):M112–M117.
36. Ray WA, Thapa PB, Gideon P. Benzodiazepines and the risk of falls in nursing home residents. J Am Geriatr Soc 2000;48:682–685.
37. Schneeweiss S, Wang PS. Claims data studies of sedative-hypnotics and hip fractures in older people: exploring residual confounding using survey information. J Am Geriatr Soc 2005;53:948–954.
38. Martin JL, Alessi CA. Limited validity of MDS items on sleep and hypnotic use in predicting falls and hip fracture among nursing home residents. J Am Geriatr Soc 2006;54:1150–1152.
39. National Institutes of Health. Manifestations and management of chronic insomnia in adults. Sleep 2005;28:1049–1057.
40. Alessi CA, Martin JL, Webber AP, et al. Randomized controlled trial of a nonpharmacological intervention to improve abnormal sleep/wake patterns in nursing home residents. J Am Geriatr Soc 2005;53:619–626.
41. Van Someren EJW, Kessler A, Mirmiran M, et al. Indirect bright light improves circadian rest–activity rhythm disturbances in demented patients. Biol Psychiatry 1997;41:955–963.
42. Alessi CA, Yoon EJ, Schnelle JF, et al. A randomized trial of a combined physical activity and environmental intervention in nursing home residents: do sleep and agitation improve? J Am Geriatr Soc 1999;47:784–791.
43. Schnelle JF, Alessi CA, Al-Samarrai NR, et al. The nursing home at night: effects of an intervention on noise, light and sleep. J Am Geriatr Soc 1999;47:430–438.

Sleep in the Older Woman

Sumi Misra

Division of General Internal Medicine, Vanderbilt University Medical Center and Geriatric Primary Care Clinic, Tennessee Valley Health Care System, Veterans Affairs Hospital, Nashville, Tennessee, U.S.A.

Beth Malow

Department of Neurology, Vanderbilt University Medical Center, and Vanderbilt Sleep Disorders Center, Vanderbilt University Medical Center, Nashville, Tennessee, U.S.A.

INTRODUCTION

Menopause is defined in the literature as the one year following cessation of menstrual periods. The premenopausal period precedes menopause by several years, as the hormonal changes begin 7 to 10 years before clinical menopause. During this period, there is a decrease in estradiol and inhibin with an increase in follicle-stimulating hormone (FSH) and luteinizing hormone (LH). There is a shift in circulation from estradiol to estrone (1), predominantly by conversion of extraglandular androstenidione, with minimal decrease in the production of testosterone.

Sleep in perimenopausal, menopausal, and postmenopausal women is often affected in a multitude of ways (Table 1) and to varying degrees. The hormonal, physiologic, and psychologic changes add layers of complexity to the conditions as well.

As women age, physical and hormonal changes make sleep lighter and less sound. Sleep disturbances become more common during menopause. Women wake up more often at night and are more tired during the day. Hot flashes and night sweats linked to lower levels of estrogen may contribute to these problems. During the menopausal years, snoring becomes more frequent. After menopause, women get less deep sleep and are more likely to awaken at night than during menopause. In older postmenopausal women, periodic limb movement disorder (PLMD) and sleep-disordered breathing (SDB) may cause excessive daytime sleepiness. In addition, pain, grief, worry, certain medical conditions, medications, and breathing disorders may disturb sleep in menopausal and postmenopausal women (2,3).

CAUSES OF SLEEP DISTURBANCE IN WOMEN

Four main causes of sleep disruption during the perimenopausal and postmenopausal states have been studied and described in the literature: hot flashes, insomnia, mood disorders, and SDB (13).

A Brazilian study was conducted in 2005 (14) to evaluate the prevalence of reported sleep disturbances through polysomnographic recording (PSG) in a sample of postmenopausal women. Thirty-three postmenopausal women, with a mean age of 56 years, a mean body mass index (BMI) of 27 kg/m^2, with 7.7 years of

TABLE 1 Common Sleep Disorders in Women Across the Life Cycle from Adulthood to Menopause

Disorders of sleep related to the menstrual cycle	I. Premenstrual [International Classification of Sleep Disorders Related to Menstrual Cycle (2005)] Hypersomia, insomnia, parasomnia
	II. Normal Menstrual Cycles
	Luteal phase associated with longer sleep latency, lower sleep efficiency and poorer quality, compared with follicular phase (4).
	III. Premenstrual Syndrome (PMS) and Postmenstrual Dysphoric Disorder (PMDD) (5)
	Insomnia, hypersomnia, tiredness and fatigue, nightmares, restless sleep, nonrestorative sleep
	IV. Dysmenorrhea
	Increased subjective fatigue, decreased rapid-eye movement (REM) sleep (6)
Disorders of sleep during pregnancy	Night waking and insomnia (1st and 3rd trimesters) (7)
	Napping, sleep apnea (8)
	Restless leg, snoring, leg twitching/jerking, poor sleep (9)
Disorders of sleep post partum	Frequent awakenings and increase in stage 4 sleep (10)
	Lower sleep efficiency, shorter latency to REM sleep (11)
	Decreased total sleep time (12)
Disorders of sleep during menopause (details in text)	I. Premenopausal/Perimenopausal
	Primary menopausal insomnia, nocturnal awakenings associated with hot flashes
	II. Postmenopausal
	Nocturnal awakenings associated with hot flashes
	Decreased sleep efficiency
	Impaired subjective sleep quality
	Restless leg syndrome (RLS)
	Periodic limb movements of sleep (PLMS)
	Sleep disordered breathing
	Nonrestorative sleep
	Excessive daytime somnolence

recognized postmenopausal period, and a mean Kupperman index of 17, were selected. The inclusion criteria were the following: age ranging from 50 to 65 years, at least 1 year of amenorrhea and an FSH that equaled or exceeded 30 mU/mL, not undergoing hormone therapy, and normal laboratory test results. The patients followed a routine climacteric checkup, answered a questionnaire about sleep, and underwent an all-night PSG recording. Frequencies in percentage of emerging sleep complaints based on the questionnaire and those pertaining to PSG diagnosis were then calculated separately. The subjective prevalence of insomnia was 61%, against 83% in PSG recordings. The prevalence of apnea reported was 23%, against 27% in the PSG. The subjective restless legs syndrome (RLS) prevalence was 45%, and the objective, 27%. Clearly, there was a high prevalence of sleep disturbance in post-menopausal patients, especially insomnia, apnea, and restless legs.

SLEEP DISTURBANCES IN THE PERIMENOPAUSAL, MENOPAUSAL, AND POSTMENOPAUSAL PERIODS

Insomnia

Peri- and postmenopausal women frequently complain of insomnia or poor sleep quality. The finding that women are between 1.2 and 2.0 times more likely than men to report insomnia regardless of definition is one of the most consistent findings in sleep epidemiologic research. Two studies (15,16) offer possible explanations for this difference:(1) biologic differences between men and women, most notably those related to menstrual cycles or menopause symptoms, drive the difference in prevalence; and (2) social differences, particularly women's roles, generate greater sleep disturbance, including insomnia.

Strine et al. (15) used the 2002 National Health Interview Survey (a nationally representative survey of noninstitutionalized adults aged 18 years and older in the United States) to estimate the association of menstrual-related problems with insomnia or regular trouble falling asleep among women 18 to 55 years of age. It was estimated that 31% of the women who had menstrual-related problems had insomnia, compared with 16% of those who did not have such problems. After adjustments were made for age, race, ethnicity, education, marital status, and employment status, women who had menstrual-related problems were 2.4 times more likely to report insomnia than were women who did not have such problems. The 16% prevalence of insomnia among women who did not have menstrual-related insomnia is similar to the estimates of prevalence of regular insomnia among men in other epidemiological studies (16). These findings are consistent with a number of studies identifying factors related to the menstrual cycle as associated with insomnia and sleep disturbance symptoms, and bolster the hypothesis that these factors contribute to the difference in rates of insomnia by sex (17).

A total of 521 women were studied by Owens et al. (18), and insomnia was associated with higher levels of anxiety, depression, stress, higher systolic and diastolic blood pressures, and greater waist-to-hip ratios. Although cross-sectional analyses indicate that sleep disturbance may be independent of menopausal status, transition into postmenopausal status is associated with deleterious changes in sleep among women not receiving hormone replacement therapy (HRT) (18). Interestingly, when subjective and objective sleep measures were compared in peri- and postmenopausal women, these women, relative to premenopausal women, were less satisfied with their sleep, but did not have diminished sleep quality, as measured by polysomnography (19).

Of note, a recent large polysomnography-based study, the Wisconsin Sleep Cohort Study, showed that postmenopausal women were less satisfied with their sleep than premenopausal women, but actually had better sleep documented on an all-night PSG, with longer total sleep times, increases in amounts of short-wave sleep (SWS), and less time awake, in bed (20).

There is significant discussion in the literature regarding the entity of primary menopausal insomnia. The underlying premise is that a symptom of menopause, such as hot flashes or mood disorders, initiates the insomnia. However, even when the symptom is treated, the insomnia persists. General consensus is that the insomnia should then be treated as primary insomnia, with the usual proven interventions of sleep and nap restrictions during the daytime, sleep hygiene principles, and relaxation techniques (21).

HRT has also been found to lead to improvement in both polysomnographic evidence of insomnia and vasomotor symptoms (22,23). In contrast, subjective complaints of insomnia not associated with polysomnographic evidence of increased frequency of arousals tend not to respond to hormonal therapy, as is also the case for nonvasomotor symptoms. Therefore, these may not be due to diminished hormone production (22–24). This nonhormonally related insomnia is of unclear origin, and there are a number of possible etiologies, including (*i*) a period of insomnia due to vasomotor events that led to behavioral conditioning, causing a persistent psycho-physiologic insomnia independent of the vasomotor events (21); (*ii*) unresolved grief associated with menopausal changes (2,3); or (*iii*) insomnia not related to the menopausal status (21).

In a 2007 study by Freedman et al. (25), 102 women (aged 44–56 years) reporting disrupted sleep were recruited through newspaper advertisements. They were assessed with the Pittsburgh Sleep Quality Index and the Hamilton Anxiety and Depression Rating Scales and completed one night of polysomnography in a controlled laboratory setting. Fifty-three percent of the women were found to have a primary sleep disorder (sleep apnea, RLS, or both). The best predictors of *objective* sleep quality (laboratory sleep efficiency) were apneas, periodic limb movements, and brief arousals, whereas those of *subjective* sleep quality (as measured by the Pittsburgh Sleep Quality Index global score) were the Hamilton anxiety score and the number of hot flashes in the first half of the night. These findings suggest that while nocturnal hot flashes may be the cause of sleep disruption in many peri- and postmenopausal women, many of these women have an underlying primary sleep disorder, such as RLS or sleep apnea. Thus, interventions that are intended to reduce the frequency and severity of hot flashes may not be fully effective for a significant number of women.

Hot Flashes

Sleep disorders related to hot flashes affect a majority (75–85%) of peri- and postmenopausal women, with most experiencing them for 12 to 16 months, some for over 5 years (25%) (26), and others have these symptoms even longer. Associated symptoms could include nocturnal awakenings, nausea, dizziness, headache, flushing of face, diaphoresis, and palpitations, all symptoms not conducive to a restful sleep experience. The nocturnal awakenings typically precede the peripheral vasomotor manifestations, possibly associated with the LH pulses and surges (27,28).

The current available body of literature is inconclusive as to the clear correlation of hot flashes and menopause-related sleep disorders. There is conflicting data regarding correlation of subjectively reported hot flashes, sleep efficiency, nocturnal awakenings, and the objective findings on polysomnographic measures of poor sleep (28–31).

Restless Leg Syndrome RLS and Periodic Limb Movements of Sleep in the Older Woman

RLS and periodic limb movement disorder (PLMD) can disturb sleep profoundly. The causes of these conditions are unknown. RLS occurs before sleep starts and causes calf discomfort and restlessness in the legs, which is relieved by movement. PLMD causes periodic leg movements that may awaken the person from sleep. RLS may cause insomnia, while PLMD may cause excessive sleepiness. Both conditions are more common in older people. RLS, one of the most common sleep disorders, was first described in 1672. It is characterized by uncomfortable, tingling, crawling, burning, and prickly limb sensations associated with an irresistible urge to move the limbs to obtain relief, typically occurring while sedentary or at sleep onset (32). In their series of studies done in 2003, Hanson et al. found a female-to-male ratio of 2:1 (32). These results were replicated in the United Kingdom by Van De Vijver et al. in 2004 (33). Similarly, increased prevalence of RLS in women was found in several other studies (34,35). Clark et al. (36) conducted a survey of middle-aged women and noted an incidence of self-reported RLS in almost 50% of the women studied, but did not document whether these women were in a peri- or postmenopausal state.

Sleep-Disordered Breathing

Sleep-disordered breathing (SDB) is common in postmenopausal women. Multiple breathing cessations during sleep occur with sleep apnea. The resulting breathing difficulty disturbs sleep and may cause daytime fatigue. Sleep apnea is linked to high blood pressure and cardiovascular disease.

Although earlier it was believed that SDB was more common in males than in females (8:1, a ratio calculated from a clinic population) (37), more recent polysomnographic studies of a large general population, the Wisconsin Sleep Cohort Study (20), suggest that the male/female ratio is approximately 2.67:1 (38). The overall prevalence in women aged 30 to 60 years is 9%, and further analysis of the Wisconsin data confirmed that menopause itself is an independent risk factor for SDB. After controlling for age, BMI, and several lifestyle factors (19), postmenopausal women were 2.6 times more likely than premenopausal women to have an apnea–hypopnea index greater than 5, and 3.5 times more likely to have the index greater than 15. According to a similar large study in 2001 by Bixler (39), which was also polysomnography based, the exact prevalence of SDB – defined as an apnea–hypopnea index greater than or equal to 15 per hour of sleep – was estimated at 3.9% in postmenopausal women, compared with 0.6% found in premenopausal women.

The study by Bixler et al. further discussed the gender difference in the prevalence of obstructive sleep apnea and SDB (an AHI score of 10 or higher and daytime hypersomnolence). The overall incidence for women was 1.2% and for men, 3.9%. Premenopausal women had a prevalence of 0.6% and postmenopausal women, 1.9%. When they further subdivided postmenopausal women into two groups, one on HRT and one not on HRT, they discovered that the prevalence in the first group was only 0.5% versus 2.7% in the second one (39). This difference between those with and without HRT (especially estrogen) was demonstrated in another study in 2003 (40). Age also plays a role in the prevalence of sleep apnea in women. In the same landmark study, Bixler et al. demonstrated that the prevalence in women aged 20 to 44 years was 0.7%, in women aged 45 to 64 years it was 1.1%, and in the 65- to 100-year-old age group it was 3.1% (39).

Mechanisms underlying this phenomenon during menopause have included a change in the body fat distribution, with an increase in the waist–hip circumference (41) and a decrease in progesterone (42). Women tend to increase abdominal fat with menopause (43). It is hypothesized that this fat redistribution may play an independent role in the development of SDB.

As mentioned earlier, one of the proposed mechanisms for SDB in menopause may be hormone related, specifically progesterone. Progesterone is a known respiratory stimulant in awake women (44). A large cross-sectional, polysomnography-based study of 1315 women not using HRT found an increase in the prevalence and severity of SDB in postmenopausal versus menopausal women (45).

The research and literature on the effectiveness of hormone therapy in the treatment and management of SDB is challenging to summarize, given the variation in hormonal regimens used, and is beyond the scope of this chapter. Overall, however, epidemiologic data suggest a therapeutic effect of HRT (19,46).

CONCLUSION

Sleep disorders are common in older women. The complaints of both insomnia and hypersomnia are more prevalent in postmenopausal women. Of the two most common sleep syndromes, obstructive sleep apnea syndrome is relatively rare in premenopausal nonpregnant women, whereas its prevalence increases during pregnancy and menopause. RLS is more prevalent in women as compared to men, and this prevalence amplifies as women get pregnant and when they reach menopause. The authors recommend that for peri- and postmenopausal women presenting with sleep problems, clinicians must take a comprehensive sleep history to rule out a primary sleep disorder and, if necessary, obtain polysomnography to confirm the diagnosis, and then follow appropriate therapeutic interventions.

ACKNOWLEDGEMENTS

This project has been supported by funds from the Bureau of Health Professions (BHPr), Health Resources and Services Administration (HRSA), and Department of Health and Human Services (DHHS), under grant number HP 00174, Geriatric Academic Career Award. The information or content and conclusions are those of the author and should not be construed as the official position or policy of nor should any endorsements be inferred by the BHPR, HRSA, DHHS, or the U.S. Government.

Our grateful acknowledgements to Donna Rosenstiel, Program Manager for the Vanderbilt Reynolds Geriatric Education Center, for ther invaluable help in preparing the chapter.

REFERENCES

1. Rousseau ME. Women's midlife health: reframing menopause. J Nurse Midwifery 1998;43:208–223.
2. Thomson J, Oswald I. Effect of estrogen on the sleep, mood, and anxiety of menopausal women. Br Med J 1977;2(6098):1317–1319.
3. U. S. Department of Health and Human Services. Depression Guideline Panel. Depression in Primary Care. Vol. 1: Detection and Diagnosis Clinical Practice Guideline. Rockville, MD: Health and Human Services. AHCPR Pub. No. 93-0550.
4. Manber R, Bootzin RR. Sleep and the menstrual cycle. Health Psychol 1997;16:209–214.
5. Mauri M. Sleep and the reproductive cycle: a review. Health Care Women Int 1990;11:409–421.
6. Baker FC, Driver HA, Rogers GG, et al. High nocturnal body temperatures and disturbed sleep in women with primary dysmenorrhea. Am J Physiol 1999;(Endocrinol Metab 40):E1013–E1021.

7. Mindell JA, Jacobsen BJ. Sleep disturbances in pregnancy. Am J Obstet Gynecol Neonatal Nurs 2000;29:590–597.
8. Hedman C, Pohjasvara T, Tolonen U, et al. Effects of pregnancy on mothers' sleep. Sleep Med 2002;3:37–42.
9. Schweiger MS. Sleep disturbances in pregnancy. Am J Obstet Gynecol 1972;114:879–882.
10. Karcan I, Williams RL, Hursch CJ, et al. Characteristics of sleep patterns during late pregnancy and the postpartum periods. Am J Obstet Gynecol 1968;101:579–586.
11. Zaffke ME, Lee KA. Sleep architecture in a postpartum sample: a comparative analysis. Sleep Res 1992; 21:327.
12. Nishihara K, Horiuchi S, Eto H, et al. The development of infants' circadian rest activity rhythm and mothers' rhythm. Physiol Behav 2002;77:91–98.
13. Moline ML, Broch L, Zak, R. Sleep in women across the life cycle from adulthood through menopause. Med Clin N Am 2004; 88:705–736.
14. de Campos HH, Bittencourt LRA, Haidar MA, et al. Sleep disturbance prevalence in postmenopausal women. Rev Bras Ginecol Obstet 2005; 27(12):731–736.
15. Strine TW, Chapman DP, Ahluwalia IB. Menstrual related problems and psychological distress among women in the United States. J Women's Health (Larchmt) 2005;14(4):316–323.
16. Ohayon MM. Epidemiology of insomnia: what we know and what we still need to learn. Sleep Med Rev 2002;6:97–111.
17. Halbreich U, Bornstein J, Pearlstein T, et al. The prevalence, impairment, impact and burden of premenstrual dysphoric disorder (PMS/PMDD). Psychoneuroendocrinology 2003;28(suppl 3):1.
18. Owens JF, Matthews KA. Sleep disturbance in healthy middle-aged women. Maturitas 1998; 30(1):41–50.
19. Young T, Finn L, Austin D, et al. Menopausal status and sleep-disordered breathing in the Wisconsin Sleep Cohort Study. Am J Respir Crit Care Med 2003;167(9):1181–1185.
20. Young T, Rabago D, Zgierska A, et al. Objective and subjective sleep quality in pre, peri and post menopausal women in the Wisconsin Sleep Cohort Study. Sleep 2003;26(6):667–672.
21. Krystal AD, Edinger J, Wohlgemuth W, et al. Sleep in peri-menopausal and post-menopausal women. Sleep Med Rev 1998;2:243–253.
22. Campbell S. Double blind psychometric studies on the effects of natural estrogens on post-menopausal women. In: Campbell S, ed. The Management of the Menopause and Post-Menopausal Years. Baltimore: University Park Press, 1976:149–158.
23. Regestein QR, Schiff I, Tulchinsky D, et al. Relationship among estrogen-induced psycho physiological changes in hypogonadal women. Psychosom Med 1981; 43(2):147–155.
24. Fry JM. Sleep disorders. Med Clin North Am 1987; 71(1):95–110.
25. Freedman RR, Roehrs TA. Sleep disturbance in menopause. Menopause 2007; 14;826–829.
26. Hammond CB, Scott JR, DiSaia PJ, et al. Climacteric. In: Danforths Obstetrics and Gynecology. 8th ed. Philadelphia: Lippincott Williams &Wilkins, 1999:677–697.
27. Belchetz PE. Drug therapy: hormonal treatment of postmenopausal women. N Eng J of Med 1994;330:1062–1071.
28. Freedman RR, Norton D, Woodward S, et al. Core body temperature and circadian rhythm of hot flashes in menopausal women. J Clin Endocrinol Metab 1995; 80:2354–2358.
29. Woodward S, Arfken CL, Ditri DW, et al. Ambient temperature effects on sleep and mood in menopausal women. Sleep 1999; 22(suppl 1): S224–S225.
30. Shaver J, Giblin E, Lentz M, et al. Sleep patterns and stability in perimenopausal women. Sleep 1998;11:556–561.
31. Polo-Kantola P, Errkola R, Irjala K, et al. Climacteric symptoms and sleep quality. Obstet Gynecol 1999;94:219–224.
32. Hanson M, Honour M, Singleton A, et al. Analysis of familial and sporadic restless legs syndrome in age of onset, gender, and severity features. J Neurol 2004; 251(11):1398–1401.

33. van de Vijver DA, Walley T, Petri H. Epidemiology of restless legs syndrome as diagnosed in UK primary care. Sleep Med 2004; 5(5):435–440.
34. Ohayon MM, Roth T. Prevalence of restless legs syndrome and periodic limb movement disorder in the general population. J Psychosom Res 2002; 53(1):547–554.
35. Nichols DA, Allen RP, Grauke JH, et al. Restless legs syndrome symptoms in primary care: a prevalence study. Arch Intern Med 2003; 163(19):2323–2329.
36. Clark AJ, Flowers J, Boots L, et al. Sleep disturbances in midlife women. J Adv Nursing 1995; 22:662–668.
37. Guilleminault C, Quera Sallva M-A, Partnen M, et al. Women and the obstructive sleep apnea syndrome. Chest 1998; 93:104–109.
38. Young T, Palta M, Dempsey J, et al. The occurrence of sleep disordered breathing among middle aged adults. N Eng J Med 1993; 328:1230–1235.
39. Bixler EO, Vgontzas AN, Lin HM, et al. Prevalence of sleep-disordered breathing in women: effects of gender. Am J Respir Crit Care Med 2001; 163(3 pt 1):608–613.
40. Manber R, Kuo TF, Cataldo N, et al. The effects of hormone replacement therapy on sleep-disordered breathing in postmenopausal women: a pilot study. Sleep 2003; 26(2):163–168.
41. Young T. Analytic epidemiology studies of sleep disordered breathing – what explains the gender difference in SDB? Sleep 1993; 16:S1–S2.
42. Manber R, Armitage R. Sex, steroids and sleep: a review. Sleep 1999; 22:540–555.
43. Rousseau ME. Womens midlife health: reframing menopause. J Nurse Midwifery 1998; 43:208–223.
44. Regensteiner JG, Woodard WD, Hagermann DD, et al. Combined effects of female hormones and metabolic rate on ventilatory drives in women. J Appl Physiol 1989; 66:808–813.
45. Dancey DR, Hanly PJ, Soong C, et al. Impact of menopause on the prevalence and severity of sleep apnea. Chest 2001; 120:151–155.
46. Sahar E, Redline S, Young T, et al. Hormone replacement therapy and sleep disordered breathing. Am J Resp Crit Car Med 2003; 167:1186–1192.

14 Napping in Older Adults

Katie L. Stone

Research Institute, California Pacific Medical Center, San Francisco, California, U.S.A.

Sonia Ancoli-Israel

Department of Psychiatry, University of California, San Diego, California, U.S.A.

INTRODUCTION

The prevalence of napping increases with advancing age. A variety of factors contribute to increased napping and sleepiness in older adults, including disruption in nighttime sleep, changes in circadian rhythms, lifestyle factors, and medical and psychiatric comorbidities. The extent to which napping affects sleep at night, functioning during the day, or health in general remains unclear.

Several epidemiologic studies have found that napping is associated with negative health outcomes such as cognitive impairment, increased risk of falls and fractures, and increased risk of mortality. On the other hand, some studies have reported benefits associated with daytime naps in terms of improved evening alertness and memory. There is some evidence suggesting that while brief sleep periods during the day may provide benefit, longer naps may negatively impact nighttime sleep quality. Furthermore, longer naps may lead to a period of sleep inertia following the nap, which may increase the risk for injury due to falls and other adverse outcomes. Additional studies are needed to more fully describe the risks and benefits according to the timing and duration of daytime sleeping among older people. Experimental studies are also needed to determine the mechanisms underlying the relationship between napping and health outcomes. In this chapter, we will review existing literature on the prevalence, causes, and consequences of napping and daytime sleepiness among older adults.

PREVALENCE OF NAPPING AND DAYTIME SLEEPINESS IN OLDER ADULTS

Prevalence of Napping

Prevalence rates for self-reported habitual napping in older adults range from 10% to 61% depending upon the characteristics of the study population, and the definition of napping employed. As described in more detail in the following text, the prevalence of napping assessed objectively (e.g., using wrist actigraphy, a methodology for distinguishing wake from sleep) tends to be higher than that of subjectively reported napping. This is likely due to two reasons. First, many older adults often nap without realizing it; therefore, objective technology would record napping intervals that would not necessarily be reported by the individual. Second, periods of extreme inactivity, which can be considerably more common in older adults, may be scored as naps by objective measures using movement to estimate sleep.

Older adults consistently report more napping than younger adults (1–5). For example, based on a population of healthy younger and older adults in the United States, Buysse et al. (3) found that over a two-week period, younger adults (mean age, 30 years) reported taking an average of 1.1 naps, while older adults (mean age, 78 years) reported taking 3.4 naps. Metz and Bunnell (4) found that "older old" subjects (mean age, 80 years) took an average of five naps per week, while "younger old" subjects (mean age, 65 years) took an average of four naps per week ($p<0.05$). "Older old" subjects also took significantly longer naps (mean, 67.5 minutes) compared with "younger old" subjects (mean, 51.3 minutes; $p<0.05$). Results of the 2003 National Sleep Foundation survey showed that 10% of respondents aged 55 to 64 years reported taking naps regularly (defined as 4–7 times/wk), compared with 24% of respondents aged 75 to 84 years (2). In a U.S. multi-center cohort of 8101 older community-dwelling Caucasian women with a mean age of 77.0 years, Stone et al. (6) found that approximately 11% reported napping daily. In addition, those who reported daily napping were on average older than those who were not daily nappers (79.5 years vs. 76.7 years, respectively; $p<0.001$).

In another study of 413 older men and women aged 60 to 96 years residing in two U.S. communities, approximately 18% reported napping >6 times per week, whereas nearly half (47.5%) reported napping >3 times per week (7). Napping was significantly more common among older adults with sleep complaints, regardless of insomnia symptoms. Using wrist actigraphy to assess daytime napping, Yoon et al. (8) found that even very healthy older adults were somewhat more likely to nap during the day than younger (college-aged) adults (77% vs. 62% of participants, respectively; $p = 0.064$), but did not sleep more in total during the daytime hours compared with younger adults ($p>0.10$). There were also differences in the timing of naps between younger and older subjects, with older adults being more likely to nap in the evening, within two hours of bedtime. In a community-based observational actigraphy study of 2932 very elderly women (mean age, 83.5 years), Blackwell et al. (9) found a large percentage (19%) with recorded napping periods of more than two hours per day.

It is uncertain whether there are gender differences in napping prevalence among older adults. A few studies have suggested that older men may nap more frequently than older women. In one Icelandic study ($N = 800$, aged 65–84 years) (10), it was reported that 50% of men napped regularly compared with 31% of women ($p<0.001$). Similarly, a Swedish study ($N = 876$, aged 65–79 years) (11) found higher napping prevalence among older men than older women (29% versus 15%, respectively; $p<0.001$). However, most other studies conducted elsewhere have found similar prevalence of napping in men and women. Combined prevalence rates have been published in most studies (1,3,4).

Many older adults take unintentional naps (i.e., naps of which they are unaware) such as falling asleep while watching television or reading. Few studies have distinguished between intentional and unintentional naps. It is therefore likely that epidemiological studies may underestimate the total amount of sleep obtained during the daytime hours. Objective actigraphic studies have shown that older adults doze for brief periods during the day, which they may not report as "napping" (8). While both intentional and unintentional naps may have negative consequences, their etiology may differ. Intentional planned naps could be due to customary practices of the population being studied, changes in daily routine (e.g., retirement) that allows for sleep during the daytime hours, or sleepiness. However, unintentional naps are more likely related to pathological daytime sleepiness due to poor health, sleep disorders, or insufficient nighttime sleep. A pattern of inadvertent, frequent, brief sleep episodes intruding upon wakefulness throughout the day may represent serious underlying sleep pathology (12).

Prevalence of Daytime Sleepiness

The constructs of daytime sleepiness and napping are not synonymous, but are clearly related. Individuals who feel sleepy during the day are presumably more likely to actually sleep during the day. In a study of daytime sleepiness and napping, Hays et al. (13) found that 25.2% of older adults over age 65 reported feeling so sleepy during the day or evening that they had to nap. However, it is also important to consider that some older adults may experience sleepiness during the daytime hours without actually sleeping during the day. This sleepiness may have negative consequences even if the person does not actually nap on a regular basis.

Subjective daytime sleepiness is an important clinical issue, as it may reflect either an underlying sleep disturbance or pathology [such as sleep-disordered breathing (SDB)], or medical or psychiatric comorbidity (including the use of sedating medications during the day). While sleep propensity is one important aspect of the subjective experience of sleepiness, other factors are also likely to play a role, including mood and habitual expectations about sleepiness.

Daytime sleepiness is most often assessed by self-reported questionnaires such as the Epworth Sleepiness Scale (ESS) (14), a 24-point scale which assesses an individual's reported likelihood of falling asleep in eight different situations. Typically, a score of ≥ 10 is considered to represent excessive daytime sleepiness (EDS). This measure, however, may be problematic for use among older adults, some of whom may not engage in one or more of the eight activities queried in the ESS (e.g., driving). In addition, this measure was developed for use in sleep clinic populations and has not been validated with older adults in the community (15,16). Other subjective measures assess sleepiness in slightly different ways, for example, by asking about how the individual feels at the moment, or on a typical day (17).

Studies that have examined the prevalence of reports of daytime sleepiness among older adults have reported prevalence estimates ranging from 6% to about 20%. Ohayon and Vecchierini (18) interviewed over 1000 older adults in France and found that 13.6% of the sample reported EDS. Using data from the Cardiovascular Health Study, Whitney et al. (19) studied 4578 older adults (aged 65 and older) in the United States and found that 20% reported significant daytime sleepiness on the ESS.

Despite the increasing prevalence of napping with age, it is uncertain whether the prevalence of EDS is higher (or lower) in older adults compared with their younger counterparts. In a recent study of 2301 Norwegian adults, Pallesen et al. (20) reported significantly lower prevalence of daytime sleepiness in adults aged 60 and older compared with those aged 18 to 29. In addition, EDS was more prevalent among older men than older women (17.5% vs. 10.8%, respectively). Similarly, a study by Bixler et al. of 16,583 central Pennsylvania residents aged 20 and older found that EDS prevalence declined from about 10% in 20-year olds to about 6% in 75-year olds (21). The interpretation of these findings is difficult, however, given that the instruments to assess sleepiness based on subjective report have not been validated in older adults. In addition, younger adults may have limited opportunity to alleviate EDS by taking brief naps during the day as compared with older adults.

Finally, it is difficult to compare prevalence estimates across studies and populations because of the variation in the questionnaires used to assess sleepiness.

Daytime sleepiness can also be considered as the propensity to fall asleep, a construct which is often assessed objectively with laboratory studies such as the Multiple Sleep Latency Test (MSLT) (22). During an MSLT, the individual is given the opportunity to try to sleep at two-hour intervals throughout the day, and the time to sleep onset is recorded. Another objective measure of sleep propensity is the Maintenance of Wakefulness Test (MWT) (23), during which the individual is instructed to try and remain awake while in a dark, quiet environment, and the amount of wake time is recorded. Both the MSLT and the MWT are considered reliable measures of daytime sleep propensity, although the results of these tests do differ for some individuals (24). In addition, use of these tests in large population-based studies of older adults may not be feasible, given the cost, the time required to complete the assessment (one full day), and the need for participants to be in a sleep laboratory or other controlled environment during the testing.

CAUSES OF DAYTIME SLEEPINESS AND NAPPING
The causes of daytime sleepiness and napping are multifactorial, and several possible underlying causes may interact to increase the likelihood that an older person will sleep during the day. Some factors that could result in daytime sleepiness include disruption of nighttime sleep, age-related changes in circadian rhythms, and medical and psychiatric comorbidities. Although sleepiness is a major underlying factor that may lead to napping, sociocultural factors also play a role in determining whether the older adult will actually nap during the day (e.g., customary "siesta" in some cultures, changes in daily activities such as retirement).

Disruption of Nighttime Sleep and Sleep Disorders
Numerous studies have linked napping behaviors to nighttime sleep disruption, including symptoms of insomnia (10,25,26), sleep fragmentation (27–29), poor sleep quality (30), use of long-acting hypnotics or other sedating medications (4,28), and circadian rhythm disturbance (e.g., advanced sleep phase) (4,28,31,32). However, the relationship between nighttime sleep and daytime sleepiness and napping may be bidirectional. Disruption of nighttime sleep may lead some older people to become sleep deprived, therefore impairing their ability to sustain wakefulness throughout the day. These individuals may begin napping to make up for lost sleep at night. On the other hand, others may begin napping, and then as a result, develop difficulties with nighttime sleep. Gislason et al. showed that those who report regular napping are more likely to report chronic difficulty maintaining sleep at night compared with individuals who do not nap (40% vs. 28%, respectively; $p<0.05$) (10). Frisoni et al. (25) found that individuals who napped regularly were more likely to report feeling unrested in the morning. In contrast, other studies found no significant relationship between the severity of nighttime sleep disruption and daytime sleepiness (1,3,11,33,34). However, some of these studies were limited by the small sample size and may have had insufficient statistical power to detect relationships.

In a recent overnight polysomnography study conducted in 174 nursing home residents, Endeshaw et al. (35) found that the only factor significantly associated with daytime sleepiness was the percentage of time spent in rapid eye movement (REM) sleep during the night. Similarly, in a study of older adults aged 65 to 98 years, Pack et al. (36) classified participants according to EDS ($n = 149$ with EDS and $n = 144$ without EDS). Increased percentage time in REM sleep and self-report of poor sleep quality were associated with higher risk of EDS. Sleep disorders, particularly SDB, which increases in prevalence with age (37), may contribute to daytime sleepiness and increase the likelihood of napping. Several large, population-based studies of older adults have shown an association between SDB severity and daytime sleepiness (19,37–39). In the previously mentioned study by Pack et al. (36), it was reported that severe SDB (AHI > 30 episodes/hr) was associated with EDS, whereas presence of periodic limb movements showed no association with EDS. Surprisingly, no studies have explored the association between SDB and napping among older adults. However, in a recent cross-sectional study using polysomnography in 90 habitual nappers and 88 nonnappers aged 18 to 75 years, habitual napping was associated with an increased prevalence of sleep apnea (5.5-fold increase in the risk of having apnea–hypopnea index $\geq$ 15) (40).

Circadian Rhythm Changes

Changes in circadian rhythms with advancing age represent another important factor leading to sleepiness and napping during the daytime. Older adults typically show lower amplitude in circadian rhythms. In addition, there is frequently an advance (i.e., shift earlier) of endogenous circadian rhythms, which may lead older adults to feel sleepier earlier in the evening and awaken earlier in the morning. This phase shift can impact daytime sleepiness and napping in two ways. First, it can lead to insufficient nighttime sleep if the older adult attempts to stay up late, but is "biologically" awakened early in the morning, resulting in insufficient sleep. Second, advanced circadian rhythms can lead to evening napping.

Medical and Psychiatric Factors

Some medical conditions and psychiatric disorders increase fatigue and daytime alertness, which may result in increased napping. Based on data from the 2003 National Sleep Foundation survey of 1506 adults aged 55 to 84 years mentioned earlier, pain, depression, diabetes, stroke, and lung diseases were associated with daytime sleepiness (41). More recently, using data from the same survey, Foley et al. (5) reported that depression, bodily pain, and nocturia were significantly related to daytime napping. Bixler et al. reported that depression is the most important contributor to EDS in older adults, showing stronger relationship even than SDB (21). However, a significant interaction with age was observed such that depression remained a significant factor predicting EDS, but was more weakly related in older adults than younger adults.

Because most of these studies have been cross-sectional and temporal associations could not be established, it cannot be determined whether medical and psychiatric conditions preceded the sleepiness, or vice versa. In addition, it remains uncertain whether medical and psychiatric disorders directly impact daytime sleepiness or whether daytime sleepiness is increased due to reduced ability to obtain sufficient sleep at night.

CORRELATES AND CONSEQUENCES OF NAPPING AND DAYTIME SLEEPINESS

Napping and Nighttime Sleep Quality

Theoretically, napping may increase sleep fragmentation and decrease sleep efficiency, leading to a cycle of increased fatigue and subsequent napping (26,28). Several studies have found that extended daytime napping can negatively impact nighttime sleep. For example, a small laboratory-based study by Monk et al. (42) found that a 1.5-hour daytime nap shortened nighttime sleep, decreased sleep efficiency, and led to earlier morning awakening among nine healthy older adults. Yoon et al. (8,32) found that healthy older adults who napped in the evening hours awoke and got out of bed earlier in the morning, spent less time in bed, and had a shorter sleep period. They also fell asleep more quickly in the evening. One possibility is that, because these older adults napped close to bedtime, they had obtained sufficient total sleep by their morning rise time. As discussed earlier, another possibility is that these older adults had more phase advanced circadian rhythms, which led to an overall earlier sleep period.

Studies examining the general population of older adults have reported an association between napping and nocturnal sleep difficulties, although the duration of daytime naps appears to be a key factor. Metz and Bunnell (4) reported a potential association (not statistically significant) between increased sleep onset latency and nap duration in a group of older adults and suggested that duration of naps had more influence than frequency of naps on difficulty initiating sleep. Longer naps have also been implicated as contributing to frequent nocturnal awakenings among older adults (42,43).

Findings across studies of napping and nighttime sleep quality, however, have not been consistent. Bliwise (34) examined factors related to sleep quality in healthy older women (mean age, 68 years), identifying themselves as good ($n = 22$) or poor ($n = 16$) sleepers. Poor sleepers were characterized by shorter objectively measured nighttime total sleep time and more subjective nonrestorative sleep; however, no differences were found between good and poor sleepers in the number of daily naps. Mallon and Hetta (11) found no difference in total sleep time or sleep problems between individuals who napped and those who did not nap ($n = 876$ adults aged 65–79 years), and Metz and Bunnell (4) found no significant relationship between napping and number of nocturnal awakenings, sleep onset latency, total sleep time, or quality of sleep, although a trend was noted toward more sleep onset difficulty and longer duration of napping. Hsu (44) also found no correlation between naps and quality of sleep among 80 community-dwelling Chinese elders, and Campbell and Dawson (45) found that an afternoon nap had no effect on subsequent nighttime sleep.

Napping and Health Outcomes

Napping has been associated with a variety of health outcomes, including mortality, cardiovascular disease, falls and fractures, and cognitive impairment. Several studies have found that daytime sleepiness and napping are related to increased risk for mortality, whereas the association between napping and risk of cardiovascular disease and coronary mortality has been equivocal. Although few studies have yet to examine the association between napping and risk of falls, this is an area that deserves further study.

In a large study of nearly 6000 older adults (mean age, 73 years), Newman et al. (46) found that reported napping was associated with increased risk for both mortality and cardiovascular disease after controlling for other known risk factors (adjusted odds ratio, 2.34; 95% confidence interval, 1.66–3.29). Campos and Siles (47) studied a cohort of 505 survivors of myocardial infarction (MI) and compared their siesta-taking behavior with a cohort of 522 matched controls without a history of MI. They found that individuals with a history of MI were more likely to take daily siestas and to take longer siestas on an average than those without a history of MI. Individuals with the shortest siesta period were least likely to have a subsequent MI after controlling for known MI risk factors, including lipids, smoking, body mass index, light physical activity, night sleep, and history of diabetes, hypertension, and angina. The prevalence of daily siestas among MI survivors was 44%, compared with 35% in controls ($p = 0.01$). This study, however, did not control for depression or cognitive impairment, both of which may be confounding variables.

Burazeri et al. (48) studied a cohort of older adults (over age 50 years) in Israel using self-reported amount of sleep per 24 hours (including nighttime sleep and daytime sleep). They found that reported sleep duration of more than 8 hours per 24 hours was related to increased mortality risk among men. This finding suggests that longer reported sleeping, whether at night or during the day, is associated with higher mortality risk. In the study mentioned earlier by Hays et al. (13), the authors found that older adults who reported frequent daytime napping were more likely to report problems with nighttime sleep, and had a higher mortality risk than those who napped less frequently. Bursztyn et al. (49–51) found that mortality rates were doubled among older adults in Israel who slept during the day compared with those who rested but did not sleep and to those who did not rest or sleep during the day. They also found that individuals who slept during the day had higher rates of MI and were more likely to have cancer or vascular causes of death compared with those who did not sleep during the day.

A recent study by Naska et al. (52) found that (among 23,681 Greek men and women aged 20–84 with no prior diagnosis of CHD, stroke, or cancer) coronary mortality risk was significantly lower among those reporting regular siesta naps as compared with others. The strongest reduction in risk was observed among working men (mortality ratio, 0.36; 95% confidence interval, 0.16–0.80). Results remained significant when restricted to men aged 60 and above. Importantly, when those with preexisting comorbidities (CHD, stroke, cancer) were not excluded from the analysis, the authors found a significant elevation in risk of coronary mortality among those taking long siesta naps (2 hours or longer). This suggests that the association between increased napping and coronary outcomes reported in some studies may be explained by poor health and preexisting comorbidities among nappers.

A possible association has also been observed between napping and risk of falls. Brassington et al. (53) found that although there was a significant bivariate correlation between reported daytime sleepiness that led to napping and risk of falling, after controlling for other known fall risk factors, there was no additional increase in the risk associated with reported napping. In contrast, Stone et al. (6) studied 8101 community-dwelling women aged 69 and older and found that women who reported napping at least seven times per week were significantly more likely to experience two or more falls in the subsequent year compared with women who took fewer naps (adjusted odds ratio, 1.32; 95% confidence interval, 1.03–1.69). Furthermore, women who napped daily were more likely to suffer an incident hip fracture during six years of follow-up (adjusted hazard ratio, 1.33; 95% confidence interval, 0.99–1.78). The duration of napping was also an important factor in this study. Older women who reported napping at least three hours per week had a significant increase in the odds of suffering two or more falls compared with women napping less than three hours per week in the multivariate model (adjusted odds ratio, 1.33; 95% confidence interval, 1.10–1.60). These associations were independent of other fall risk factors, including use of benzodiazepines. One possible mechanism for this association is that older women may experience a period of sleep inertia upon awakening from a nap, particularly for longer naps. During this time, the risk of accidents and injuries such as falls and fractures may be increased. It is also possible that napping is an indicator of daytime sleepiness due to a nighttime sleep disturbance.

Napping may also increase the risk of cognitive impairment. In a recent actigraphy study, Blackwell et al. (9) studied 2932 older community-dwelling women (mean age, 83.5 years) residing in four communities within the United States. In this study, napping two or more hours per day was associated with greater odds of cognitive impairment. Results were strongest for executive function. Older women who had actigraphic nap durations of ≥2 hours per day were at 1.74-fold increased odds of cognitive impairment compared with those with shorter nap durations (adjusted odds ratio, 1.74; 95% confidence interval, 1.26–2.40). Because this study was cross-sectional, it was not possible to determine the directionality of this association (i.e., whether napping led to cognitive impairment, or vice versa).

Clearly, direct causal links between napping and negative health outcomes cannot be drawn based on available data. It is likely that older people with underlying health conditions are both more likely to sleep during the day and to have shorter survival. It is also possible, however, that daytime sleeping may lead to reduced daytime activities, less exposure to light during the day, fewer social interactions, and other changes that may increase mortality risk. Studies are needed to understand the potential mechanisms underlying the relationship between napping and health outcomes in older adults.

Daytime Sleepiness and Health Outcomes

Daytime sleepiness, independent of napping, can pose serious risks of injuries and premature death. This is reflected in the findings from a 1991 National Sleep Foundation survey, in which 5% of respondents with difficulty sleeping at night reported having an automobile accident due to daytime sleepiness, compared with 2% of those with no problems sleeping (54). Fifty percent reported frequently waking up feeling drowsy or tired. These findings also highlight the impact of nighttime sleep disturbance on increased daytime sleepiness.

Older adults who experience daytime sleepiness have also been shown to be at increased risk of other aging-related outcomes, such as poor physical and cognitive function, and increased cardiovascular risk factors. Gooneratne et al. (55) found that, in a group of older adults (>65 years) in an assisted living facility, those reporting daytime sleepiness were more likely to report functional impairments related to their sleepiness than individuals who did not report daytime sleepiness. This study assessed the subjective experience of sleepiness, but did not assess whether or not the individual slept during the daytime hours, and it is unclear whether the effect of sleepiness on functional impairment was related to actual sleeping during the daytime hours or to other factors that led to the subjective feeling of sleepiness. Nonetheless, these findings do suggest that reported sleepiness could be an important indicator for risk of functional impairment. Other studies have also shown that daytime sleepiness is associated with poor functional status. In the National Sleep Foundation's Sleep in America Poll in older adults mentioned earlier, those who reported the most severe symptoms of sleepiness were less likely to exercise regularly and more likely to have functional impairments (e.g., mobility, fine motor skills, pushing/pulling objects) after controlling for age, body mass index, income, and number of comorbid conditions (56). Another study by Lee et al. (57) examined sleepiness in 137 Alzheimer patients and found that higher levels of daytime sleepiness were associated with greater impairments in instrumental activities of daily living, even apart from cognitive deficits. Daytime sleepiness may also be related to cognitive deficits. Ohayon and Vecchierini (18) found that older adults who reported EDS were more likely to report cognitive impairment across several dimensions, even after controlling for other known risk factors for cognitive impairment. A study by Asada et al. (58) examined reported napping and later development of Alzheimer's disease (AD) and found that while napping under one hour had some protective effects, napping over one hour per day was associated with higher risk of AD among individuals with the APOEε 4 genotype (which is associated with elevated AD risk). A few studies have also suggested an independent link between daytime sleepiness and cardiovascular risk factors. In a study by Choi et al. (59), among 86 patients (mean age, 47 years) with suspected sleep apnea, daytime sleepiness was associated with decreased cardiac function. Goldstein et al. (60) studied 157 healthy men and women aged 55 to 80 who were not hypertensive upon enrollment. EDS (Epworth score > 10) was associated with diagnosis of hypertension five years later, suggesting that simple clinical evaluation for EDS may have prognostic value for identifying older adults at risk for hypertension. In a study by Lindberg et al., women aged 20 to 99 were classified according to EDS and snoring (two major symptoms of obstructive sleep apnea syndrome). Among women aged > 50, increased sleepiness is associated with more than two-fold increased risk of prevalent diabetes, with similar associations observed among those with and without snoring. The presence of snoring and sleepiness together was a strong risk factor for prevalent hypertension among women <50 years (adjusted odds ratio, 3.41; 95% confidence interval, 1.78–6.54), but less so among older women (adjusted odds ratio, 1.50; 95% confidence interval, 1.02–2.19) (61).

BENEFICIAL EFFECTS OF NAPPING AMONG OLDER ADULTS

While this issue has received relatively little attention in the research literature, there is some evidence that relatively short naps can be beneficial under certain circumstances. Theoretically, there may be a U-shaped association between napping and health outcomes, such that those who take brief naps are at the lowest risk of health outcomes, compared with those who take no naps or longer naps. Short naps may increase evening alertness and performance, and improve memory, while lengthy daytime sleep may have adverse consequences (e.g., shortened or fragmented nighttime sleep, period of sleep inertia following the nap).

Most research on the beneficial effects of napping has been conducted with younger adults, shift workers, and long-distance drivers. Findings do suggest beneficial effects of napping on performance and alertness in these populations

(62–65). In young adults, short naps have been shown to reduce subjective sleepiness, increase daytime alertness, improve neurobehavioral performance (particularly in sleep-deprived subjects) (66), and improve mood (67). Furthermore, Vgontzas et al. (65) showed that daytime napping following a night of sleep loss resulted in beneficial changes in cortisol and interleukin-6 secretion. However, the duration of the nap may be critical. For example, in a study by Brooks and Lack, a 30-minute nap resulted in impaired alertness and performance immediately after the nap (indicative of sleep inertia), followed by improvement in these functions. A 10-minute nap produced immediate improvements in cognitive performance as well as sleepiness and fatigue (68). In older adults, a period of sleep inertia following a nap may have very detrimental effects, increasing the risk for injurious falls and other accidents.

Takahashi (69) reviewed the literature on prescribed napping in sleep medicine and concluded that laboratory findings suggest napping can, in fact, be beneficial if properly timed and short in duration. One study showed that older adults may benefit in terms of increased alertness and reduced fatigue from a short (about 30 minutes) nap in the early afternoon. The authors did not find that this short daytime nap negatively impacted nighttime sleep (70). In fact, Asada et al. (58) found that a reported history of short naps (<1 hour) was associated with lower risk of AD among individuals with the APOEε 4 genotype.

In a laboratory study of naps among 32 healthy older adults, Campbell and Dawson (45) found that an afternoon nap (mean duration, 81 minutes) had no negative effect on subsequent nighttime sleep, but increased total sleep time per 24 hours and enhanced cognitive and psychomotor performance immediately after the nap and throughout the next day.

It is somewhat unclear whether napping has beneficial effects in terms of health outcomes. Data from two case–control studies of Greek men across age groups suggested a protective effect of afternoon rests or naps against coronary heart disease (71,72). Findings from these studies have not been confirmed or duplicated in other countries and contradict the numerous recent reports of increased cardiovascular mortality associated with daytime sleepiness or napping(13,46,47, 49–51).

DISCUSSION

In summary, napping and subjective feelings of daytime sleepiness are more common among older than among younger adults. This increase in napping is likely caused by changes in nighttime sleep, circadian rhythms, and lifestyle factors. While a brief sleep period during the day may have some benefit in terms of increased evening alertness, longer periods of daytime sleep may negatively impact nighttime sleep quality and may be associated with negative health outcomes such as cognitive impairment, risk of falls and fractures, cardiovascular complications, and increased mortality risk among older persons. While several studies have examined issues of timing and duration of naps in younger subjects, additional research is needed on the timing and characteristics of napping among older people. Further studies are also needed to explore the mechanisms underlying the relationship between napping and negative health outcomes. Longitudinal studies would be particularly useful to determine if napping and sleepiness precede the onset of adverse health outcomes, or are merely a consequence of illness and other conditions among older adults.

ACKNOWLEDGEMENTS

Supported by Public Health Service Grants AG05407, AR35582, AG05394, AR35584, AR35583, AG08415.

REFERENCES

1. Dinges DF. Napping patterns and effects in human adults. In: Dinges DF, Broughton RJ, eds. Sleep and Alertness: Chronobiological, Behavioral and Medical Aspects of Napping. New York: Raven Press, 1989:171–204.
2. 2003 Sleep in America Poll. National Sleep Foundation (Accessed at www.sleepfoundation.org/polls/2003SleepPollExecutiveSumm.pdf.)
3. Buysse DJ, Browman KE, Monk TH, et al. Napping and 24-hour sleep/wake patterns in healthy elderly and young adults. J Am Geriatr Soc 1992; 40(8):779–786.
4. Metz ME, Bunnell DE. Napping and sleep disturbances in the elderly. Fam Pract Res J 1990; 10(1):47–56.
5. Foley DJ, Vitiello MV, Bliwise DL, et al. Frequent napping is associated with excessive daytime sleepiness, depression, pain, and nocturia in older adults: findings from the National Sleep Foundation '2003 Sleep in America' Poll. Am J Geriatr Psychiatry 2007; 15(4):344–350.
6. Stone KL, Ewing SK, Lui LY, et al. Self-reported sleep and nap habits and risk of falls and fractures in older women: the study of osteoporotic fractures. J Am Geriatr Soc 2006; 54(8):1177–1183.
7. McCrae CS, Rowe MA, Dautovich ND, et al. Sleep hygiene practices in two community dwelling samples of older adults. Sleep 2006; 29(12):1551–1560.
8. Yoon IY, Kripke DF, Youngstedt SD, et al. Actigraphy suggests age-related differences in napping and nocturnal sleep. J Sleep Res 2003; 12(2):87–93.
9. Blackwell T, Yaffe K, Ancoli-Israel S, et al. Poor sleep is associated with impaired cognitive function in older women: the study of osteoporotic fractures. J Gerontol A Biol Sci Med Sci 2006; 61(4):405–410.
10. Gislason T, Reynisdottir H, Kristbjarnarson H, et al. Sleep habits and sleep disturbances among the elderly – an epidemiological survey. J Intern Med 1993; 234(1):31–39.
11. Mallon L, Hetta J. A survey of sleep habits and sleeping difficulties in an elderly Swedish population. Ups J Med Sci 1997; 102(3):185–197.
12. Schmitt FA, Phillips BA, Cook YR, et al. Self report on sleep symptoms in older adults: correlates of daytime sleepiness and health. Sleep 1996; 19(1):59–64.
13. Hays JC, Blazer DG, Foley DJ. Risk of napping: excessive daytime sleepiness and mortality in an older community population. J Am Geriatr Soc 1996; 44(6):693–698.
14. Johns MW. A new method for measuring daytime sleepiness: the Epworth sleepiness scale. Sleep 1991; 14(6):540–545.
15. Martin JL, Ancoli-Israel S. Napping in older adults. Sleep Med Clin 2006; 1:177–186.
16. Ancoli-Israel S, Martin JL. Insomnia and daytime napping in older adults. J Clin Sleep Med 2006; 2:333–342.
17. Mitler MM, Carskadon MA, Hirshkowitz M. Evaluating sleepiness. In: Kryger MH, Roth T, Dement WC, eds. Principles and Practice of Sleep Medicine. Philadelphia: Elsevier Saunders, 2005:1417–1423.
18. Ohayon MM, Vecchierini MF. Daytime sleepiness and cognitive impairment in the elderly population. Arch Intern Med 2002; 162(2):201–208.
19. Whitney CW, Enright PL, Newman AB, et al. Correlates of daytime sleepiness in 4578 elderly people: the Cardiovascular Health Study. Sleep 1998; 21(1):27–36.
20. Pallesen S, Nordhus IH, Omvik S, et al. Prevalence and risk factors of subjective sleepiness in the general adult population. Sleep 2007; 30(5):619–624.
21. Bixler EO, Vgontzas AN, Lin HM, et al. Excessive daytime sleepiness in a general population sample: the role of sleep apnea, age, obesity, diabetes, and depression. J Clin Endocrinol Metab 2005; 90(8):4510–4515.

22. Carskadon MA, Dement WC, Mitler MM, et al. Guidelines for the multiple sleep latency test (MSLT): a standard measure of sleepiness. Sleep 1986; 9(4):519–524.
23. Mitler MM, Gujavarty KS, Browman CP. Maintenance of wakefulness test: a polysomnographic technique for evaluating treatment efficacy in patients with excessive somnolence. Electroencephalogr Clin Neurophysiol 1982; 53:658–661.
24. Sangal RB, Thomas L, Mitler MM. Disorders of excessive sleepiness. Treatment improves ability to stay awake but does not reduce sleepiness. Chest 1992; 102(3):699–703.
25. Frisoni GB, De Leo D, Rozzini R, et al. Napping in the elderly and its associations wtih night sleep and psychological status. Int Psychogeriatr 1996; 8:477–487.
26. Carskadon MA, Brown ED, Dement WC. Sleep fragmentation in the elderly: relationship to daytime sleep tendency. Neurobiol Aging 1982; 3(4):321–327.
27. Foley D, Monjan A, Masaki K, et al. Daytime sleepiness is associated with 3-year incident dementia and cognitive decline in older Japanese-American men. J Am Geriatr Soc 2001; 49(12):1628–1632.
28. Ancoli-Israel S, Kripke DF. Prevalent sleep problems in the aged. Biofeedback Self Regul 1991; 16(4):349–359.
29. Ohayon MM, Caulet M, Philip P, et al. How sleep and mental disorders are related to complaints of daytime sleepiness. Arch Intern Med 1997; 157(22):2645–2652.
30. Pilcher JJ, Schoeling SE, Prosansky CM. Self-report sleep habits as predictors of subjective sleepiness. Behav Med 2000; 25(4):161–168.
31. Ancoli-Israel S. Insomnia in the elderly: a review for the primary care practitioner. Sleep 2000; 23(suppl 1):S23–S30; discussion S6–S8.
32. Yoon IY, Kripke DF, Elliott JA, et al. Age-related changes of circadian rhythms and sleep–wake cycles. J Am Geriatr Soc 2003; 51(8):1085–1091.
33. Asplund R. Sleep disorders in the elderly. Drugs Aging 1999; 14(2):91–103.
34. Bliwise NG. Factors related to sleep quality in healthy elderly women. Psychol Aging 1992; 7(1):83–88.
35. Endeshaw YW, Ouslander JG, Schnelle JF, et al. Polysomnographic and clinical correlates of behaviorally observed daytime sleep in nursing home residents. J Gerontol A Biol Sci Med Sci 2007; 62(1):55–61.
36. Pack AI, Dinges DF, Gehrman PR, et al. Risk factors for excessive sleepiness in older adults. Ann Neurol 2006; 59(6):893–904.
37. Ancoli-Israel S, Kripke DF, Klauber MR, et al. Sleep-disordered breathing in community-dwelling elderly. Sleep 1991; 14(6):486–495.
38. Foley DJ, Masaki K, White L, et al. Sleep-disordered breathing and cognitive impairment in elderly Japanese-American men. Sleep 2003; 26(5):596–599.
39. Gottlieb DJ, Whitney CW, Bonekat WH, et al. Relation of sleepiness to respiratory disturbance index: the Sleep Heart Health Study. Am J Respir Crit Care Med 1999; 159(2):502–507.
40. Masa JF, Rubio M, Perez P, et al. Association between habitual naps and sleep apnea. Sleep 2006; 29(11):1463–1468.
41. Foley D, Ancoli-Israel S, Britz P, et al. Sleep disturbances and chronic disease in older adults: results of the 2003 National Sleep Foundation Sleep in America Survey. J Psychosom Res 2004; 56(5):497–502.
42. Monk TH, Buysse DJ, Carrier J, et al. Effects of afternoon "siesta" naps on sleep, alertness, performance, and circadian rhythms in the elderly. Sleep 2001; 24(6):680–687.
43. Floyd JA. Sleep and aging. Nurs Clin North Am 2002; 37(4):719–731.
44. Hsu HC. Relationships between quality of sleep and its related factors among elderly Chinese immigrants in the Seattle area. J Nurs Res 2001; 9(5):179–190.
45. Campbell SS, Dawson D. Aging young sleep: a test of the phase advance hypothesis of sleep disturbance in the elderly. J Sleep Res 1992; 1(3):205–210.
46. Newman AB, Spiekerman CF, Enright P, et al. Daytime sleepiness predicts mortality and cardiovascular disease in older adults. The Cardiovascular Health Study Research Group. J Am Geriatr Soc 2000; 48(2):115–123.

47. Campos H, Siles X. Siesta and the risk of coronary heart disease: results from a population-based, case–control study in Costa Rica. Int J Epidemiol 2000; 29:429–437.

48. Burazeri G, Gofin J, Kark JD. Over 8 hours of sleep–marker of increased mortality in Mediterranean population: follow-up population study. Croat Med J 2003; 44(2):193–198.

49. Bursztyn M, Ginsberg G, Stessman J. The siesta and mortality in the elderly: effect of rest without sleep and daytime sleep duration. Sleep 2002; 25(2):187–191.

50. Bursztyn M, Ginsberg G, Hammerman-Rozenberg R, et al. The siesta in the elderly: risk factor for mortality? Arch Intern Med 1999; 159(14):1582–1586.

51. Bursztyn M, Stessman J. The siesta and mortality: twelve years of prospective observations in 70-year-olds. Sleep 2005; 28(3):345–347.

52. Naska A, Oikonomou E, Trichopoulou A, et al. Siesta in healthy adults and coronary mortality in the general population. Arch Intern Med 2007; 167(3):296–301.

53. Brassington GS, King AC, Bliwise DL. Sleep problems as a risk factor for falls in a sample of community-dwelling adults aged 64–99 years. J Am Geriatr Soc 2000; 48(10):1234–1240.

54. Roth T, Ancoli-Israel S. Daytime consequences and correlates of insomnia in the United States: results of the 1991 National Sleep Foundation Survey. II. Sleep 1999; 22(suppl 2):S354–S358.

55. Gooneratne NS, Weaver TE, Cater JR, et al. Functional outcomes of excessive daytime sleepiness in older adults. J Am Geriatr Soc 2003; 51(5):642–649.

56. Chasens ER, Sereika SM, Weaver TE, et al. Daytime sleepiness, exercise, and physical function in older adults. J Sleep Res 2007; 16(1):60–65.

57. Lee JH, Bliwise DL, Ansari FP, et al. Daytime sleepiness and functional impairment in Alzheimer disease. Am J Geriatr Psychiatry 2007; 15(7):620–626.

58. Asada T, Motonaga T, Yamagata Z, et al. Associations between retrospectively recalled napping behavior and later development of Alzheimer's disease: association with APOE genotypes. Sleep 2000; 23(5):629–634.

59. Choi JB, Nelesen R, Loredo JS, et al. Sleepiness in obstructive sleep apnea: a harbinger of impaired cardiac function? Sleep 2006; 29(12):1531–1536.

60. Goldstein IB, Ancoli-Israel S, Shapiro D. Relationship between daytime sleepiness and blood pressure in healthy older adults. Am J Hypertens 2004; 17(9):787–792.

61. Lindberg E, Berne C, Franklin KA, et al. Snoring and daytime sleepiness as risk factors for hypertension and diabetes in women – a population-based study. Respir Med 2007; 101(6):1283–1290.

62. Purnell MT, Feyer AM, Herbison GP. The impact of a nap opportunity during the night shift on the performance and alertness of 12-h shift workers. J Sleep Res 2002; 11(3):219–2227.

63. Macchi MM, Boulos Z, Ranney T, et al. Effects of an afternoon nap on nighttime alertness and performance in long-haul drivers. Accid Anal Prev 2002; 34(6):825–834.

64. Takahashi M, Arito H. Maintenance of alertness and performance by a brief nap after lunch under prior sleep deficit. Sleep 2000; 23(6):813–819.

65. Vgontzas AN, Pejovic S, Zoumakis E, et al. Daytime napping after a night of sleep loss decreases sleepiness, improves performance, and causes beneficial changes in cortisol and interleukin-6 secretion. Am J Physiol Endocrinol Metab 2007; 292(1):E253–E261.

66. Taub JM. Effects of scheduled afternoon naps and bedrest on daytime alertness. Int J Neurosci 1982; 16(2):107–127.

67. Daiss SR, Bertelson AD, Benjamin LT, Jr. Napping versus resting: effects on performance and mood. Psychophysiology 1986; 23(1):82–88.

68. Brooks A, Lack L. A brief afternoon nap following nocturnal sleep restriction: which nap duration is most recuperative? Sleep 2006; 29(6):831–840.

69. Takahashi M. The role of prescribed napping in sleep medicine. Sleep Med Rev 2003; 7(3):227–235.

70. Tamaki M, Shirota A, Hayashi M, et al. Restorative effects of a short afternoon nap (<30 min) in the elderly on subjective mood, performance and eeg activity. Sleep Res Online 2000; 3(3):131–139.
71. Trichopoulos D, Tzonou A, Christopoulos C, et al. Does a siesta protect from coronary heart disease? Lancet 1987; 2(8553):269–270.
72. Kalandidi A, Tzonou A, Toupadaki N, et al. A case–control study of coronary heart disease in Athens, Greece. Int J Epidemiol 1992; 21(6):1074–1080.

15 Sleep in Late-Stage Dementia and End of Life

Shoab A. Nazir

Division of Pulmonary, Critical Care and Sleep Medicine, University of Arkansas for Medical Sciences, and Central Arkansas Veterans Health Care System, Little Rock, Arkansas, U.S.A.

Kathy C. Richards

Polisher Research Institute, Madlyn and Leonard Abramson Center for Jewish Life, and School of Nursing, University of Pennsylvania, Philadelphia, Pennsylvania, U.S.A.

INTRODUCTION

Dementia is characterized by a global decline in cognitive abilities that results in an impairment of performance of previously learned activities of daily living. The types of dementias can be categorized according to clinical presentation, neuropathology, and etiology. Although sleep disturbances are common in older adults compared with younger adults, sleep is much more disturbed in persons with dementia (1–3). Nineteen to forty-four percent of community-dwelling persons with dementia have some form of sleep disturbance (4–6). Many disorders causing dementia result in degenerative changes in regions of the brain involved in the regulation of sleep and wakefulness. A pattern common to all dementias includes sleep fragmentation and disruption of the sleep–wake cycle. Sleep disturbances have serious consequences such as increased aggression, daytime cognitive impairment, falls, and institutionalization (7–11). Sleep disturbances mirror the severity of dementia and may even accelerate cognitive and functional decline (12,13). Sleep disturbances increase caregiver burden and interrupt caregivers' sleep, which might also result in institutionalization (14).

EPIDEMIOLOGY OF DEMENTIA

Alzheimer's disease (AD) is the most common type of dementia, with an estimated 4.5 million Americans with the disease, and the number is projected to reach 13.2 million by 2050 (15). Vascular dementia is the second most common type of dementia, with a prevalence of 1% to 4% in individuals over age 65 years (16). Dementia with Lewy bodies (DLB) is the third most common type of dementia, with an estimated prevalence of 0.7%, and has been reported in 15% to 25% of hospital-based cases at autopsy (17). Up to 80% of patients with Parkinson's disease (PD) may develop dementia within 8 years of diagnosis, and male gender and the presence of visual hallucinations are highly predictive of dementia in PD (18,19). Other less common forms of dementia include progressive supranuclear palsy (PSP), Huntington's disease (HD), Creutzfeldt–Jakob disease, and frontotemporal dementia (FTD). The prevalence of dementia is higher among nursing home residents, with about 50% of newly admitted residents having dementia (20).

MANIFESTATIONS

Sleep disturbances in dementia may manifest as insomnia, hypersomnia, excessive motor activity at night, and behavioral problems. In addition, patients may have other coexisting primary sleep disorders such as sleep-disordered breathing.

Hypersomnia

Excessive daytime sleepiness (EDS) has been shown to be an early indicator of dementia and has a positive correlation with the severity of dementia (21,22). Patients with PD and those with parkinsonian syndromes such as DLB, multisystem atrophy, and Shy–Drager syndrome suffer from EDS. EDS itself may be associated with an increased risk for the development of PD and is more common in PD with dementia than in AD (23,24). AD patients with more reported daytime napping seem to have more parkinsonian motor signs, suggesting that this subgroup may have an increased propensity for sleepiness resembling PD (25). DLB patients have more daytime hypersomnia than patients with AD (26).

Circadian Rhythm Disorders

Circadian function may be normal in mild or early forms of dementia (27,28). Changes in the sleep–wake cycles seem to parallel the severity of dementia (12,29–32). The ability to maintain daily cortisol rhythms in association with disturbed rest/activity and sleep cycles in early dementia suggests lack of global circadian dysfunction, but perhaps focal abnormalities in elements that control sleep and activity rhythms (10). Cyclic worsening of agitation and confusion in the evening hours, commonly referred to as "sundowning" in demented persons, are thought to occur because of circadian disturbances, particularly due to a phase delay of the core body temperature (33–35). Circadian abnormalities in patients with AD are manifested by increased frequency and duration of nocturnal awakenings and daytime naps, and increased nighttime and decreased daytime motor activity (4,12,36). Circadian abnormalities, including agitation, may be perpetuated by decreased exposure to morning bright light, particularly in the nursing home setting (37,38). Sleep is known to be more fragmented in DLB than in AD and may partly be related to greater disturbances of locomotor activity circadian rhythms (26,39). Disrupted day–night activities related to abnormalities in the circadian molecular machinery have also been shown in animal models of HD (40). However, precise mechanisms underlying the sleep disturbances in humans with HD are still not clear (41).

REM Behavior Disorder

REM behavior disorder (RBD) is characterized by the loss of rapid eye movement (REM) sleep-associated skeletal muscle atonia and is related to dysfunction of REM sleep control. The association of RBD with PD, DLB, and other disorders with Lewy body pathology is well established (42). RBD is now considered a suggestive feature in the clinical diagnostic criteria for DLB (43). RBD tends to precede the onset of PD or dementia by years or decades in up to 40% to 60% of the cases (44–51). RBD is not common in AD. One reported case was subsequently found to be associated with Lewy bodies on neuropathologic examination (52,53).

Periodic Limb Movements and Restless Legs Syndrome

Periodic limb movements in sleep (PLMS) and restless legs syndrome (RLS) are widely prevalent in the elderly, with estimates of 9% to 24% for RLS and up to 45%

for PLMS (54–56). Many patients with dementia are also on other medications such as dopamine antagonists and antidepressants that may potentially worsen these movement disorders. It is possible that these disorders play a significant role in perpetuating nocturnal agitation, wandering, and insomnia in patients with dementia.

Sleep-Disordered Breathing
Demented patients are more likely to have sleep-disordered breathing (SDB) such as obstructive sleep apnea (OSA) (57). In addition, a higher prevalence of dementia has been noted in patients with OSA compared with those without OSA (58). Seventy to ninety percent of patients with AD have OSA, and there is a significant positive correlation with the apnea index and the severity of dementia and the degree of agitation (59–62). The apolipoprotein E-epsilon 4/4 gene (ApoE ε4), which is a well-known risk factor for AD, is now thought to be a risk factor for OSA as well (63,64). The severity of OSA in nondemented subjects has a positive correlation with the degree of memory dysfunction only in ApoE ε4 carriers (65). A preliminary study showed that patients with AD with SDB have less REM sleep compared with those without SDB, but there was no difference in other sleep stages (66). SDB could thus compound cognitive dysfunction since REM sleep is also known to be important for memory consolidation. Patients with vascular dementia have an even higher incidence of OSA compared with patients with AD (67).

EEG ABNORMALITIES AND POLYSOMNOGRAPHIC FINDINGS IN DEMENTIA
Almost all dementias are associated with many abnormal but nonspecific EEG and polysomnographic (PSG) findings. PSG recordings in persons with AD show sleep fragmentation, EEG slowing during REM sleep, decreased percentage of REM sleep time, decreased number of REM periods, increased REM latency, and decreased slow-wave sleep in comparison with age-matched healthy controls or patients with depression (31,68–71).

NEUROBIOLOGY OF SLEEP IN DEMENTIA
Melatonin levels have been found to be lower in patients with AD and are thought to mediate changes in circadian rhythms (72,73). The melatonin decrease was specifically profound in AD patients carrying the ApoE ε4 genotype which is a predictor of early onset AD (72,74). However, in a longitudinal study, patients with AD who were ApoE ε4 negative were shown to have worse sleep efficiency and increased time awake after sleep onset (75). A more recent study showed that polymorphic variations in the enzyme monoamine oxidase A decreased the amount of serotonin available for conversion to melatonin and increased the propensity for sleep disruption in AD, while ApoE ε4 status had no effect (76). In AD, the decreased ability of the hippocampus to suppress the hypothalamic–pituitary–adrenal axis via its negative feedback on the paraventricular nucleus is proposed to play a role in the reduction of slow-wave sleep and declarative memory loss (77). Although RBD is frequently associated with synucleinopathies like DLB, it has also been reported in patients with parkinsonism with parkin gene Park2 mutations who have a lower incidence of synuclein deposition, indicating that mechanisms other than synuclein deposition may cause RBD (78).

ASSESSMENT OF SLEEP IN DEMENTIA

The evaluation of sleep in the demented patient can be quite challenging. Although PSG is a standard tool to study sleep, it can be highly intrusive and difficult to conduct in patients with moderate to severe dementia. Less invasive and more ambulatory tools such as actigraphy and the minimally invasive telemetric actigraphy devices provide additional information about circadian rhythms and sleep/wake patterns that cannot be determined by PSG (3,36,79). Behavioral observations, although labor intensive, are added tools to study sleep in this difficult population (80). The frequency of the behavioral observations affects their sensitivity, and they are more effective when observations are made more frequently (81). Sleep reports of live-in caregivers correlate with measures of nighttime sleep disturbance measured by actigraphy (82), but this correlation seems to be influenced by a number of patient and caregiver factors. McCurry et al. showed that less demented and less depressed patients sleep well despite caregiver reports of poor sleep, and caregivers who used criticism as a behavioral management strategy were more likely to make discrepant reports (83).

The diagnosis of RLS is particularly problematic in the elderly with dementia due to the cognitive impairment; there are no valid objective methods of diagnosing RLS in this patient population. Abnormal behaviors such as rubbing or pounding the legs or excessive motor activity observed by caregivers have been proposed as possible countermeasures to overcome the unpleasant sensations associated with RLS (84). Finally, although PSG is the "gold standard" for the diagnosis of SDB, the use of portable monitoring devices may aid in making the diagnosis in a less invasive manner and under more familiar surroundings. This approach is, however, not well validated, and with the rising prevalence of SDB, well-conducted studies are urgently needed (85,86). The assessment of sleep in patients with dementia is best served with a complementary approach using various modalities.

MANAGEMENT OF SLEEP DISORDERS IN DEMENTIA

Management of sleep disturbances in dementia should be individualized and guided by the underlying specific sleep disorder. Care must be taken to recognize and identify acute causes of delirium, which may cause sleep disturbance in patients with dementia. Management strategies may be divided into pharmacologic and nonpharmacologic approaches.

Nonpharmacologic Approaches
Environmental and Behavioral Interventions

Environmental factors have a profound impact on sleep, particularly in the nursing home setting. Nighttime noise, light changes, and scheduled incontinence care practices are important factors that result in sleep fragmentation (87,88). However, interventions to minimize nighttime noise levels and light exposures may not significantly improve sleep in nursing home residents if the noise reduction is not potent enough, since there is good correlation between the change in noise levels and the change in sleep (89). In one study, changes in nighttime care schedules decreased the frequency of awakenings but affected no other sleep variable (87). A pilot study evaluating structured daytime activity showed improvements in nighttime sleep efficiency and decreased daytime napping (90). A larger follow-up study with a control group showed that individualized social activity based on the severity of dementia increased nighttime sleep and decreased the day/night sleep ratio (91). A combination of increased daytime physical activity and nighttime interventions to decrease noise and disruptive nighttime nursing home care may improve nighttime sleep and agitation (92). However, two large controlled trials evaluating a multidimensional approach of increased daytime activity, daytime or evening bright light exposure, structured bedtime, and nondisruptive nighttime care showed reductions in daytime sleep but no significant improvements in nighttime sleep quality in institutionalized patients (93,94). A comprehensive program was more successful in improving sleep parameters in patients with AD who lived at home, suggesting that the sleep environment may play an important role (95). More robust interventions combined with judicious use of pharmacotherapy may yield better results in severely demented patients living in nursing homes.

Light Therapy
Patients with dementia, particularly those living in nursing homes, have inadequate light exposure and abnormal circadian rhythms. Studies evaluating the utility of light therapy in patients with dementia have shown mixed results. Light therapy seems to have no effect on agitation in institutionalized patients (96). In a heterogeneous group of patients with different types of dementia, exposure to bright light in the morning and evening delayed the acrophase of activity rhythms and strengthened the circadian rhythms, but had no effect on other sleep parameters (97). Applying the same protocol to patients with AD, light therapy consolidated nighttime sleep without affecting either the duration of daytime and nighttime sleep or the acrophase of activity rhythms (98). In one study, morning bright light therapy for 4 weeks in patients with AD not only improved nighttime sleep percentage and decreased daytime napping, but also improved cognition measured by the Mini-Mental State Examination (MMSE) (99). This and other studies suggest that a longer duration of treatment may result in better sleep parameters that may persist for some time after treatment (100–102).

Continuous Positive Airway Pressure
Patients with dementia and concurrent OSA tolerate continuous positive airway pressure (CPAP) fairly well, and noncompliance is usually associated with depression (103). Treatment with CPAP also decreases subjective daytime sleepiness in patients with AD (104). Age and the presence of dementia should not hinder the utilization of CPAP.

Alternative Modalities
Passive body heating by immersion in hot water before bedtime has shown to improve sleep efficiency and decrease sleep onset latency and wake time after sleep onset in elderly insomniacs with vascular dementia without affecting the endogenous circadian rhythm (105). Other modalities such as acupressure (106), massage (107), aromatherapy (108), and exercise programs (92) may help improve sleep in patients with dementia. Active intervention to provide caregivers with assistance to implement good sleep hygiene measures in patients with dementia results in better sleep and exercise schedules and less daytime napping (109).

Pharmacologic Approaches

The use of sedative-hypnotics to improve sleep in the elderly is controversial due to the risk of falls associated with their use, both in the community and in the nursing home setting (110,111). The newer nonbenzodiazepine agents seem to be no safer (112). However, it has also been shown that sleep disturbance itself is an independent predictor of falls, and it is unclear if pharmacotherapy imparts a greater risk (113). Cholinesterase inhibitors are commonly used for the cognitive decline in patients with dementia. Since they increase the levels of acetylcholine in the brain, increased REM sleep has been associated with their use (114). Along with the increase in REM sleep, a higher incidence of nightmares have been reported (115). Among the three acetylcholinesterase inhibitors currently approved for dementia, donepezil increases stage 2 sleep compared with galantamine and rivastigmine (116). Galantamine and rivastigmine have less of an effect on sleep overall (117–120). Modafinil may be a useful drug to treat excessive daytime sleepiness in PD and in other forms of dementia (121–123). Presently, there is no evidence to support the use of melatonin for sleep disturbances or cognitive impairment in people with dementia (124–126). Atypical antipsychotics have been shown to be effective in treating the behavioral disturbances of dementia. Some are also effective in improving sleep. Risperidone and quetiapine are effective in decreasing nighttime aggressiveness and wandering and in increasing sleep efficiency due to their dose-related hypnotic effects (127–130). Dopamine agonists are the preferred medications for the treatment of PLMS and RLS (131,132). These include the Food and Drug Administration–approved agents ropinirole and pramipexole, but other agents such as carbidopa-levodopa and pergolide are also effective.

SLEEP IN THE CAREGIVER

Poor sleep patterns in caregivers of patients with dementia are very common. Disrupted sleep routines, caregiver burden, poor physical and mental health, and poor family functioning are contributory (133,134). Sleep tends to be shorter, particularly in the elderly caregiver (135). Caregiver sleep significantly improves with institutional respite care of demented patients, but sleep quality in the demented subjects worsens during the respite care (136). Adult daycare services may decrease the time that dementia caregivers have to deal with behavioral issues, giving them valuable time to recuperate (137). Poor sleep in older caregivers of patients with dementia may be associated with increased levels of catecholamines and markers for inflammation and coagulation, potentially predisposing them to a higher risk of cardiovascular disease (138,139).

SLEEP IN END OF LIFE

Pain is often reported by many dying elderly, and patients with dementia are just as likely to experience pain towards the end of their lives (140). The assessment of pain in advanced dementia is a challenge and the ability of health care providers to evaluate pain may be suboptimal, particularly in those with advanced dementia (141). Various evaluation tools have been developed for the assessment of pain in persons with cognitive impairment (142,143). Demented patients are less likely to be referred to a hospice, although hospice care has been shown to improve psychiatric and behavioral symptoms and perhaps lessen pain and improve sleep in this patient population (144,145). Older benzodiazepines are just as effective as the newer nonbenzodiazepine hypnotics such as zolpidem for the treatment of insomnia in a hospice setting (146).

SUMMARY

Sleep disturbances are common in persons with dementia. They may manifest as insomnia, hypersomnia, circadian rhythm disorders, parasomnias, and SDB. Sleep disturbances are one of the leading causes for institutionalization. The assessment of sleep disorders in dementia needs to be multifaceted. Yet, current methodologies may be inadequate in the evaluation of certain disorders such as RLS, which are prevalent in the elderly. A multicomponent approach including judicious use of pharmacotherapy for the treatment of these sleep disturbances will have the greatest yield. Hospice care may be a viable option toward the end of life to lessen the impact of poor sleep and behavioral problems. Finally, it is important to address the sleep needs of the burdened caregiver of persons with dementia.

REFERENCES

1. Foley DJ, Monjan AA, Brown SL, et al. Sleep complaints among elderly persons: an epidemiologic study of three communities. Sleep 1995; 18(6):425–432.
2. Motohashi Y, Maeda A, Wakamatsu H, et al. Circadian rhythm abnormalities of wrist activity of institutionalized dependent elderly persons with dementia. J Gerontol A Biol Sci Med Sci 2000; 55(12):M740–M743.
3. Sullivan SC, Richards KC. Predictors of circadian sleep–wake rhythm maintenance in elders with dementia. Aging Ment Health 2004; 8(2):143–152.
4. McCurry SM, Logsdon RG, Teri L, et al. Characteristics of sleep disturbance in community-dwelling Alzheimer's disease patients. J Geriatr Psychiatry Neurol 1999; 12(2):53–59.
5. Ritchie K. Behavioral disturbances of dementia in ambulatory care settings. Int Psychogeriatr 1996; 8(suppl 3):439–442.
6. Lyketsos CG, Lopez O, Jones B, et al. Prevalence of neuropsychiatric symptoms in dementia and mild cognitive impairment: results from the cardiovascular health study. JAMA 2002; 288(12):1475–1483.
7. Avidan AY, Fries BE, James ML, et al. Insomnia and hypnotic use, recorded in the minimum data set, as predictors of falls and hip fractures in Michigan nursing homes. J Am Geriatr Soc 2005; 53(6):955–962.
8. Moran M, Lynch CA, Walsh C, et al. Sleep disturbance in mild to moderate Alzheimer's disease. Sleep Med 2005; 6(4):347–352.
9. Blackwell T, Ancoli-Israel S, Gehrman PR, et al. Actigraphy scoring reliability in the study of osteoporotic fractures. Sleep 2005; 28(12):1599–1605.
10. Hatfield CF, Herbert J, van Someren EJ, et al. Disrupted daily activity/rest cycles in relation to daily cortisol rhythms of home-dwelling patients with early Alzheimer's dementia. Brain 2004; 127(Pt 5):1061–1074.
11. Steeman E, Abraham IL, Godderis J. Risk profiles for institutionalization in a cohort of elderly people with dementia or depression. Arch Psychiatr Nurs 1997; 11(6):295–303.
12. Pat-Horenczyk R, Klauber MR, Shochat T, et al. Hourly profiles of sleep and wakefulness in severely versus mild-moderately demented nursing home patients. Aging (Milano) 1998; 10(4):308–315.
13. Pollak CP, Stokes PE. Circadian rest–activity rhythms in demented and nondemented older community residents and their caregivers. J Am Geriatr Soc 1997; 45(4):446–452.

14. Gaugler JE, Edwards AB, Femia EE, et al. Predictors of institutionalization of cognitively impaired elders: family help and the timing of placement. J Gerontol B Psychol Sci Soc Sci 2000; 55(4):P247–P255.
15. Hebert LE, Scherr PA, Bienias JL, et al. Alzheimer disease in the US population: prevalence estimates using the 2000 census. Arch Neurol 2003; 60(8):1119–1122.
16. Hebert R, Brayne C. Epidemiology of vascular dementia. Neuroepidemiology 1995; 14(5):240–257.
17. McKeith IG, Galasko D, Kosaka K, et al. Consensus guidelines for the clinical and pathologic diagnosis of dementia with Lewy bodies (DLB): report of the consortium on DLB international workshop. Neurology 1996; 47(5):1113–1124.
18. Aarsland D, Andersen K, Larsen JP, et al. Prevalence and characteristics of dementia in Parkinson disease: an 8-year prospective study. Arch Neurol 2003; 60(3):387–392.
19. Galvin JE, Pollack J, Morris JC. Clinical phenotype of Parkinson disease dementia. Neurology 2006; 67(9):1605–1611.
20. German PS, Rovner BW, Burton LC, et al. The role of mental morbidity in the nursing home experience. Gerontologist 1992; 32(2):152–158.
21. Foley D, Monjan A, Masaki K, et al. Daytime sleepiness is associated with 3-year incident dementia and cognitive decline in older Japanese-American men. J Am Geriatr Soc 2001; 49(12):1628–1632.
22. Fetveit A, Bjorvatn B. Sleep duration during the 24-hour day is associated with the severity of dementia in nursing home patients. Int J Geriatr Psychiatry 2006; 21(10):945–950.
23. Abbott RD, Ross GW, White LR, et al. Excessive daytime sleepiness and subsequent development of Parkinson disease. Neurology 2005; 65(9):1442–1446.
24. Boddy F, Rowan EN, Lett D, et al. Subjectively reported sleep quality and excessive daytime somnolence in Parkinson's disease with and without dementia, dementia with Lewy bodies and Alzheimer's disease. Int J Geriatr Psychiatry 2006.
25. Park M, Comella CL, Leurgans SE, et al. Association of daytime napping and Parkinsonian signs in Alzheimer's disease. Sleep Med 2006; 7(8):614–618.
26. Grace JB, Walker MP, McKeith IG. A comparison of sleep profiles in patients with dementia with Lewy bodies and Alzheimer's disease. Int J Geriatr Psychiatry 2000; 15(11):1028–1033.
27. Okawa M, Mishima K, Hishikawa Y, et al. Circadian rhythm disorders in sleep–waking and body temperature in elderly patients with dementia and their treatment. Sleep 1991; 14(6):478–485.
28. Prinz PN, Christie C, Smallwood R, et al. Circadian temperature variation in healthy aged and in Alzheimer's disease. J Gerontol 1984; 39(1):30–35.
29. Bliwise DL, Carroll JS, Dement WC. Predictors of observed sleep/wakefulness in residents in long-term care. J Gerontol 1990; 45(4):M126–M130.
30. Meguro K, Ueda M, Kobayashi I, et al. Sleep disturbance in elderly patients with cognitive impairment, decreased daily activity and periventricular white matter lesions. Sleep 1995; 18(2):109–114.
31. Prinz PN, Peskind ER, Vitaliano PP, et al. Changes in the sleep and waking EEGs of nondemented and demented elderly subjects. J Am Geriatr Soc 1982; 30(2):86–93.
32. Prinz PN, Vitaliano PP, Vitiello MV, et al. Sleep, EEG and mental function changes in senile dementia of the Alzheimer's type. Neurobiol Aging 1982; 3(4):361–370.
33. Harper DG, Stopa EG, McKee AC, et al. Differential circadian rhythm disturbances in men with Alzheimer disease and frontotemporal degeneration. Arch Gen Psychiatry 2001; 58(4):353–360.
34. Harper DG, Volicer L, Stopa EG, et al. Disturbance of endogenous circadian rhythm in aging and Alzheimer disease. Am J Geriatr Psychiatry 2005; 13(5):359–368.
35. Volicer L, Harper DG, Manning BC, et al. Sundowning and circadian rhythms in Alzheimer's disease. Am J Psychiatry 2001; 158(5):704–711.
36. Paavilainen P, Korhonen I, Lotjonen J, et al. Circadian activity rhythm in demented and non-demented nursing-home residents measured by telemetric actigraphy. J Sleep Res 2005; 14(1):61–68.

37. Ancoli-Israel S, Klauber MR, Jones DW, et al. Variations in circadian rhythms of activity, sleep, and light exposure related to dementia in nursing-home patients. Sleep 1997; 20(1):18–23.
38. Martin J, Marler M, Shochat T, et al. Circadian rhythms of agitation in institutionalized patients with Alzheimer's disease. Chronobiol Int 2000; 17(3):405–418.
39. Harper DG, Stopa EG, McKee AC, et al. Dementia severity and Lewy bodies affect circadian rhythms in Alzheimer disease. Neurobiol Aging 2004; 25(6):771–781.
40. Morton AJ, Wood NI, Hastings MH, et al. Disintegration of the sleep–wake cycle and circadian timing in Huntington's disease. J Neurosci 2005; 25(1):157–163.
41. Petersen A, Bjorkqvist M. Hypothalamic-endocrine aspects in Huntington's disease. Eur J Neurosci 2006; 24(4):961–967.
42. Boeve BF, Silber MH, Saper CB, et al. Pathophysiology of REM sleep behaviour disorder and relevance to neurodegenerative disease. Brain 2007.
43. McKeith IG, Dickson DW, Lowe J, et al. Diagnosis and management of dementia with Lewy bodies: third report of the DLB Consortium. Neurology 2005; 65(12):1863–1872.
44. Boeve BF, Silber MH, Ferman TJ, et al. Association of REM sleep behavior disorder and neurodegenerative disease may reflect an underlying synucleinopathy. Mov Disord 2001; 16(4):622–630.
45. Olson EJ, Boeve BF, Silber MH. Rapid eye movement sleep behaviour disorder: demographic, clinical and laboratory findings in 93 cases. Brain 2000; 123 (Pt 2):331–339.
46. Schenck CH, Bundlie SR, Mahowald MW. Delayed emergence of a parkinsonian disorder in 38% of 29 older men initially diagnosed with idiopathic rapid eye movement sleep behaviour disorder. Neurology 1996; 46(2):388–393.
47. Turner RS, Chervin RD, Frey KA, et al. Probable diffuse Lewy body disease presenting as REM sleep behavior disorder. Neurology 1997; 49(2):523–527.
48. Turner RS, D'Amato CJ, Chervin RD, et al. The pathology of REM sleep behavior disorder with comorbid Lewy body dementia. Neurology 2000; 55(11):1730–1732.
49. Boeve BF, Silber MH, Parisi JE, et al. Synucleinopathy pathology and REM sleep behavior disorder plus dementia or Parkinsonism. Neurology 2003; 61(1):40–45.
50. Hickey MG, Demaerschalk BM, Caselli RJ, et al. "Idiopathic" rapid-eye-movement (REM) sleep behavior disorder is associated with future development of neurodegenerative diseases. Neurologist 2007; 13(2):98–101.
51. Iranzo A, Molinuevo JL, Santamaria J, et al. Rapid-eye-movement sleep behaviour disorder as an early marker for a neurodegenerative disorder: a descriptive study. Lancet Neurol 2006; 5(7):572–577.
52. Schenck CH, Garcia-Rill E, Skinner RD, et al. A case of REM sleep behavior disorder with autopsy-confirmed Alzheimer's disease: postmortem brain stem histochemical analyses. Biol Psychiatry 1996; 40(5):422–425.
53. Schenck CH, Mahowald MW, Anderson ML, et al. Lewy body variant of Alzheimer's disease (AD) identified by postmortem ubiquitin staining in a previously reported case of AD associated with REM sleep behavior disorder. Biol Psychiatry 1997; 42(6):527–528.
54. Rothdach AJ, Trenkwalder C, Haberstock J, et al. Prevalence and risk factors of RLS in an elderly population: the MEMO study. Memory and morbidity in Augsburg elderly. Neurology 2000; 54(5):1064–1068.
55. Nichols DA, Allen RP, Grauke JH, et al. Restless legs syndrome symptoms in primary care: a prevalence study. Arch Intern Med 2003; 163(19):2323–2329.
56. Ancoli-Israel S, Kripke DF, Klauber MR, et al. Periodic limb movements in sleep in community-dwelling elderly. Sleep 1991; 14(6):496–500.
57. Bader GG, Turesson K, Wallin A. Sleep-related breathing and movement disorders in healthy elderly and demented subjects. Dementia 1996; 7(5):279–287.
58. Sharafkhaneh A, Giray N, Richardson P, et al. Association of psychiatric disorders and sleep apnea in a large cohort. Sleep 2005; 28(11):1405–1411.
59. Gehrman PR, Martin JL, Shochat T, et al. Sleep-disordered breathing and agitation in institutionalized adults with Alzheimer disease. Am J Geriatr Psychiatry 2003; 11(4):426–433.

60. Ancoli-Israel S, Klauber MR, Butters N, et al. Dementia in institutionalized elderly: relation to sleep apnea. J Am Geriatr Soc 1991; 39(3):258–263.
61. Hoch CC, Reynolds CF 3rd, Kupfer DJ, et al. Sleep-disordered breathing in normal and pathologic aging. J Clin Psychiatry 1986; 47(10):499–503.
62. Reynolds CF 3rd, Kupfer DJ, Taska LS, et al. Sleep apnea in Alzheimer's dementia: correlation with mental deterioration. J Clin Psychiatry 1985; 46(7):257–261.
63. Gottlieb DJ, DeStefano AL, Foley DJ, et al. APOE epsilon4 is associated with obstructive sleep apnea/hypopnea: the Sleep Heart Health Study. Neurology 2004; 63(4):664–668.
64. Kadotani H, Kadotani T, Young T, et al. Association between apolipoprotein E epsilon 4 and sleep-disordered breathing in adults. JAMA 2001; 285(22):2888–2890.
65. O'Hara R, Schroder CM, Kraemer HC, et al. Nocturnal sleep apnea/hypopnea is associated with lower memory performance in APOE epsilon4 carriers. Neurology 2005; 65(4):642–644.
66. Cooke JR, Liu L, Natarajan L, et al. The effect of sleep-disordered breathing on stages of sleep in patients with Alzheimer's disease. Behav Sleep Med 2006; 4(4):219–227.
67. Erkinjuntti T, Partinen M, Sulkava R, et al. Sleep apnea in multiinfarct dementia and Alzheimer's disease. Sleep 1987; 10(5):419–425.
68. Bliwise DL, Tinklenberg J, Yesavage JA, et al. REM latency in Alzheimer's disease. Biol Psychiatry 1989; 25(3):320–328.
69. Montplaisir J, Petit D, Gauthier S, et al. Sleep disturbances and EEG slowing in Alzheimer's disease. Sleep Res Online 1998; 1(4):147–151.
70. Reynolds CF 3rd, Kupfer DJ, Houck PR, et al. Reliable discrimination of elderly depressed and demented patients by electroencephalographic sleep data. Arch Gen Psychiatry 1988; 45(3):258–264.
71. Vitiello MV, Bokan JA, Kukull WA, et al. Rapid eye movement sleep measures of Alzheimer's-type dementia patients and optimally healthy aged individuals. Biol Psychiatry 1984; 19(5):721–734.
72. Liu RY, Zhou JN, van Heerikhuize J, et al. Decreased melatonin levels in postmortem cerebrospinal fluid in relation to aging, Alzheimer's disease, and apolipoprotein E-epsilon 4/4 genotype. J Clin Endocrinol Metab 1999; 84(1):323–327.
73. Mishima K, Tozawa T, Satoh K, et al. Melatonin secretion rhythm disorders in patients with senile dementia of Alzheimer's type with disturbed sleep–waking. Biol Psychiatry 1999; 45(4):417–421.
74. Strittmatter WJ, Roses AD. Apolipoprotein E and Alzheimer's disease. Annu Rev Neurosci 1996; 19:53–77.
75. Yesavage JA, Friedman L, Kraemer H, et al. Sleep/wake disruption in Alzheimer's disease: APOE status and longitudinal course. J Geriatr Psychiatry Neurol 2004; 17(1):20–24.
76. Craig D, Hart DJ, Passmore AP. Genetically increased risk of sleep disruption in Alzheimer's disease. Sleep 2006; 29(8):1003–1007.
77. Buckley TM, Schatzberg AF. Aging and the role of the HPA axis and rhythm in sleep and memory-consolidation. Am J Geriatr Psychiatry 2005; 13(5):344–352.
78. Kumru H, Santamaria J, Tolosa E, et al. Rapid eye movement sleep behavior disorder in Parkinsonism with Parkin mutations. Ann Neurol 2004; 56(4):599–603.
79. Ancoli-Israel S, Clopton P, Klauber MR, et al. Use of wrist activity for monitoring sleep/wake in demented nursing-home patients. Sleep 1997; 20(1):24–27.
80. Bliwise DL, Hughes M, McMahon PM, et al. Observed sleep/wakefulness and severity of dementia in an Alzheimer's disease special care unit. J Gerontol A Biol Sci Med Sci 1995; 50(6):M303–M306.
81. Cohen-Mansfield J, Waldhorn R, Werner P, et al. Validation of sleep observations in a nursing home. Sleep 1990; 13(6):512–525.
82. Tractenberg RE, Singer CM, Cummings JL, et al. The Sleep Disorders Inventory: an instrument for studies of sleep disturbance in persons with Alzheimer's disease. J Sleep Res 2003; 12(4):331–337.

83. McCurry SM, Vitiello MV, Gibbons LE, et al. Factors associated with caregiver reports of sleep disturbances in persons with dementia. Am J Geriatr Psychiatry 2006; 14(2):112–120.

84. Allen RP, Picchietti D, Hening WA, et al. Restless legs syndrome: diagnostic criteria, special considerations, and epidemiology. A report from the restless legs syndrome diagnosis and epidemiology workshop at the National Institutes of Health. Sleep Med 2003; 4(2):101–119.

85. Executive summary on the systematic review and practice parameters for portable monitoring in the investigation of suspected sleep apnea in adults. Am J Respir Crit Care Med 2004; 169(10):1160–1163.

86. Portable monitoring in the diagnosis of obstructive sleep apnea. J Clin Sleep Med 2006; 2(3):333.

87. Cruise PA, Schnelle JF, Alessi CA, et al. The nighttime environment and incontinence care practices in nursing homes. J Am Geriatr Soc 1998; 46(2):181–186.

88. Gentili A, Weiner DK, Kuchibhatil M, et al. Factors that disturb sleep in nursing home residents. Aging (Milano) 1997; 9(3):207–213.

89. Schnelle JF, Alessi CA, Al-Samarrai NR, et al. The nursing home at night: effects of an intervention on noise, light, and sleep. J Am Geriatr Soc 1999; 47(4):430–438.

90. Richards KC, Sullivan SC, Phillips RL, et al. The effect of individualized activities on the sleep of nursing home residents who are cognitively impaired: a pilot study. J Gerontol Nurs 2001; 27(9):30–37.

91. Richards KC, Beck C, O'Sullivan PS, et al. Effect of individualized social activity on sleep in nursing home residents with dementia. J Am Geriatr Soc 2005; 53(9):1510–1517.

92. Alessi CA, Yoon EJ, Schnelle JF, et al. A randomized trial of a combined physical activity and environmental intervention in nursing home residents: do sleep and agitation improve? J Am Geriatr Soc 1999; 47(7):784–791.

93. Alessi CA, Martin JL, Webber AP, et al. Randomized, controlled trial of a nonpharmacological intervention to improve abnormal sleep/wake patterns in nursing home residents. J Am Geriatr Soc 2005; 53(5):803–810.

94. Ouslander JG, Connell BR, Bliwise DL, et al. A nonpharmacological intervention to improve sleep in nursing home patients: results of a controlled clinical trial. J Am Geriatr Soc 2006; 54(1):38–47.

95. McCurry SM, Gibbons LE, Logsdon RG, et al. Nighttime insomnia treatment and education for Alzheimer's disease: a randomized, controlled trial. J Am Geriatr Soc 2005; 53(5):793–802.

96. Ancoli-Israel S, Martin JL, Gehrman P, et al. Effect of light on agitation in institutionalized patients with severe Alzheimer disease. Am J Geriatr Psychiatry 2003; 11(2):194–203.

97. Ancoli-Israel S, Martin JL, Kripke DF, et al. Effect of light treatment on sleep and circadian rhythms in demented nursing home patients. J Am Geriatr Soc 2002; 50(2):282–289.

98. Ancoli-Israel S, Gehrman P, Martin JL, et al. Increased light exposure consolidates sleep and strengthens circadian rhythms in severe Alzheimer's disease patients. Behav Sleep Med 2003; 1(1):22–36.

99. Yamadera H, Ito T, Suzuki H, et al. Effects of bright light on cognitive and sleep–wake (circadian) rhythm disturbances in Alzheimer-type dementia. Psychiatry Clin Neurosci 2000; 54(3):352–353.

100. Fetveit A, Bjorvatn B. Bright-light treatment reduces actigraphic-measured daytime sleep in nursing home patients with dementia: a pilot study. Am J Geriatr Psychiatry 2005; 13(5):420–423.

101. Fontana Gasio P, Krauchi K, Cajochen C, et al. Dawn–dusk simulation light therapy of disturbed circadian rest–activity cycles in demented elderly. Exp Gerontol 2003; 38(1–2):207–216.

102. Fetveit A, Bjorvatn B. The effects of bright-light therapy on actigraphical measured sleep last for several weeks post-treatment. A study in a nursing home population. J Sleep Res 2004; 13(2):153–158.

103. Ayalon L, Ancoli-Israel S, Stepnowsky C, et al. Adherence to continuous positive airway pressure treatment in patients with Alzheimer's disease and obstructive sleep apnea. Am J Geriatr Psychiatry 2006; 14(2):176–180.
104. Chong MS, Ayalon L, Marler M, et al. Continuous positive airway pressure reduces subjective daytime sleepiness in patients with mild to moderate Alzheimer's disease with sleep disordered breathing. J Am Geriatr Soc 2006; 54(5):777–781.
105. Mishima Y, Hozumi S, Shimizu T, et al. Passive body heating ameliorates sleep disturbances in patients with vascular dementia without circadian phase-shifting. Am J Geriatr Psychiatry 2005; 13(5):369–376.
106. Yang MH, Wu SC, Lin JG, et al. The efficacy of acupressure for decreasing agitated behaviour in dementia: a pilot study. J Clin Nurs 2007; 16(2):308–315.
107. McDowell JA, Mion LC, Lydon TJ, et al. A nonpharmacologic sleep protocol for hospitalized older patients. J Am Geriatr Soc 1998; 46(6):700–705.
108. Ballard CG, O'Brien JT, Reichelt K, et al. Aromatherapy as a safe and effective treatment for the management of agitation in severe dementia: the results of a double-blind, placebo-controlled trial with Melissa. J Clin Psychiatry 2002; 63(7):553–558.
109. McCurry SM, Gibbons LE, Logsdon RG, et al. Training caregivers to change the sleep hygiene practices of patients with dementia: the NITE-AD project. J Am Geriatr Soc 2003; 51(10):1455–1460.
110. Ray WA, Thapa PB, Gideon P. Benzodiazepines and the risk of falls in nursing home residents. J Am Geriatr Soc 2000; 48(6):682–685.
111. Ray WA, Griffin MR, Schaffner W, et al. Psychotropic drug use and the risk of hip fracture. N Engl J Med 1987; 316(7):363–369.
112. Wang PS, Bohn RL, Glynn RJ, et al. Zolpidem use and hip fractures in older people. J Am Geriatr Soc 2001; 49(12):1685–1690.
113. Brassington GS, King AC, Bliwise DL. Sleep problems as a risk factor for falls in a sample of community-dwelling adults aged 64–99 years. J Am Geriatr Soc 2000; 48(10):1234–1240.
114. Moraes Wdos S, Poyares DR, Guilleminault C, et al. The effect of donepezil on sleep and REM sleep EEG in patients with Alzheimer disease: a double-blind placebo-controlled study. Sleep 2006;29(2):199–205.
115. Kitabayashi Y, Ueda H, Tsuchida H, et al. Donepezil-induced nightmares in mild cognitive impairment. Psychiatry Clin Neurosci 2006; 60(1):123–124.
116. Cooke JR, Loredo JS, Liu L, et al. Acetylcholinesterase inhibitors and sleep architecture in patients with Alzheimer's disease. Drugs Aging 2006; 23(6):503–511.
117. Markowitz JS, Gutterman EM, Lilienfeld S, et al. Sleep-related outcomes in persons with mild to moderate Alzheimer disease in a placebo-controlled trial of galantamine. Sleep 2003; 26(5):602–606.
118. Stahl SM, Markowitz JS, Papadopoulos G, et al. Examination of nighttime sleep-related problems during double-blind, placebo-controlled trials of galantamine in patients with Alzheimer's disease. Curr Med Res Opin 2004; 20(4):517–524.
119. Ancoli-Israel S, Amatniek J, Ascher S, et al. Effects of galantamine versus donepezil on sleep in patients with mild to moderate Alzheimer disease and their caregivers: a double-blind, head-to-head, randomized pilot study. Alzheimer Dis Assoc Disord 2005; 19(4):240–245.
120. McKeith I, Del Ser T, Spano P, et al. Efficacy of rivastigmine in dementia with Lewy bodies: a randomised, double-blind, placebo-controlled international study. Lancet 2000; 356(9247):2031–2036.
121. Adler CH, Caviness JN, Hentz JG, et al. Randomized trial of modafinil for treating subjective daytime sleepiness in patients with Parkinson's disease. Mov Disord 2003; 18(3):287–293.
122. Hogl B, Saletu M, Brandauer E, et al. Modafinil for the treatment of daytime sleepiness in Parkinson's disease: a double-blind, randomized, crossover, placebo-controlled polygraphic trial. Sleep 2002; 25(8):905–909.
123. Howcroft DJ, Jones RW. Does modafinil have the potential to improve disrupted sleep patterns in patients with dementia? Int J Geriatr Psychiatry 2005; 20(5):492–495.

124. Jansen SL, Forbes DA, Duncan V, et al. Melatonin for cognitive impairment. Cochrane Database Syst Rev 2006(1):CD003802.
125. Serfaty M, Kennell-Webb S, Warner J, et al. Double blind randomised placebo controlled trial of low dose melatonin for sleep disorders in dementia. Int J Geriatr Psychiatry 2002; 17(12):1120–1127.
126. Singer C, Tractenberg RE, Kaye J, et al. A multicenter, placebo-controlled trial of melatonin for sleep disturbance in Alzheimer's disease. Sleep 2003; 26(7):893–901.
127. Meguro K, Meguro M, Tanaka Y, et al. Risperidone is effective for wandering and disturbed sleep/wake patterns in Alzheimer's disease. J Geriatr Psychiatry Neurol 2004; 17(2):61–67.
128. Onor ML, Saina M, Trevisiol M, et al. Clinical experience with risperidone in the treatment of behavioral and psychological symptoms of dementia. Prog Neuropsychopharmacol Biol Psychiatry 2007; 31(1):205–209.
129. Onor ML, Saina M, Aguglia E. Efficacy and tolerability of quetiapine in the treatment of behavioral and psychological symptoms of dementia. Am J Alzheimers Dis Other Demen 2006; 21(6):448–453.
130. Savaskan E, Schnitzler C, Schroder C, et al. Treatment of behavioural, cognitive and circadian rest–activity cycle disturbances in Alzheimer's disease: haloperidol vs. quetiapine. Int J Neuropsychopharmacol 2006; 9(5):507–516.
131. Hening WA, Allen RP, Earley CJ, et al. An update on the dopaminergic treatment of restless legs syndrome and periodic limb movement disorder. Sleep 2004; 27(3):560–583.
132. Littner MR, Kushida C, Anderson WM, et al. Practice parameters for the dopaminergic treatment of restless legs syndrome and periodic limb movement disorder. Sleep 2004; 27(3):557–559.
133. Tremont G, Davis JD, Bishop DS. Unique contribution of family functioning in caregivers of patients with mild to moderate dementia. Dement Geriatr Cogn Disord 2006; 21(3):170–174.
134. McCurry SM, Logsdon RG, Teri L, et al. Sleep disturbances in caregivers of persons with dementia: contributing factors and treatment implications. Sleep Med Rev 2007; 11(2):143–153.
135. McKibbin CL, Ancoli-Israel S, Dimsdale J, et al. Sleep in spousal caregivers of people with Alzheimer's disease. Sleep 2005; 28(10):1245–1250.
136. Lee D, Morgan K, Lindesay J. Effect of institutional respite care on the sleep of people with dementia and their primary caregivers. J Am Geriatr Soc 2007; 55(2):252–258.
137. Gaugler JE, Jarrott SE, Zarit SH, et al. Respite for dementia caregivers: the effects of adult day service use on caregiving hours and care demands. Int Psychogeriatr 2003; 15(1):37–58.
138. von Kanel R, Dimsdale JE, Ancoli-Israel S, et al. Poor sleep is associated with higher plasma proinflammatory cytokine interleukin-6 and procoagulant marker fibrin D-dimer in older caregivers of people with Alzheimer's disease. J Am Geriatr Soc 2006; 54(3):431–437.
139. Mausbach BT, Ancoli-Israel S, von Kanel R, et al. Sleep disturbance, norepinephrine, and D-dimer are all related in elderly caregivers of people with Alzheimer disease. Sleep 2006; 29(10):1347–1352.
140. Leong IY, Nuo TH. Prevalence of pain in nursing home residents with different cognitive and communicative abilities. Clin J Pain 2007; 23(2):119–127.
141. Cohen-Mansfield J, Lipson S. Pain in cognitively impaired nursing home residents: how well are physicians diagnosing it? J Am Geriatr Soc 2002; 50(6):1039–1044.
142. Warden V, Hurley AC, Volicer L. Development and psychometric evaluation of the Pain Assessment in Advanced Dementia (PAINAD) scale. J Am Med Dir Assoc 2003; 4(1):9–15.
143. Zwakhalen SM, Hamers JP, Berger MP. The psychometric quality and clinical usefulness of three pain assessment tools for elderly people with dementia. Pain 2006; 126(1–3):210–220.
144. Bekelman DB, Black BS, Shore AD, et al. Hospice care in a cohort of elders with dementia and mild cognitive impairment. J Pain Symptom Manage 2005; 30(3):208–214.

145. Munn JC, Hanson LC, Zimmerman S, et al. Is hospice associated with improved end-of-life care in nursing homes and assisted living facilities? J Am Geriatr Soc 2006; 54(3):490–495.
146. Bain KT, Weschules DJ, Knowlton CH, et al. Toward evidence-based prescribing at end of life: a comparative review of temazepam and zolpidem for the treatment of insomnia. Am J Hosp Palliat Care 2003; 20(5):382–388.

Index